AF560768

# Facial Soft Tissue Reconstruction

## Thomas Procedures in Facial Plastic Surgery

# Facial Soft Tissue Reconstruction

## Thomas Procedures in Facial Plastic Surgery

**Gregory H. Branham** MD FACS
Professor and Chief—Facial Plastic and Reconstructive Surgery
Department of Otolaryngology
Washington University School of Medicine
St. Louis, Missouri, USA

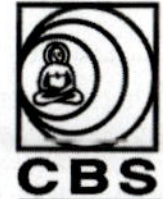

**CBS Publishers & Distributors** Pvt Ltd

New Delhi • Bengaluru • Pune • Kochi • Chennai
Mumbai • Kolkata • Hyderabad • Patna • Manipal

People's Medical Publishing House—USA, Shelton, Connecticut

People's Medical Publishing House-USA
2 Enterprise Drive, Suite 509
Shelton, CT 06484
Tel: 203-402-0646
Fax: 203-402-0854
E-mail: info@pmph-usa.com

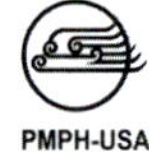




11 12 13 14/PMPH/9 8 7 6 5 4 3 2 1
ISBN-13: 978-1-60795-149-0
ISBN-10: 1-60795-149-5

This Edition has been published by special arrangement with PMPH-USA, Ltd
**CBS ISBN:** 978-81-239-2246-1

**Special Indian Edition: 2013**

Published by Satish Kumar Jain for
**CBS Publishers & Distributors** Pvt Ltd
4819/XI Prahlad Street, 24 Ansari Road, Daryaganj, New Delhi 110 002, India.
Ph: 23289259, 23266861, 23266867 Fax: 011-23243014 Website: www.cbspd.com
e-mail: delhi@cbspd.com; cbspubs@airtelmail.in

*Corporate Office:* 204 FIE, Industrial Area, Patparganj, Delhi 110 092
Ph: 4934 4934 Fax: 4934 4935 e-mail: publishing@cbspd.com; publicity@cbspd.com

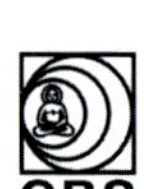


*Branches*

- **Bengaluru:** Seema House 2975, 17th Cross, K.R. Road, Banasankari 2nd Stage, Bengaluru 560 070, Karnataka
  Ph: +91-80-26771678/79 Fax: +91-80-26771680 e-mail: bangalore@cbspd.com
- **Pune:** Bhuruk Prestige, Sr. No. 52/12/2+1+3/2 Narhe, Haveli (Near Katraj-Dehu Road Bypass), Pune 411 041, Maharashtra
  Ph: +91-20-64704058, 64704059, 32342277 Fax: +91-20-24300160 e-mail: pune@cbspd.com
- **Kochi:** 36/14 Kalluvilakam, Lissie Hospital Road, Kochi 682 018, Kerala
  Ph: +91-484-4059061-65 Fax: +91-484-4059065 e-mail: cochin@cbspd.com
- **Chennai:** 20, West Park Road, Shenoy Nagar, Chennai 600 030, Tamil Nadu
  Ph: +91-44-26260666, 26208620 Fax: +91-44-45530020 e-mail: chennai@cbspd.com

*Representatives*

- **Mumbai** 0-9833017933
- **Kolkata** 0-9831437309
- **Hyderabad** 0-9885175004
- **Patna** 0-9334159340
- **Manipal** 0-9742022075

Printed at R P Printers, Noida

To my coauthors whose contributions have enriched this text in immeasurable ways

To Regan Thomas, my mentor and fellowship director

To my wife, Cindy, and my three wonderful children,
Allison, Matthew and Grace for their love and support

To my mother, Theodocia Hearon Branham, who taught me
the value of hard work, perseverance and a good education.

# PREFACE

Facial Soft Tissue Reconstruction is a multi-step process that begins with a thoughtful and detailed preoperative plan followed by meticulous execution. Attentive postoperative care followed by scar enhancement/camouflage techniques will achieve the best result. A mindset of critical analysis of results, acquisition of new knowledge and refinement of techniques is imperative to hone the surgeon's skills and provide the best possible care to patients.

Facial Soft Tissue Reconstruction is a very rewarding discipline and offers many unique opportunities and challenges. Whether dealing with a Moh's surgical defect following skin cancer or repairing a soft tissue loss from trauma, the ability to "think on your feet" and problem solve is essential. Being prepared and acquiring experience are essential to success. An understanding of the healing process and how it impacts soft tissues through such forces as contracture and scar formation allow us to plan for these as we reconstruct a defect. By understanding the vascular anatomy of the skin and the physiology of the flaps that we raise we are able to avoid complications that plagued the early reconstructive surgeons.

While there are many possibilities for the reconstruction of a soft tissue defect, not all are equivalent. Education and experience are the best teachers with regard to which technique is best for a particular patient's defect. This text provides a useful beginning to the educational portion and experience over time will guide you forward. This text is not an encyclopedic or exhaustive review of every possible flap that has ever been used, nor is it an historical review of the origins of the local flaps and soft tissue reconstructive techniques.

Rather, in this text the authors have taken a pragmatic approach to the reconstruction of these defects and as such have attempted to outline commonly used techniques that yield consistent and reproducible results. We have emphasized the techniques and procedural aspects of this discipline providing step by step illustrations of the techniques.

I hope that you will find the text helpful and that it contributes to your success as a facial soft tissue reconstructive surgeon whether you are still in residency training, beginning your practice or are a seasoned veteran in the operating room.

Gregory H. Branham, MD, FACS

# CONTRIBUTORS

**Gregory H. Branham, MD, FACS**
Associate Professor and Chief-Facial Surgery
Department of Otolaryngology
Washington University School of Medicine
St. Louis, MO

**Michael J. Brenner, MD, FACS**
Facial Plastic & Reconstructive Surgery
Assistant Professor
Southern Illinois University School of Medicine
Springfield, IL

**Mark A. Checcone, MD**
Assistant Professor, Facial Plastic and Reconstructive Surgery
Washington University School of Medicine
St. Louis, MO

**Jill L. Hessler, MD**
Adjunct Clinical Assistant Professor Stanford University
Premier Plastic Surgery
Palo Alto, CA

**John B. Holds, MD, FACS**
Clinical Professor
Departments of Ophthalmology and Otolaryngology
Head and Neck Surgery
Saint Louis University School of Medicine
St. Louis, MO

**Christina K. Magill, MD**
Resident in Otolaryngology
Washington University School of Medicine
St. Louis, MO

**Jasmine Mohadjer, MD**
Ophthalmic Plastic and Reconstructive Surgery
The Eye Institute of West Florida
Largo, Florida

**Arash Moradzadeh, MD**
Resident in Otolaryngology
Washington University School of Medicine
St Louis, MO

**Chad J. Sukut, MD**
Fellow, Mohs Micrographic Surgery
Division of Dermatology
Southern Illinois University School of Medicine
Springfield, IL

# Table of Contents

# 1

# Anatomy and Physiology of the Skin

Gregory H. Branham, MD, FACS

The skin is the largest organ of the body and provides an amazing protective barrier to disease and ultraviolet radiation. The skin is exposed to ionizing radiation and insults to the DNA. Most of these insults are able to be repaired at the cellular level, but after substantial chronic exposure, some are undetected and thus unrepaired and result in a cutaneous malignancy. The mainstay of treatment for these cutaneous malignancies remains surgical excision. Once the tumor has been completely removed, definitive reconstruction can be planned and executed.

It is essential that the surgeon understand the anatomy and biologic processes occurring in the skin before reconstructing a defect. The ultimate success of any flap or graft is dependent on its ability to maintain or quickly establish a reliable blood supply. Knowledge of the vascular anatomy of the skin allows us to plan a flap that will have a reliable vascular supply. In addition, understanding the biochemical processes that occur at the cellular level in the skin following injury provides us with an understanding of flap physiology. Such understanding allows us to ameliorate the effects of injury in the newly placed flap or graft as healing begins. This chapter focuses first on the relevant skin anatomy and concludes with a basic discussion of the physiology of the skin.

## Histology of the Skin

The skin is comprised of several layers and cell types **(Figure 1-1)**. The epidermis is the most superficial layer and is comprised primarily of keratinocytes but also contains melanocytes, Langerhans' cells, and Merckel cells. The most superficial layer of the epidermis is nonliving tissue called the stratum corneum **(see inset in Figure 1-1)**. This layer is primarily keratinocytes that are flattened and devoid of nuclei and keratin granules and provides the first layer of protection. The next deeper layer of the epidermis is the stratum granulosum. This layer is several cells thick and these cells contain keratin and keratohyalin granules within the cytoplasm. This layer terminates in the prickle cell layer or stratum spinosum. This layer derives its name from the desmosomes that attach the cells to one another and appear as spines. Below the stratum spinosum lays the basal cell layer or stratum germinativum. It is this layer that is responsible for the regeneration of the layers above. The basal cell layer is one cell layer thick and rests on the basement membrane. Melanocytes are intermixed at varying ratios.

The dermal-epidermal junction divides the epidermis from the dermis. This area, known as the basement membrane, is a highly specialized area that is responsible for the attachment of the epidermis to the underlying dermis. The dermis is comprised of the papillary and reticular dermis. The papillary dermis is a loose network of collagen, blood vessels, and fibroblasts. The fibroblasts are responsible for the production of collagen. The reticular dermis is a thicker layer comprised primarily of collagen with some elastin fibers and a few fibroblasts. Embedded in the dermis are glandular elements such as hair follicles or pilosebaceous units and eccrine and

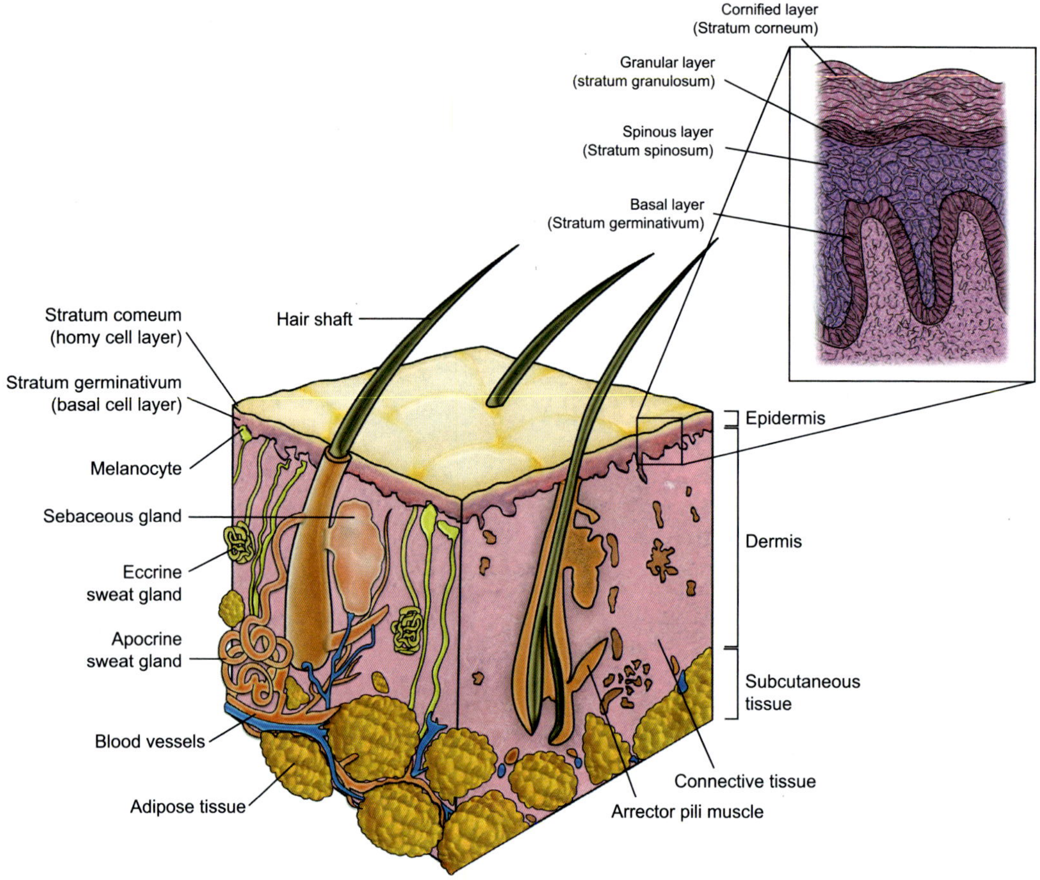


**Figure 1-1.** Anatomy of the skin. Inset shows layers of the epidermis.

apocrine sweat glands. These provide sources for basal cells that assist in reepithelialization following injury. Just below the dermis is the superficial fascial layer or subcutaneous layer that consists of fat and fascia.

## Vascular Anatomy

Piercing the subcutaneous or superficial fascial layer are the musculocutaneous perforating vessels that arise from named arteries and terminate in the subdermal plexus (**see Figure 1-2**). The subdermal plexus is a network of arteries and veins that run along the junction of the subcutaneous fat layer and the dermis. The small vessels of the subdermal plexus pierce the dermis to terminate at the junction of the papillary and reticular dermis in an arcade known as the subpapillary plexus or the papillary dermal plexus (**see inset in Figure 1-2**). It is the subpapillary plexus that gives rise to the vertically oriented capillary loops that extend into the dermal papillae. In summary, there is a vascular arcade of the skin that is located at the subdermal layer (subdermal plexus) and another within the dermis at the junction of the papillary and reticular dermis (subpapillary plexus).

## Neural Anatomy

The nerves in the skin follow the pattern of the vascular anatomy and, as such, form part of the neurovascular bundle or pedicle. Histologically, nerves in the skin are similar to those throughout the peripheral nervous system. Cutaneous nerves are sensory or autonomic, as there is no need for motor nerves at the skin level. Cranial nerves V, VII, IX, and the cervical nerves are the sensory afferent fibers of the head and neck. There is a number of specialized

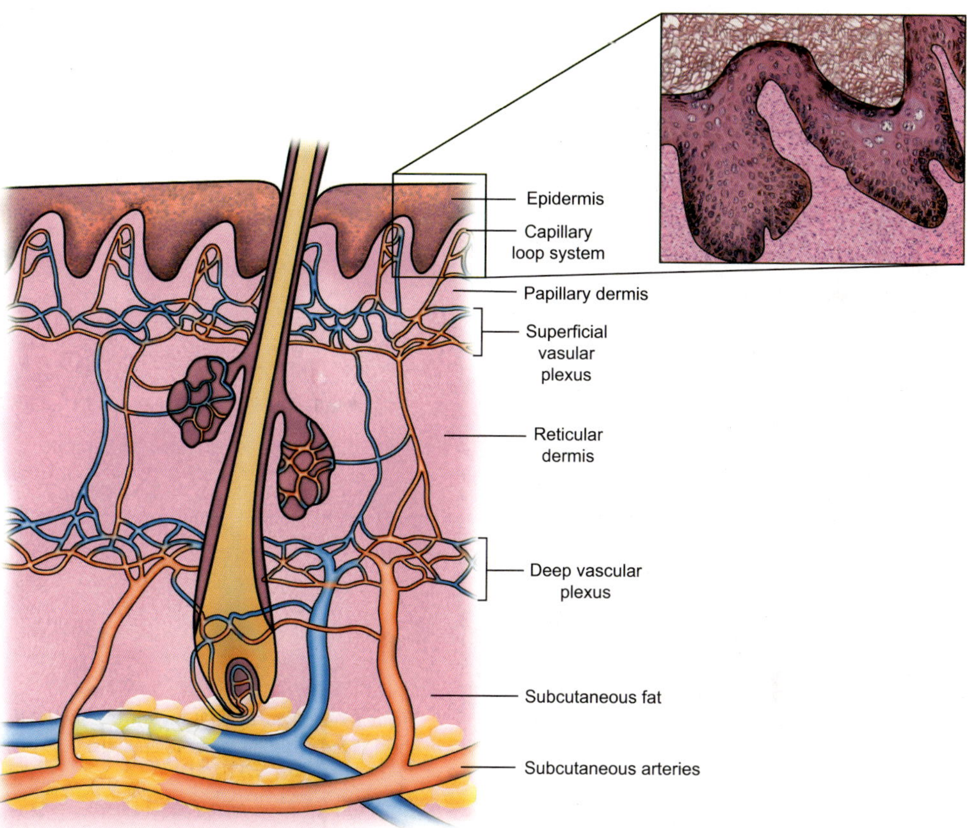


**Figure 1-2.** Vascular anatomy of the skin. Inset shows the papillary dermal plexus.

nerve endings located in the skin, and these are responsible for the perception of pain, temperature, proprioception, pressure, and itching (**Figure 1-3**). Meissner's corpuscles are encapsulated receptors that mediate touch and are located superficially in the dermal papillae. The Vater–Pacini corpuscles mediate pressure and are located at the fascial level. Many nonencapsulated nerve endings lie in the end organs of the skin, hair follicles, and dermal papillae. The efferent fibers are primarily autonomic in nature and innervate the smooth muscle of the blood vessels, glomus bodies, sweat glands, and the erector pili muscles that are associated with hair follicles.

## Pilosebaceous Units

Most of the skin throughout the body is covered with hair. Some areas have only a fine or vellus hair, whereas other areas such as the scalp and beard in males are covered with thick hair of varying degrees of coarseness. The rate of growth of the hair varies with the area of the body. In males, some scalp follicles are programmed to respond to testosterone by becoming quiescent, resulting in male pattern baldness. Each hair follicle, whether containing a fine or a coarse hair, is contained within a pilosebaceous unit (**see Figure 1-4**). The pilosebaceous unit consists of the hair, hair follicle, and associated erector pili muscle and the sebaceous gland and sensory end organ. Pilosebaceous units are absent in mucosa and on the palms and soles. The presence of hair must be considered when designing a flap with consideration given to its ultimate location. A prime example of this would be to use a paramedian forehead flap for nasal defects. If the flap extends into the scalp, then hair bearing tissue will be transposed onto the nose and this must be addressed.

## Random Pattern Flaps

Local or random pattern flaps are the most common type of flap used in facial reconstruction for

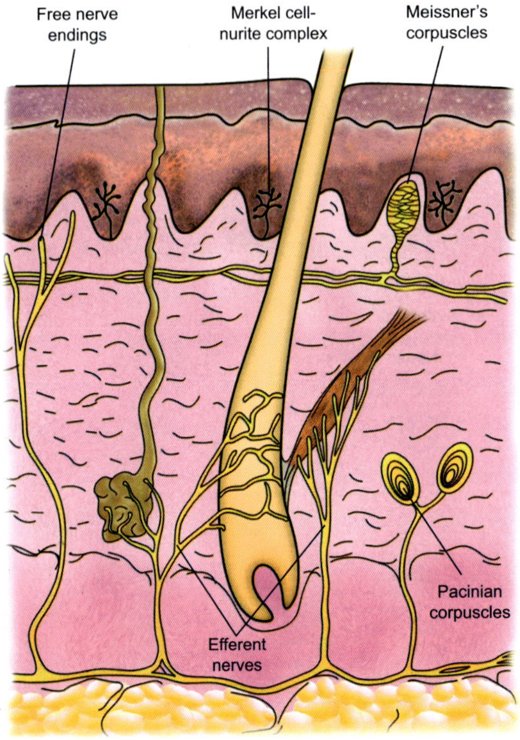


**Figure 1-3.** Neural anatomy of the skin with specialized cutaneous nerve endings.

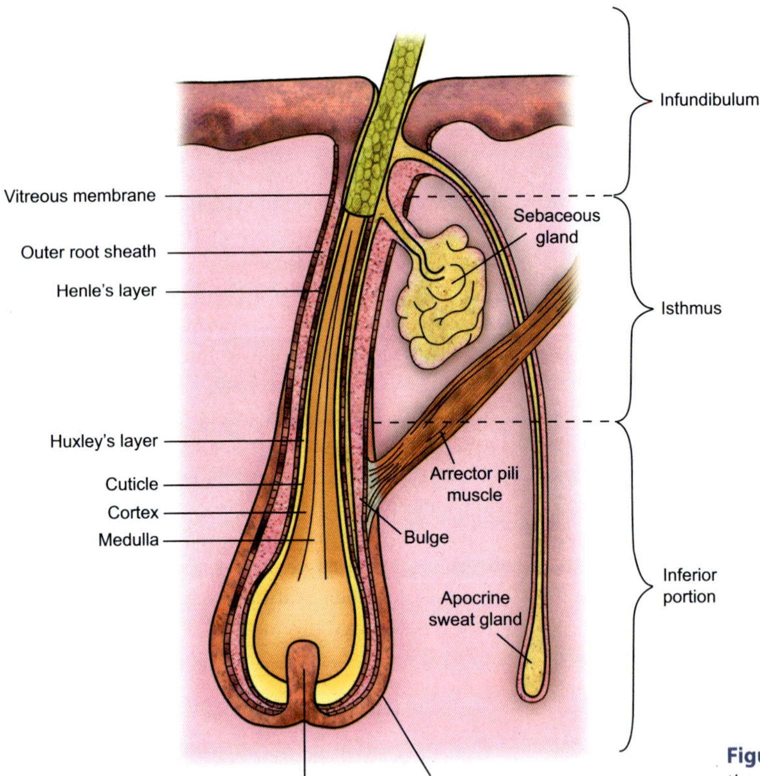


**Figure 1-4.** Pilosebaceous unit of the skin.

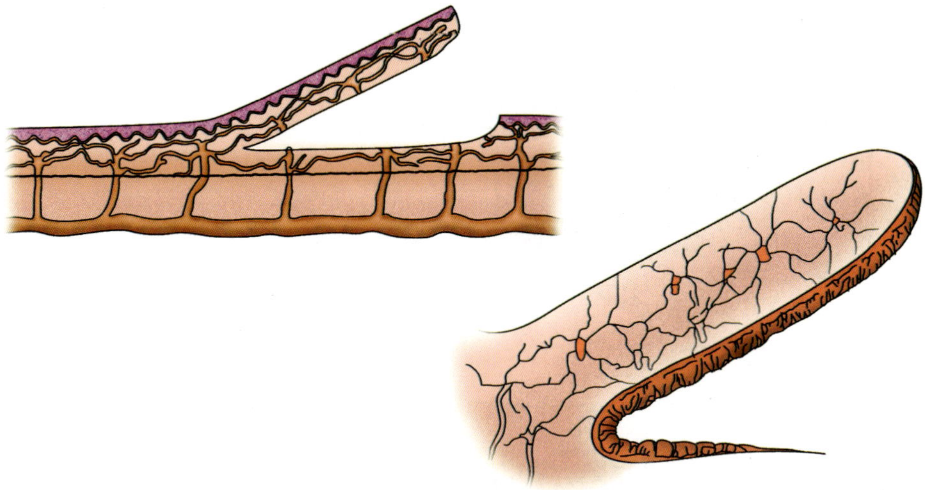

**Figure 1-5.** Random pattern flaps. Random pattern flaps are elevated in the subcutaneous plane and the musculocutaneous perforating vessels are divided leaving only the most proximal perforating vessels intact to supply circulation to the flap.

small- to moderate-sized defects. Such flaps are often called local flaps because tissue that is local or adjacent to the defect is used. This local or adjacent tissue often provides a superior color/texture match. The term "random pattern" is used to describe the vascular supply to the flap. These flaps rely on the musculocutaneous perforating branches for their blood supply as well as the anastomotic connections to the subdermal and subpapillary plexi (**see Figure 1-5**). Because these flaps are raised at the level of the subcutaneous plane, the musculocutaneous perforating vessels are divided, and only the most proximal perforating vessels remain intact to supply microcirculation of the subdermal and subpapillary plexi. It was long felt that survival of the distal end of the flap was based on a ratio of flap length to flap width, with a ratio of 21 being the maximum allowable. However, whether the flap survives is dependent on the capillary filling pressure at the distal end of the flap. This pressure gradient must overcome the pressure that is exerted by any tension on the flap and the loss of pressure that occurs as the blood flows toward the distal end of the arcade and through any network of anastomosing vessels to arrive at the capillary loops in the dermal papillae. If this critical pressure is exceeded, regardless of flap length, the flap will show signs of demarcation and subsequent necrosis. This may be manifest as a superficial epidermolysis at the distal end of the flap or a full thickness loss if vascularity is sufficiently compromised.

## Axial Pattern Flaps

Segmental vessels that lie deep to the muscle are usually termed "vessels" and give rise to direct cutaneous arteries (**Figure 1-6**). Flaps that are based on these direct cutaneous arteries are termed axial pattern flaps. The pedicle of the flap contains the artery and vein that supply the circulation for the flap. The artery is accompanied by several veins known as the venae comitantes. When the entire segmental artery and veins are elevated below the muscle, it is called a muculocutaneous flap. When the flap is elevated in the subcutaneous plane at the level of the direct cutaneous arteries, it is an axial pattern flap. These flaps are generally reserved for larger facial defects that require more tissue or perhaps a component that must be turned on itself as in the case of a forehead flap for nasal reconstruction. Survival of an axial pattern flap is dependent on maintaining an intact artery and vein or vascular pedicle. The distal end of the axial pattern flap is random in its vascular supply, and the same factors that affect the survival of the random pattern flap come into play here as well. Adequate venous outflow is essential to prevent venous congestion which is the most common cause of flap loss in

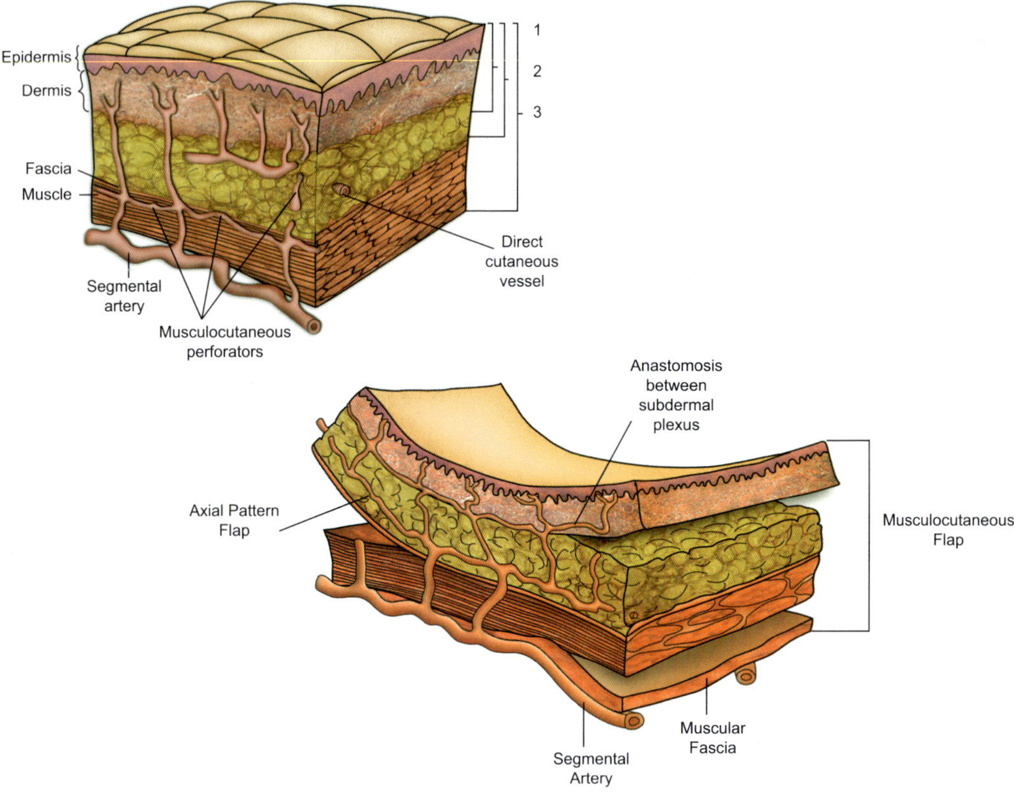


**Figure 1-6.** Axial pattern flaps. Axial pattern flaps are based on a segmental artery and vein that are elevated as a part of the flap known as the pedicle.

these flaps. Venous outflow is usually compromised by overskeletonizing or thinning of the pedicle with resulting injury to the venous outflow channels or venae comitantes.

## Factors Affecting Flap Survival

There are a number of factors that impact flap survival. These factors occur both at the macroscopic and microscopic or cellular level and represent a balance between the perfusion and the metabolic demands of the tissues. Factors at the macroscopic level impacting viability include flap design issues and mechanical factors. At the cellular level, factors such as tissue injury response, microcirculatory regulation, and comorbid disease states greatly impact the ultimate success of the reconstruction. The principles of design of local skin flaps are covered in Chapter 4 and is not discussed in detail here. However, it is intuitive to conclude that a poorly designed flap (e.g., inattention to flap length to width) will have a poorer survival rate than a well-designed flap. Mechanical factors include such considerations as tension on the flap and may be related to a flawed design or to poor execution (e.g., inadequate undermining of the donor site). Necrosis ensues when the capillary filling pressure of the capillary loops is exceeded by the extramural pressure generated by the tension of the flap.

## Tissue Injury Response

As the flap heals into its recipient site, many changes occur over time (**Figure 1-7**). These changes are well documented as a typical wound healing response; this area is covered in greater detail in Chapter 2.

## Inflammatory Phase

After the tissue is injured during transposition to its new location, there are a number of factors at the cellular level that impact flap survival. Upon injury,

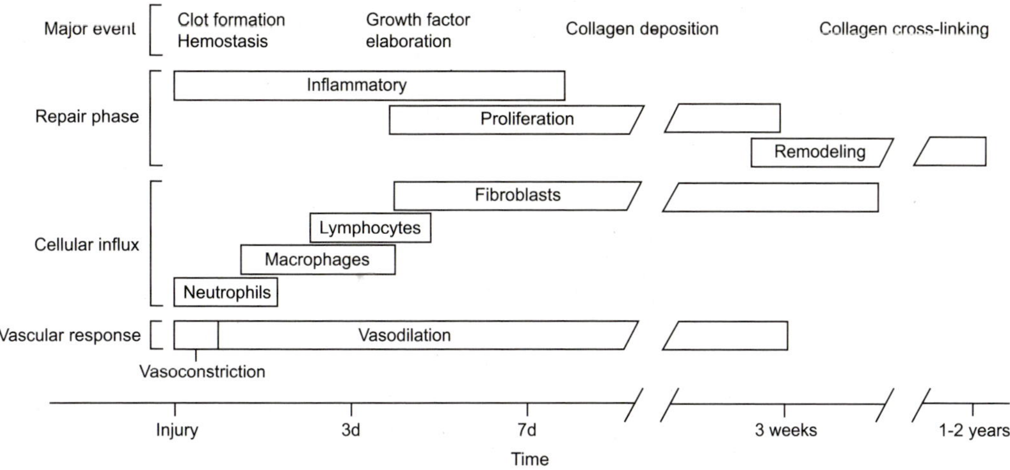


**Figure 1-7.** Timeline for wound healing and tissue repair. (Modified from Lorenz HP, Longaker MT: Wounds: biology, pathology, and management.)

the tissue immediately begins a vasoconstrictive response that is aimed first at controlling blood loss. During injury of the endothelial cells, a number of vasoactive compounds are released and the coagulation cascade is initiated. Platelet adhesion and aggregation follows from the initiation of the coagulation cascade. These activated platelets release a number of vasoactive compounds including serotonin, histamine, proteases, and thromboxane A2 (**Figure 1-8**).

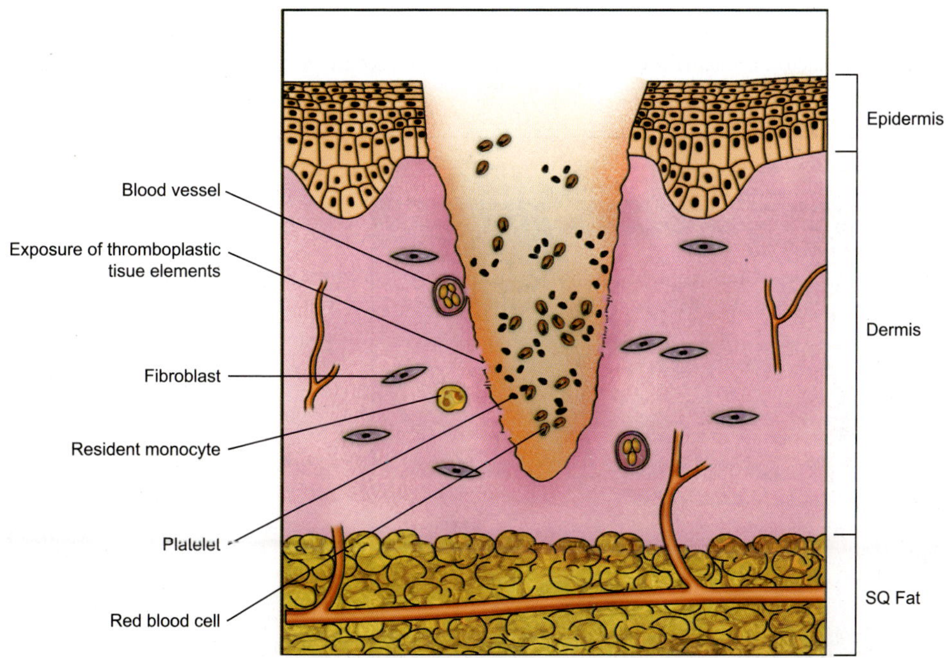


**Figure 1-8.** Wound-healing response initial phase. Hemostasis and release of vasoactive compounds is the initial step in the response of tissues to injury.

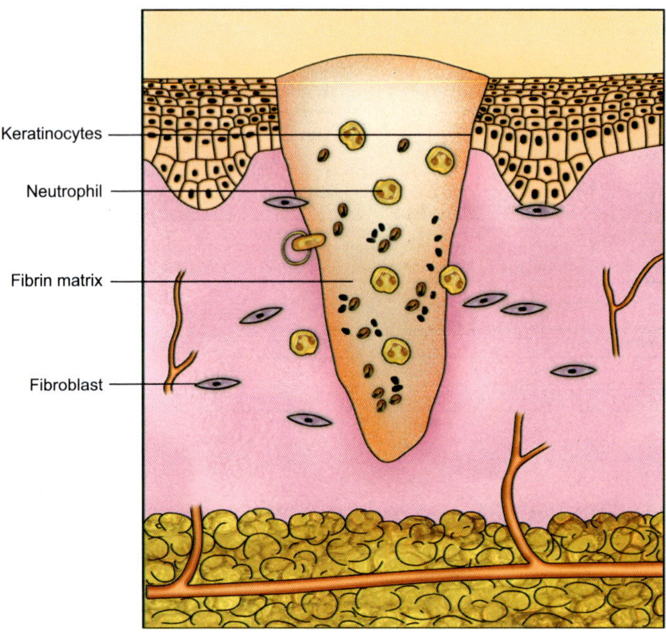


**Figure 1-9.** Wound-healing response inflammatory phase. Cellular influx into the wound and early provisional matrix formation occur in the first 2 days.

Dilated vessels result from the activation of the coagulation and complement cascades and the release of bradykinin. The vessels respond to release of C3a and C5a from the complement cascade with increased vascular permeability. In addition, other compounds that interact at the cellular level are released such as platelet-derived growth factor, epidermal growth factor, transforming growth factor beta, and fibroblast growth factor among others. These factors attract the cellular components of the repair phase to the wound, such as neutrophils, which clean up the wound (**Figure 1-9**). Later, at 2 to 3 days, circulating monocytes predominate in the wound and transform to macrophages, which further clean the wound (**Figure 1-10**). In addition, macrophages secrete numerous growth factors

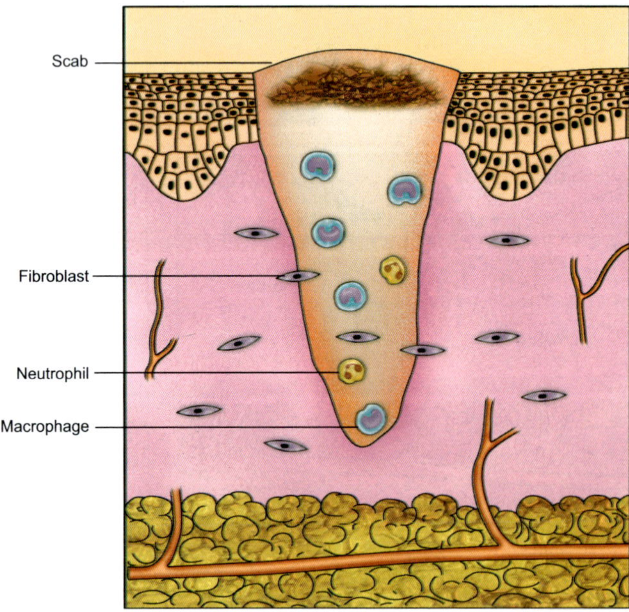


**Figure 1-10.** Wound-healing response late inflammatory phase. At 2–3 days, macrophages predominate and this marks the end of the inflammatory phase.

**TABLE 1-1 A Partial List of Growth Factors Present at the Wound Site***

| *Growth Factor* | *Cellular Source* | *Target Cells* | *Biologic Activity* |
|---|---|---|---|
| TGF-β1 and TGF-β2 | Macrophages, platelets, fibroblasts, keratinocytes | Inflammatory cells, keratinocytes, fibroblasts | Chemotaxis, proliferation, matrix production (fibrosis) |
| TGF-β3 | Macrophages | Fibroblasts | Anti-scarring? |
| TGF-α | Macrophages, platelets, keratinocytes | Keratinocytes, fibroblasts, endothelial cells | Proliferation |
| TNF-α | Neutrophils | Macrophages, keratinocytes, fibroblasts | Activation of growth factor expression |
| PDGF | Macrophages, platelets, fibroblasts, endothelial cells, vascular smooth muscle cells | Neutrophils, macrophages, fibroblasts, endothelial cells, vascular smooth muscle cells | Chemotaxis, proliferation, matrix production |
| FGF-1, FGF-2, FGF-4 | Macrophages, fibroblasts, endothelial cells | Keratinocytes, fibroblasts, endothelial cells, chondrocytes | Angiogenesis, proliferation, chemotaxis |
| FGF-7 (KGF-1), FGF-10 (KGF-2) | Fibroblasts | Keratinocytes | Proliferation, chemotaxis |
| EGF | Platelets, macrophages, keratinocytes | Keratinocytes, fibroblasts, endothelial cells | Proliferation, chemotaxis |
| IGF-1/Sm-C | Fibroblasts, macrophages, serum | Fibroblasts, endothelial cells | Proliferation, collagen synthesis |
| IL-1α and IL-1β | Macrophages, neutrophils | Macrophages, fibroblasts, keratinocytes | Proliferation, collagenase synthesis, chemotaxis |
| CTGF | Fibroblasts, endothelial cells | Fibroblasts | Downstream of TGF-β1 |
| VEGF | Macrophages, keratinocytes, fibroblasts | Endothelial cells | Angiogenesis |

*Redundant biologic effects occur through both autocrine and paracrine mechanisms.
TGl-β, transforming growth factor-β; TGF-α, transforming growth factor-α; TNF-α, tumor necrosis factor-α; PDGF, platelet-derived growth factor; FGF, fibroblast growth factor; KGF, keratinocyte growth factor; EGF, epidermal growth factor; IGF-1, insulin-like growth factor 1; Sm-C, somatostatin C; IL-1, lnterleukin-l; CTGF, connective tissue growth factor; VEGF, vascular endothelial cell growth factor.
Modified from Lorenz HP, Longaker MT: Wounds: biology, pathology, and management. In Norton JA, et al, ed.: Surgery: Scientific Basis and Current Practice, vol 1. New York, Springer-Verlag, 2000:224.

**(see Table 1-1).** This initiates the second or proliferative phase of wound healing.

## Proliferative Phase

In the second phase of response, reepithelialization begins, fibroblasts begin the process of collagen synthesis and secretion of extracellular matrix and wound contraction occurs **(Figure 1-11)**. This wound contraction must be accounted for when planning flaps and especially when using full- or split-thickness skin grafts. As neovascularization and vascular proliferation occur, the wound develops a more robust blood supply. If the wound is left to heal by secondary intention, granulation tissue develops that is characterized by vascular proliferation in this maturing wound matrix. The process of keratinization occurs as collagen and hyaluronic acid begin to replace the initial fibrin matrix and epithelial cells migrate from the periphery of the wound or from the basal cell layer of the skin appendages.

There are a number of interventions that have been espoused to assist in flap survival and healing. These interventions are based on knowledge that has been gained through research of flap physiology and wound-healing mechanisms. Dextran infusion has been shown to decrease platelet aggregation and increase fibrinolysis, thus enhancing flap survival. Other inhibitors of platelet aggregation include nitric oxide and prostacyclin. Ridrogel, a thromboxane inhibitor, has been shown to increase flow in arterially compromised flaps with low arterial flow in experimental animal models.

## Comorbid Disease and Other Factors

There are a number of disease processes that can impair wound healing **(Table 1-2)**. Diabetes is

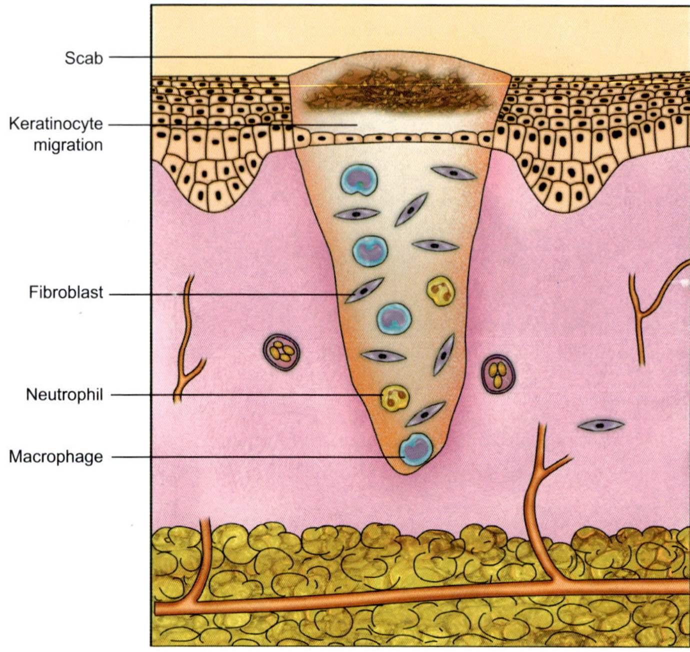


**Figure 1-11.** Wound-healing response proliferation phase. Fibroblasts predominate and matrix formation, epithelial migration, and wound contracture occur.

known to impair wound healing and flap survival as a result of the small-vessel disease that is induced. Infection is more common in this population as well. Advanced age is associated with increased atherosclerotic peripheral vascular disease and diminished arterial blood flow. Atherosclerosis has also been shown to alter the nitric oxide system. Smoking is known to decrease the oxygen saturation in the tissues secondary to the vasoconstrictive effect of nicotine on the endovascular smooth muscle. In addition, over time skin becomes chronically hypoxic and collagen and elastin in the skin are fractured causing the skin to loose its elasticity. Local anesthetics containing epinephrine cause temporary vasoconstriction and may impair flap viability in concentrations of 1100,000 or greater. Hyperbaric oxygen has been used to enhance the survival of flaps that are showing signs of distress as manifested by duskiness and poor capillary refill. There are many pharmacologic interventions that

**TABLE 1-2 Diseases Associated with Impaired Wound Healing**

| | |
|---|---|
| Hereditary | Malnutrition |
| Ehlers–Danlos syndrome | Cushing's syndrome |
| Prolidase deficiency | Hyperthyroidism |
| Coagulation disorders hemophilia, von Willebrand's disease, factor XIII deficiency, hypofibrogenemia | Immunologic Deficiency States |
| Werner's syndrome | Acquired Immunodeficiency Disease |
| Vascular Disorders | Transplantation Immunosuppression |
| Congestive heart failure | Other |
| Atherosclerosis | Chronic pulmonary disease |
| Hypertension | Chronic liver disease |
| Vasculitis | Malignancy |
| Venous stasis | Myelofibrosis and other thrombocytopenias |
| Lymphedema | Other chronic illness |
| Metabolic | Antineoplastic drugs |
| Chronic renal failure | Radiation therapy |
| Diabetes mellitus | Smoking |

Adapted from Thomas JR, Holt GR, *Facial Scars: Incision, Revision and Camouflage*, CV Mosby, St. Louis, 1989.

are being investigated to enhance flap survival; however, there is no substitute for a well-designed and meticulously executed local flap.

## References


1. Local Skin Flaps. *Facial Plast. Clin. NA* Vol 4. Number 4, 1996. Branham, GH, editor.
2. *Facial Plastic and Reconstructive Surgery* (2nd edition). Ira Papel, editor.
3. Weerda H, ed. *Reconstructive Facial Plastic Surgery A Problem-Solving Manual.* Thieme, New York, 2001
4. Ellsworth WA, Colon, GA. Management of medical morbidities and risk factors before surgery smoking, diabetes, and other complicating factors. *Semin.Plast Surg* 2006, 20, 205–213.
5. Semchyshyn N, Sengelmann RD. Surgical complications. eMedicine journal: *Dermatology*. May 2009.
6. Vander Straten M, Carrasco D, Paterson MS, et al. Tobacco use and skin disease. *South Med J* 2001 June 94(6) 621–634.
7. Ersoy A, Sevin K, Sevin A, Serel S. Effects of clopidogrel on survival of rat skin flaps. *J Plast Reconstr Aesthet Surg* 2007, 861–863.
8. Akan M, Cakir B, Misirlioglu A, Yildirim S, Taylan G, Akoz T. Effects of clopidogrel and high dose aspirin on survival of skin flaps in rats. *Scand J Plast Reconstr Surg Hand Surg* 2005, 39(1), 7–10.
9. Honrado CP, Murakami, CS. Wound healing and physiology of skin flaps. *Facial Plast Surg Clin NA* 13, 2005, 203–214.
10. Mathes, S., ed. *Plastic Surgery*. Saunders/Elsevier, New York, 2006.

2

# Basic Wound Healing

Arash Moradzadeh, MD and Jill L. Hessler, MD

## Introduction

The visible changes that take place during wound healing can be correlated to a well-orchestrated series of overlapping events involving numerous cells, cytokines, and growth factors. An understanding of these molecular events will aid the facial plastic surgeon in understanding the normal physiologic changes taking place to injured tissues. Understanding cellular events allows for more rapid identification of possible causes of suboptimal wound healing and allows for the initiation of timely strategies geared to optimizing cosmetic results.

## Phases of Wound Healing

### Hemostasis

After tissue injury, the first step in wound healing is hemostasis. The key mediators of hemostasis are blood vessels (vasoconstriction), fibrin, and platelets. A clot forms soon after injury. The clot serves as a matrix of proteins allowing for hemostasis and forms a scaffold for incoming inflammatory cells, and growth factors. Clot formation also prevents the loss of electrolytes and provides a protective layer from the environment. The blanching seen at the site of injury within minutes is a result of vasoconstriction mediated by vasoactive amines such as thromboxane and prostaglandins released from injured cells. Epinephrine released into the circulation and norepinephrine released locally also aid in vasoconstriction.

Endothelial cell injury will expose subendothelial collagen, resulting in both the adherence of platelets and the initiation of the coagulation cascade. As platelets aggregate, they will release alpha granules filled with various cytokines essential to wound healing such as platelet-derived growth factor (PDGF), transforming growth factor-B (TGF-B), and fibroblast growth factor-2 (FGF-2) **(Figure 2-1).** Fibrin is produced by the cleavage of fibrinogen by thrombin. Thrombin is a product of the extrinsic coagulation cascade. The fibrin monomers are then cross-linked by factor XIII; alternatively, fibrin can directly bind to the aggregating platelets to help form the primary clot. The matrix created will bind fibronectin released by fibroblasts, providing surface binding sites for the migration of various cells. Fibrin also binds to insulin-like growth factor (IGF-1) stimulating cell proliferation, vascular endothelial growth factor (VEGF), and fibroblast growth factor (FGF-2) to promote angiogenesis. Soon after fibrin helps form the primary clot, plasminogen, activated by tissue plasminogen activator, degrades the clot.

### Inflammatory Phase

Ten to 15 minutes after injury, there is a switch from the vasoconstrictive phase to a more persistent vasodilatation phase mediated by histamine, prostaglandins, thrombin, leukotrienes, and kinins. Physically, this phase is characterized by erythema, edema, and dolor seen at the site of injury. As platelets degranulate, cytokines and growth factors are released locally, recruiting circulating inflammatory cells and promoting angiogenesis. Polymorphonuclear cells (PMNs) are the first inflammatory cells to arrive at the site of injury.

Cytokine IL-8 and PDGF attract PMNs to the site of injury. The PMNs help remove cellular debris, bacteria, and foreign materials from the wound. These functions are mediated by phagocytosis and apoptosis stimulated in part by the many

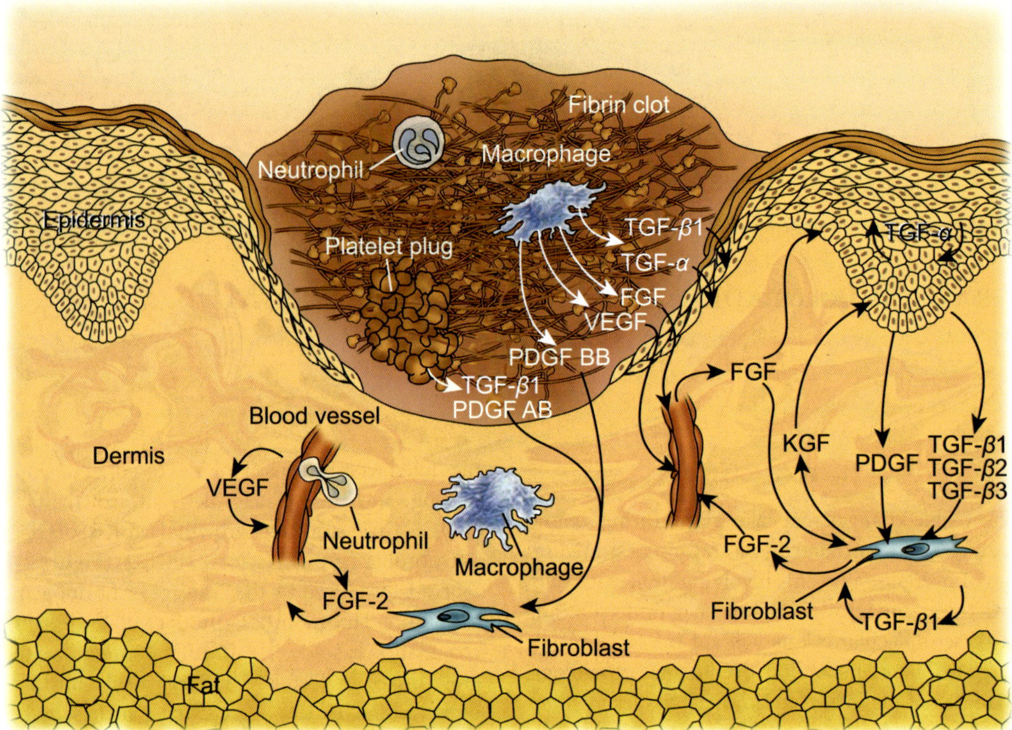


**Figure 2-1.** Inflammatory phase: cutaneous wound 3 days after injury. Growth factors thought to play an important role in cell migration into the wound are shown.

inflammatory cytokines released by PMNs: IL-1B, IL-6, and TNF-α. In a noncontaminated wound, these cells will peak early and disappear rapidly. However, in contaminated wounds, the neutrophils persist and prolong the inflammatory phase leading to delayed wound healing.

Monocytes also arrive and mature into macrophages with similar functions as the PMNs. However, the macrophage plays a more complex role in wound healing than PMNs. There are numerous chemotactic factors such as fibronectin, thrombin, TGF-β, complement C3a and C5a, and elastin, which attract monocytes into the wound. Once the macrophages reach the extracellular matrix, they will release numerous cytokines. The various cytokines and growth factors will promote inflammation (IL-1, IL-6, TNF-α), the differentiation of fibroblasts to myofibroblasts (TGF-β), and angiogenesis (VEGF, FGF-2, IGF-1) **(Figure 2-1).** The collective result of these influences is reepithelialization. TGF-α released from eosinophils will stimulate keratinocytes, an important contributor in reepithelialization.

## Proliferation Phase

The important role of macrophages is further highlighted in the proliferative phase of wound healing that begins days after injury **(Figure 2-2).** During this phase, the ECM scaffold is replaced with granulation tissue, which contains macrophages that release more cytokines and growth factors, promoting wound healing **(Figure 2-3).** The granulation tissue forms as a result of the ingress of capillaries to the site of injury and the migration of fibroblasts that produce collagen. Migration of fibroblast into a wound is stimulated by the same factors released during the inflammatory phase: PDGF, TGF-β, NGF, and fibronectin, a component of the original ECM. This highlights the overlapping nature of the phases of wound healing **(Figure 2-4).** The fibroblast will produce the collagen-rich ECM that replaces the temporary fibrin-rich ECM found in the inflammatory phase of wound healing. Collagen production begins 3–5 days after injury under the stimulus of PDG, EGF, IGF-1, TGF-β, and others.

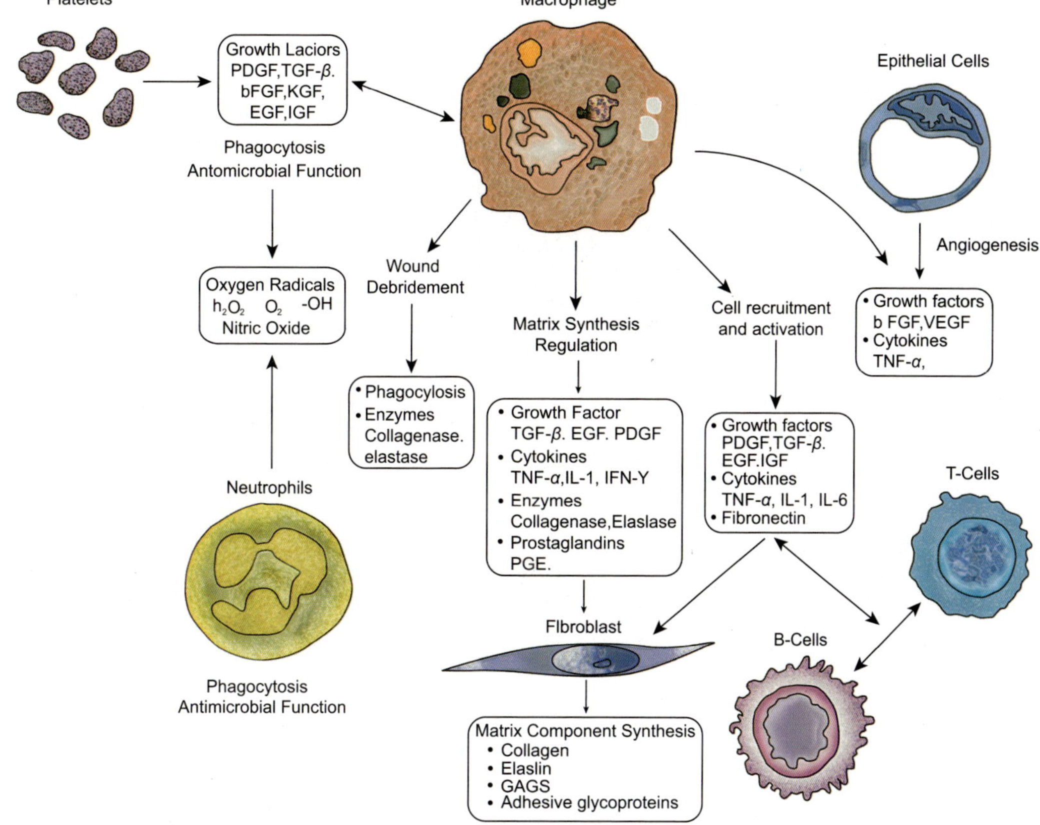


**Figure 2-2.** The important role of macrophages in wound healing.

Individual procollagen polypeptides are produced in the fibroblast, exported into the ECM, and cleaved to allow for aggregation into fibrils.

Reepithelialization begins 10 hours after injury with epithelial cells at the wound edge migrating across the fibroblast-rich ECM. To make this migration, the cells will form cytoplasmic pseudopod extensions and they will then dissolve their intracellular connections, allowing for lateral movement along the ECM across the wound. The keratinocytes will proliferate behind the migrating front of cells, allowing for complete epithelialization by contact guidance. In superficial wounds, the adnexal structures such as hair follicles will also contribute keratinocyte stem cells for reepithelialization. When the migrating cells finally meet, contact inhibition will occur and the cells will return to their normal morphology. In a wound closed primarily, the process of reepithelialization can be complete in just 24 hours.

Matrix metalloproteinases (MMPs) are important players in reepithelialization. MMPs play an essential role in angiogenesis and fibroblast migration; both required processes for wound healing **(Figure 2-3).** During migration, keratinocytes release urokinase plasminongen activator (uPA). The uPA converts plasminogen to plasmin. Plasmin will stimulate the MMPs and together plasmin, MMP-1 (collagenase), and MMP-2 will promote keratinocyte migration and ECM degradation. Experimental application of a broad MMP inhibitor such as BB-3103 has been shown to completely halt reepithelialization, demonstrating the critical role of MMPs in wound healing.

## Maturation Phase (Remodeling)

Wound maturation begins during granulation tissue production seen in the proliferative phase and may continue for weeks, even years **(Figure 2-4).** Clinical findings during wound maturation are contraction, decreased thickness, increase strength, reduced erythema, and a permanent absence of

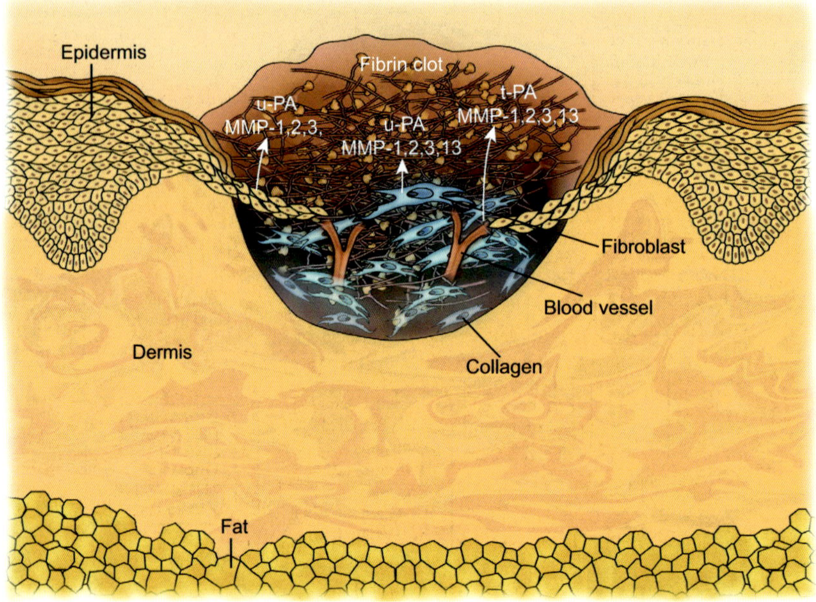


**Figure 2-3.** Proliferative phase: cutaneous wound 5 days after injury. Factors shown aid in reepithelialization and neovascularization.

skin appendages. Fibroblasts and their products, collagen and MMPs, in association with neovascularization, will be the essential players in wound maturation.

Wound contraction begins 5 days after injury and continues for several weeks depending on the condition of the wound. In an open wound, the edges of the skin will move closer to one another at a rate of 0.75 mm/day. This process takes place as a result of the contractile properties of myofibroblasts. Growth factors TGF-β and PDGF cause the fibroblasts to switch to myofibroblasts. During this same period, fibroblasts will continue to produce collagen until postinjury day 21. The increased collagen levels in the ECM negatively feedbacks to the fibroblast to slow down collagen production.

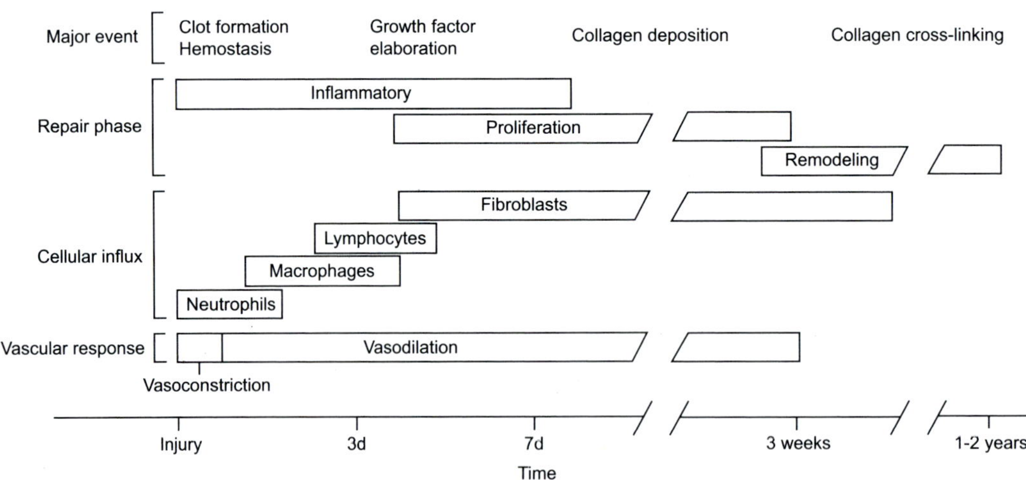


**Figure 2-4.** Time line for wound healing and tissue repair.

Collagen breakdown is under the control of the MMPs regulated by tissue inhibitors of metalloproteinases (TIMPs) activity. As this process continues the proportion of type III collagen decreases and type I collagen increases. Remodeling is a tightly controlled balance between collagen production, breakdown, and remodeling. An imbalance during this process results in aberrant wound healing discussed later. Water will also be reabsorbed from the wound, further organizing the collagen fibers, and capillaries will regress, leaving a pale avascular scar. The end result of remodeling is a more organized arrangement of thicker cross-linked collagen fibers, maximizing wound strength.

## Wound Tensile Strength

Remodeling may take up to 18 months with a return of tensile strength to a maximum of only 70–80% of the strength found in uninjured skin. At day 21, the wound has maximal amounts of collagen; however, it has only 20% of the strength seen in normal dermis. At 6 weeks tensile strength approaches 70% of normal. It usually takes 6 months to reach maximal strength as a result of collagen breakdown and rearrangement. Thus, an inverse relationship exists between wound strength and wound thickness under the control of collagen remodeling. Factors affecting wound strength are discussed as follows.

**TABLE 2-1 Local and systemic factors that impede wound healing**

| *Disease states* | *Local factors* |
|---|---|
| Hereditary | Ischemia |
| Coagulation disorders | Infection |
| Ehlers–Danlos/Marfan's | Tissue trauma |
| Prolidase deficiency | Retained foreign body |
| Werner's syndrome | Desiccation |
| Vascular disorders | Medications |
| Congestive heart failure | Glucocorticoids |
| Atherosclerosis | Anticoagulants |
| Hypertension | Antineoplastic agents |
| Vasculitis | Colchicine |
| Venous stasis | Penicillamine |
| Lymphedema | Vitamin E |
| Metabolic | Salicylates (high dose) |
| Chronic renal failure | Nonsterioidals (high dose) |
| Diabetes mellitus | Zinc sulfate (high dose) |
| Malnutrition | Vitamin A (high dose) |
| Cushing's syndrome | |
| Hyperthyroidism | |
| Immunologic deficiency states | |
| Others | |
| Chronic pulmonary disease | |
| Liver failure | |
| Malignancy | |

*Source*: Terris DJ. Dynamics of wound healing. In: Bailey BJ (ed). *Head and neck surgery-otolaryngology.* 2nd ed. Philadelphia: Lippincott-Raven Publishers, 1998, With permission.

## Factors Affecting Wound Healing

Most of the factors that are detrimental to wound healing can be separated into local factors and systemic factors (**Table 2-1**). A complete understanding of the patient's health, paired with the ability to recognize local changes associated with the phases of wound healing, will allow the surgeon to modify factors that negatively affect wound healing in a timely manner.

## Local Factors Affecting Wound Healing

Necrotic tissue in a wound impedes wound healing by preventing the physiologic process of granulation tissue formation, subsequent epithelialization, and wound contraction. The necrotic tissue also harbors bacteria, which prolongs the inflammatory phase of wound healing. Collagen deposition will not occur until the inflammation subsides. Thus, a clean, moist wound will allow for a rapid progression through the phases of healing and result in an acceptable scar.

Similarly, a desiccated wound will be covered in a scab and usually demonstrates some degree of necrosis, delaying wound reepithelialization. A clean, moist, occluded wound will allow uninterrupted cellular migration, resulting in more rapid healing. In fact, moist wounds have been shown to promote cell migration at twice the rate of desiccated wounds. The occlusive dressing allows for fluid collection that is rich in PDGF promoting keratinocyte and fibroblasts essential to the epithelialization process. However, excessive moisture like necrotic tissue provides an optimal environment for bacterial growth.

In an open or chronic wound, debridement of healthy tissue with irrigation will create a more favorable environment for wound healing. Debridement removes MMPs that inhibit wound healing, decreases bacterial load, and promotes the formation of granulation tissue, wound contraction, and epithelialization.

Local tissue perfusion and oxygen tension are also essential to normal healing. Tissue ischemia can result from foreign debris, hematoma, infection, and vascular disease or metabolic derangements. Whereas cell migration and angiogenesis are stimulated by tissue hypoxia, collagen synthesis and deposition demonstrate a need for higher oxygen tension. These findings form the basis for hyperbaric oxygen in the treatment of nonhealing wounds. Fibroblast proliferation has been shown to increase with hyperbaric oxygen.

## Systemic Factors Affecting Wound Healing

Nicotine found in cigarettes stimulates the sympathetic nervous system and causes vasoconstriction. The carbon monoxide in cigarette smoke causes tissue hypoxia. When these two poisons are coupled together, the smoker is at greater risk for tissue necrosis and wound infection, which can lead to poor aesthetic results. Patients should be advised to quit smoking a minimum of 4 weeks before and after surgery.

Malnutrition also puts the patient at risk for poor wound healing. Particularly at risk are individuals with renal, hepatic, or gastrointestinal disease and those with cancer or chronic diseases including alcoholism. Appropriate protein intake is needed for normal angiogenesis and fibroblast function, resulting in collagen production and remodeling.

Vitamins and minerals are essential to many molecular events that result in normal wound healing. A critical step in the production of procollagen is the hydroxylation of lysine and proline, a process dependent on vitamin C and iron. Zinc and copper are also important to collagen formation and crosslinking, whereas vitamin A is important in phagocyte function, cell-mediated immunity and collagen synthesis. When applied topically vitamin E inhibits wound healing via a reduction in fibroblasts, effecting collagen synthesis and tensile strength. Vitamin K is essential to the clotting cascade and the production of prothrombin, important to the formation of the primary clot.

Prescription and herbal medications can also negatively affect wound healing. Nonsteroidal antiinflammatory drugs (NSAIDs) have been linked to decreased collagen production, and aspirin to reduced platelet function. Steroids impair the inflammatory phase of wound healing, increasing the risk of infection and suppressing fibroblast function and collagen synthesis. Vitamin A can be used to protect against some of the deleterious effects of corticosteroids on wound healing, specifically, fibroblast suppression, resulting in decreased collagen production and reepithelialization. Chemotherapeutic agents similarly impair the inflammatory process in wound healing.

Diabetes impairs wound healing by disrupting angiogenesis, fibroblast function, and inflammatory cell function, predisposing these patients to chronic nonhealing wounds. Collage production is also altered, leading to diminished tensile strength in the wound. Tight glucose control and vitamin A supplementation can improve wound healing in patients with diabetes. Many other disease states beyond the scope of this chapter can also impair wound healing (Table 1-2).

## Aberrant Wound Healing: Keloids and Hypertrophic Scars

Aberrant deposition of fibrous tissue in a wound is classified as a keloid or hypertrophic scar. A hypertrophic scar demonstrates excess fibrous tissue deposition at the site of injury, within the boundaries of the wound. Hypertrophic scars commonly undergo some degree of regression within 24–48 months. In contrast, keloids show tissue deposition beyond the borders of the original wound; they do not regress and usually recur after excision. Wounds that cross skin tension lines (i.e., earlobe) in darker-skinned individuals are common sites for keloid formation.

Although the molecular basis for lesions is not completely understood, hypertrophic scars and keloids result from an imbalance between the deposition of collagen and its normal degradation. Histologically, the hypertrophic scar shows excess deposition of collagen arranged mainly parallel to the long axis of the scar. In keloids, the collagen deposition is irregular, commonly described as collagen whorls or keloid collagen bundles.

The treatment for both processes is aimed at inhibiting the overproduction of collagen. This can be accomplished with intralesional corticosteroid injections, compressive dressings, silicone gel sheeting, interferon-alpha2b, and radiation. The growth factor TGF-β1 has been shown to induce keloid collagen growth. Drugs directed at blocking the activity of TGF-β1 or upregulating TGF-β3, which reduces fibronectin and collagen deposition, are under clinical investigation for the management of aberrant scarring.

Other studies have shown a downregulation of apoptosis-related genes in hypertrophic scar. Imiquimod 5% cream has been shown to induce TNF-α and IL-8, both shown to increase the expression of apoptosis-related gene products. In one study, the daily application of Imquimod 5% for 8 weeks following scar excision resulted in no recurrence of keloids. One drawback was a 50% hyperpigmentation at the site of application.

The pulse dye laser (PDL) has received recent attention for its potential ability to reduce the size and appearance of aberrant scar tissue with minimal side effects. A normal mature scar is relatively avascular, whereas keloids and hypertrophic scars demonstrate increased vascularity. The PDL targets the chromophore hemoglobin, destroying the blood vessels feeding the keloid. A study treating median sternotomy keloids every 6–8 weeks for 6 months showed significant improvement in the appearance of the scar with benefits lasting at least 6 months.

Numerous methods have been described to treat keloids and hypertrophic scars, but to date, optimal treatment remains elusive, and recurrence remains a significant management challenge for facial plastic surgeons. Clean wounds with meticulous closure remain the best way to create favorable scars. Early identification and pathologic scar prevention remains the best approach to avoiding significant disfigurement. With continued advances in molecular biology, we are more likely to find treatments targeted at the root causes of aberrant wound healing.

## References


1. Atiyeh BS. Nonsurgical management of hypertrophic scars: Evidence-based therapies, standard practices, and emerging methods. *Aesth Plast Surg* 2007, 31, 468–492.
2. Baum CL, Arpey CJ. Normal cutaneous wound healing: Clinical correlation with cellular and molecular events. *Dermatol Surg* 2005, 31(6), 674–686.
3. Cummings CW, Flint PW, Harker LA, Haughey BH, Richardson MA, Robbins, KT, Schuller DE, Thomas JR. *Cummings Otolaryngology: Head and Neck Surgery*, 4th ed., Mosby Elsevier, Philadelphia, 2004.
4. Honrado CP, Murakami CS. Wound healing and physiology of skin flaps. *Facial Plast Surg Clin N Am* 2005, 13, 203–214.
5. Martin P. Wound healing—Aiming for perfect skin regeneration. *Science* 1997, 276, 75–81.
6. Monaco JL, Lawrence WT. Acute wound healing: An overview. *Clin Plast Surg* 2003, 30, 1–12.
7. Mutalik S. Treatment of keloids and hypertrophic scars. *Indian J Dermatol Venereol Leprol* 2005, 71, 3–8.
8. Myers WT, Leong M, Phillis LG. Optimizing the patient for surgical treatment of the wound. *Clin Plastic Surg* 2007, 34, 607–620.
9. Papel ID. *Facial Plastic and Reconstructive Surgery*, 2nd ed., New York, Thieme, 2002.
10. Singer AJ, Clark RAF. Cutaneous wound healing. *N Eng J Med* 1999, 341, 738–746.
11. Werner S, Grose R. Regulation of wound healing by growth factors and cytokines. *Physiol Rev* 2003, 83, 835–870.
12. Witte MB, Barbul A. General principles of wound healing. *Surg Clin North Am* 1997, 77,501–513.
13. Teller P. White TK. Wound healing: injury through maturation. *Surg Clin N Am* 2009, 89, 99–610.

3

# Soft Tissue Techniques

Gregory H. Branham, MD, FACS

## Instrumentation

It is essential to have the proper instrumentation when performing soft tissue reconstruction of the face and neck **(Figure 3-1)**. Ideally, the surgeon has identified a set of preferred instruments that are always available and are designated for his/her use. At a minimum, it is imperative that the surgeon be familiar with the instrumentation on various sets that are available when working in a hospital operating room setting. This is obviously not an issue when one is working in a private outpatient surgery center or office setting where there is generally more control over instrumentation.

The minimum instrumentation that should be available includes knife handles for #11 and #15/15c blades—generally a #4 knife handle will suffice unless the surgeon prefers otherwise. Two fine-tissue forceps such as a 0.5-mm Castroviejo forceps, Bishop–Harmon forceps, or other fine forceps for aligning cutaneous edges **(Figure 3-2)**. These should not be used to grasp large pieces of tissue, as they can cut through or traumatize the skin edges. Two Brown–Adson forceps are useful for grasping edges of flaps and larger pieces of tissue. The author prefers Brown–Adson forceps over standard Adson forceps, as they are less traumatic because they have multiple teeth on either side of the jaws and spread the force

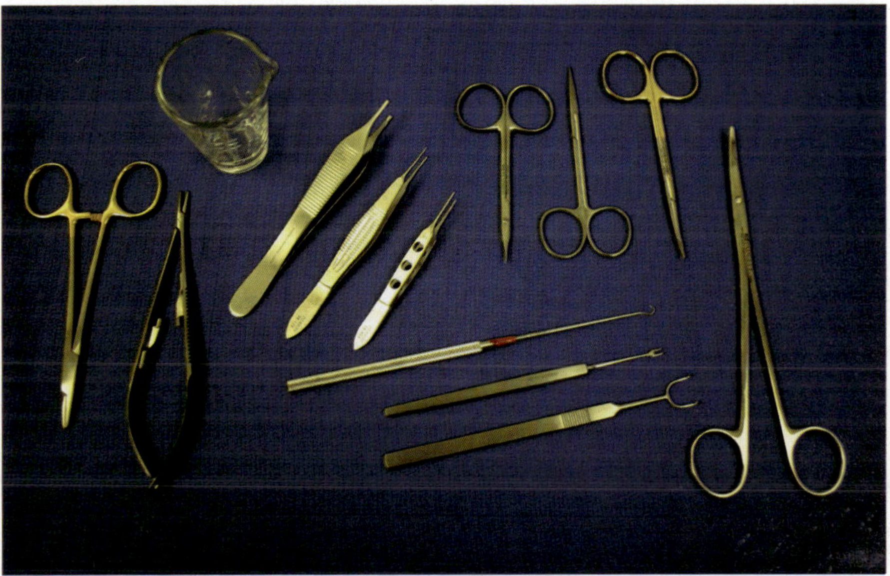

**Figure 3-1.** Surgical instruments for soft tissue reconstruction. A typical array of instruments used for most soft tissue reconstructions. Not shown is a caliper which is very useful to have and is usually kept peel packed separately and can be added as needed for any reconstruction.

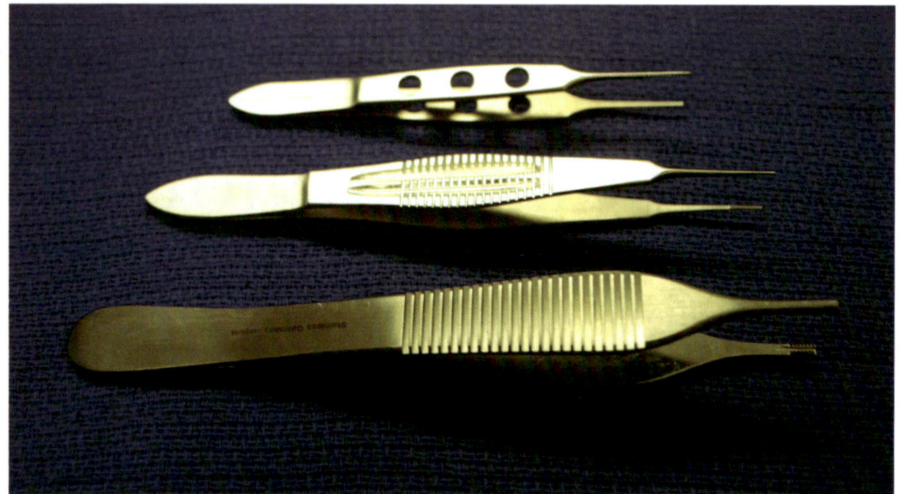

**Figure 3-2.** Soft tissue forceps. Shown are the Brown-Adson tissue forceps that have a larger platform and multiple small teeth. Also shown are the Castroviejo 0.5mm tissue forceps and the BishopHarmon tissue forceps.

of the tension across them. They are less likely to tear through the tissue.

Two needle holders with smooth platforms that will not cut through delicate 6-0 and 7-0 monofilament sutures are also recommended. Needle holders with cross-hatched platforms should only be used for larger sutures that are braided and will not be damaged by the needle holder. The author also prefers a heavier-gauge Castroviejo needle driver for most of the suturing that is done using smaller needles such as a P3 or PC1 needle. A delicate Castroviejo such as those used for microvascular anastomoses are too delicate for long-term use and should be avoided for routine cutaneous closures **(Figure 3-3).**

Two single prong hooks, two delicate microdouble pronged hooks (e.g., Guthrie) and two heavier-duty wide double-prong hooks are also necessary. Some surgeons prefer a small multiple pronged hook that is commonly referred to as a "Cat's Paw" **(Figure 3-4).** A millimeter caliper should be in each set to allow appropriate measurements for designing and planning of the reconstruction.

Finally, several scissors are needed for dissection **(Figure 3-5)**. The author prefers to have a large

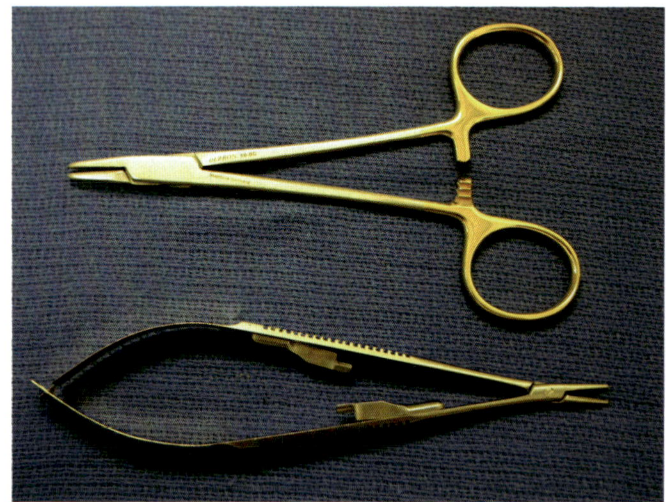

**Figure 3-3.** Needle holders for soft tissue reconstruction. The Webster needle holder has a smooth platform that will not traumatize the very small suture used in the soft tissue reconstruction. Larger standard needle holders typically have a waffled platform that can cut through the suture or weaken when it is grasped for tying or stabilizing. The Castroviejo needle holder can be held like a pencil and is ideal for delicate sutures and fine motor skills needed for facial soft tissue reconstruction.

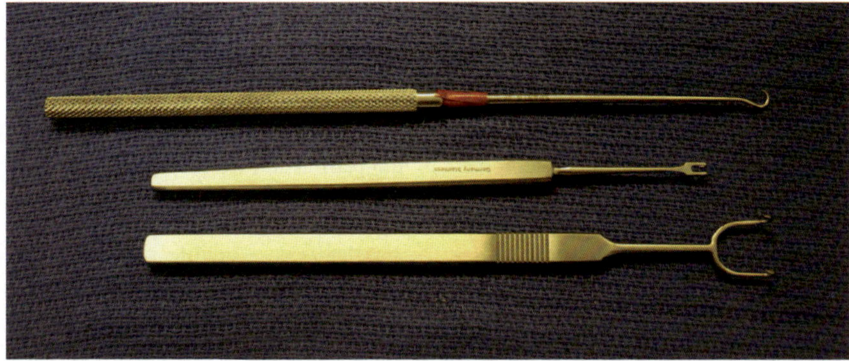

**Figure 3-4.** Tissue hooks. A single prong hook as well as a larger, sturdier double prong hook are essential for soft tissue reconstruction. A micro-double prong hook (Guthrie or sometimes referred to as a Tyrell) is also extremely useful in very delicate soft tissue handling.

facelift scissor (e.g., Freeman) in addition to the smaller tissue scissors so that only a single tray has to be opened if the surgeon is creating a larger flap such as a paramedian forehead flap or larger melolabial flap. Preferred tissue scissors are Kaye blepharoplasty scissors ,as they have a beveled edge, a slightly

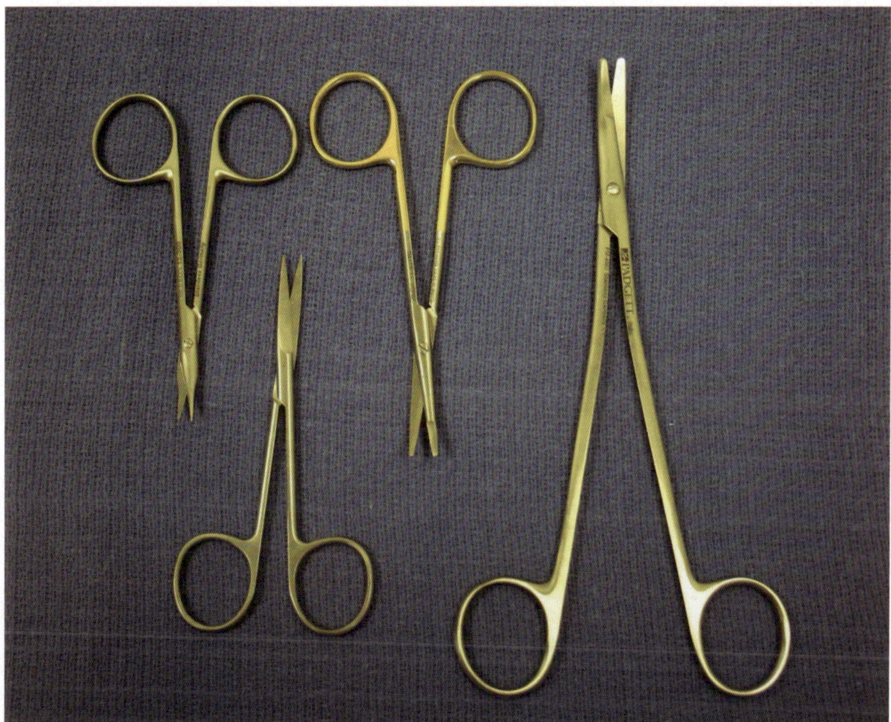

**Figure 3-5.** Scissors for soft tissue reconstruction A large Freeman Facelift scissors is useful for elevation of larger flaps. It has an outward beveled edge that facilitates undermining of the soft tissues as the scissor is opened. The angled handles are more ergonomic. The Kaye Blepharoplasty scissors are likewise beveled on the outer edge of the blades and have a serrated cutting edge that grips the tissues to prevent sliding through the scissors. Not shown are the Wescott scissors which are designed similar to the Castroviejo needle holder and can also be held like a pencil. Again the advantage is that they are suitable for delicate dissection and were originally designed for use in eye surgery. A straight Iris scissors is indispensable for suture cutting.

rounded tip, and a serrated cutting surface. The serrations allow the scissors to be used to cut tissue and prevent the tissue from slipping through the blades of the scissors as the tissue is being cut. It is essential that these scissors be sharp at all times and that they are well maintained. A small Westcott scissor is helpful when working in the periorbital area and straight sharp Iris scissors are necessary for cutting fine sutures. A larger, straight Mayo scissors is helpful for cutting dressings and larger sutures and bolsters. This group of instruments will provide the surgeon with an excellent armamentarium for performing almost any soft-tissue reconstruction using a local or regional flap.

## Local Anesthesia

Regardless of the type of anesthesia that is used, whether local, conscious sedation, or general anesthesia, local infiltration anesthetics are routinely used as an adjunct to facilitate patient comfort and safety as well as providing the surgeon adequate vasoconstriction in the surgical field. There are a number of local infiltrative anesthetics available for use, and it is essential that the surgeon understand the properties of these pharmacologic agents and their toxicities. Although there is no ideal anesthetic, consideration must be given to the following properties such as duration of action, irritation of tissue, onset of action, and a wide therapeutic window with low toxicity.

Local anesthetics are divided into two major classes: amides and esters (**Table 3-1**). Both amides and esters have a hydrophilic end and a lipophilic end. The lipophilic end is aromatic and is responsible for penetrating the nerve tissue. It is linked to the hydrophilic end with an intermediate chain. The hydrophilic end determines whether the agent is amide or ester. Esters are metabolized rapidly in the plasma and liver, whereas amides are metabolized more slowly in the liver alone. Individuals may demonstrate an allergy to one of the classes of anesthetics necessitating a switch to the other class with esters more commonly causing allergic problems. Individuals may also exhibit allergic responses to some of the preservatives used in preparing the anesthetics, both amides and esters, such as methylparaben.

The most commonly used local anesthetic for soft tissue surgery is lidocaine, which comes in several strengths (0.5–2% for injection and 2–4% for topical use). Lidocaine has a fast onset of action and duration of 1–3 hours depending on whether epinephrine has been added. Adding epinephrine can increase the duration of action by as much as 50%. Epinephrine is available in varying concentrations, the most common being 1:100,000. In facial reconstructive surgery, adding epinephrine is essential to assist in vasoconstriction in the surgical field.

The surgeon should be familiar with the toxic ranges and duration of action for each of the anesthetics used. For lidocaine, the toxic range is 3–4 mg/kg without epinephrine and 5–7 mg/kg with epinephrine. Some surgeons will choose to buffer the acidity of the lidocaine with one part of injectable sodium bicarbonate to nine parts of lidocaine. This buffering makes the injection less painful, but

**TABLE 3-1 Physical and Chemical Properties of Local Anesthetics**

| | | *% As Base at* | *LD50 Dose (mg)** | |
|---|---|---|---|---|
| *Drug* | *$pK_a$* | *pH 7.4* | *Intravenous* | *Subcutaneous* |
| **Esters** | | | | |
| Benzocaine | 3.5 | 100 | NA | NA |
| Procaine | 8.9 | 3 | 80 | 400 |
| Chloroprocaine | 8.7 | 4 | 97 | 950 |
| Tetracaine | 8.5 | 14 | 4 | 32 |
| **Amides** | | | | |
| Prilocaine | 7.9 | 24 | 62 | 820 |
| Mepivacaine | 7.6 | 39 | 35 | 280 |
| Lidocaine | 7.9 | 24 | 38 | 211 |
| Bupivacaine | 8.1 | 17 | 6 | 45 |

*Lethal dose in 50% of the mice.

Source: Covino, BG and Vassallo, HG: Local Anesthetics: mechanisms of action and clinical use. New York, 1976, Grune & Stratton.

**TABLE 3-2 Recommended Concentrations of Local Anesthetics and Maximum Doses**

| | | *Clinical Plain Solution* | | *Epinephrine Solution* | | *Infiltration* |
|---|---|---|---|---|---|---|
| *Drug (Trade Name)* | *Concentrations* | *mg* | *mg/kg* | *mg* | *mg/kg* | *Duration (min)* |
| Cocaine | 1%–4% | 200 | 1.5 | | | |
| Procaine (Novocain | 1%–10% | 500 | | 1000 | | 45–60 |
| Benzocaine | 14%–20% | | | | | |
| Tetracaine (Pontocaine | 1% | 100 | | 200 | | 60–180 |
| 2-Chloroprocaine (Nesacaine) | 1%–3% | 800 | 11 | 1000 | 14 | 30–45 |
| Lidocaine (Xylocaine) | 0.5%–5% | 300 | 4.5 | 500 | 7 | 60–120 |
| Mepivacaine (Carbocaine) | 1%–2% | 400 | | 500 | 7 | 90–180 |
| Prilocaine (Citanest) | 4% | 400 | | 500 | | 60–120 |
| Bupivacaine (Marcaine) | 0.25%–0.75% | 175 | | 250 | 3 | 240–480 |
| Etidocaine (Duranest) | 11.5% | 300 | 4 | 400 | 6 | 240–480 |
| Ropivacaine (Naropin) | 0.2%–1% | ? | ? | 200 | | 240–480 |
| Levobupivacaine | 0.25%–1% | ? | | | | 240–480 |

From White PF, ed: Ambulatory Anesthesia and Surgery. Philadelphia, WB Saunders, 1997:409.

also alters the balance of the local anesthetic between its ionized and nonionized form. The ionized form is the water-soluble form and the nonionized is the active lipophilic form that is capable of penetrating the nerve. It is the lipophilic nonionized form that determines onset of action, potency, and duration of action. There are a number of local anesthetics available to the surgeon, each with distinct advantages and disadvantages **(Table 3-2).**

## Topical Anesthetics

Use of topical anesthetics has gained in popularity and is now a widespread practice. These topical agents are primarily used in situations where there is a fear of needles (e.g., pediatric patients) or where a topical anesthetic is all that will be needed (e.g., a laser treatments such as hair removal). The first topical agent in use was eutectic mixture of local anesthetics (EMLA), which is an emulsion of lidocaine and prilocaine in a water-in-oil emulsion. It is applied to unbroken skin and is occluded. Its major disadvantage is its long onset of action requiring 90 minutes for adequate topical effect. Newer topical anesthetics have emerged that are more potent; care must be taken not to attempt to treat too large of a surface area as severe systemic toxicity and even death have been reported due to the intradermal absorption of toxic doses of the agents. BLT is currently one of the most commonly used agents and consists of benzocaine 20%, lidocaine 6% and tetracaine 4%. These agents, along with EMLA, are associated with methemoglobinemia, which causes cyanosis and diminished oxygen–carrying capacity of the blood. The mechanism is thought to occur as these agents are metabolized to ortho-toluidine, which then converts hemoglobin to methemoglobin.

## Tumescent Anesthesia

This form of anesthesia involves infusing large amounts of very dilute buffered anesthetic solutions. It was initially developed by anesthesiologist Dr. Jeffery Klein for use with body liposuction where large areas need to be anesthetized safely and where large fluid shifts occur during the procedure. Its use has migrated into facial cosmetic and reconstructive surgery for smaller procedures as well. The advantages of tumescent anesthetic techniques include the ability to hydrodissect a large amount of tissue (a process called "wetting") in the subdermal plane prior to surgery and the ability to anesthetize large areas without toxicity from an overdose of the local anesthetic. Numerous recipes exist for tumescent fluid, but they basically contain a very dilute concentration of lidocaine (0.05–0.15%) with concentrations of epinephrine of 1:1,000,000. Even though large total amounts of lidocaine are given, the absorption intravascularly is slow, peaking 10–14 hours after injection. It is thought that this is due to lidocaine's low-capacity tissue-binding affinity in subdermal fat. Whether the local anesthetic is injected or placed topically, there exists the possibility for toxicity if care is not taken. Manifestations of this toxicity begin as minor complaints such as headache and lightheadedness progressing to visual

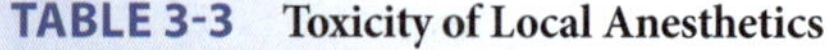

**TABLE 3-3 Toxicity of Local Anesthetics**

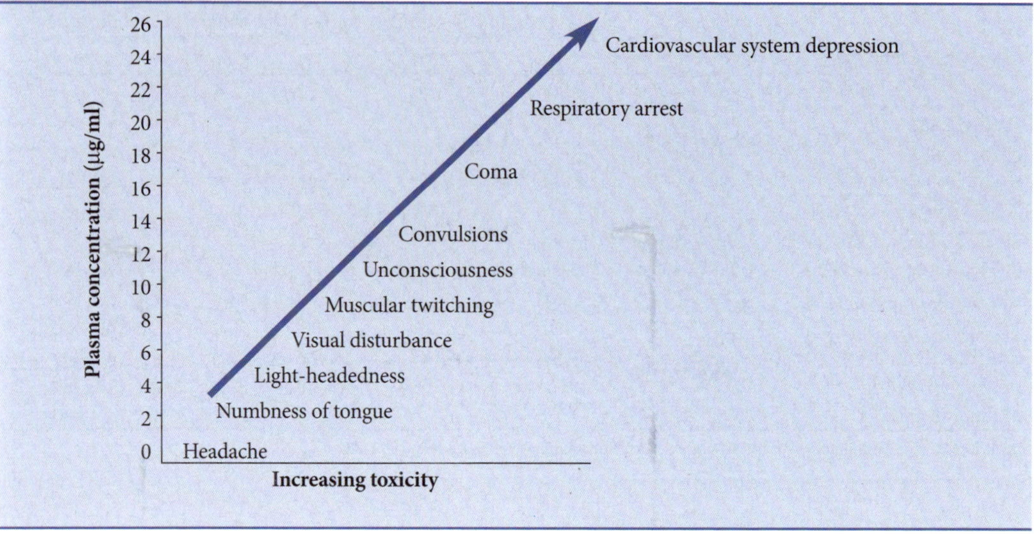


From Cousins, M.J., and Bridenbaugh, P.C.: Neural blockade in clinical anesthesia and management of pain, New York, 1980, Lippincott & Crowell.

disturbance and proceeding to seizures and loss of consciousness (**Table 3-3**).

## Incision Planning

When incisions are anticipated on the face, it is important for the scar to be the least visible that it can be. This is accomplished by adhering to several key principles including the concept of relaxed skin tension lines and facial esthetic subunits. Relaxed skin tension lines are those lines that develop over time on the face and are created by the action of the facial musculature on the skin (**Figure 3-6**). Placement of incisions along these lines or parallel to these lines will create the most favorable scar (**Figure 3-7**).

The other key concept is that of facial esthetic units. The face is naturally divided into units such as the perioral, periorbital, nasal, forehead, cheek, and chin (**Figure 3-8**). Each of these units can be further subdivided into subunits, which we discuss in later chapters.

## Undermining

When closing the wound, the edges should be undermined to relieve tension at the edge of the wound. A low tension closure is essential to create a fine and smooth scar. In general, undermining should be accomplished in the subcutaneous plane, which is relatively less vascular than the intradermal plane, which disrupts the vascular plexus causing significant bleeding and bruising. Gentle countertraction will help to define the plane as the tissues

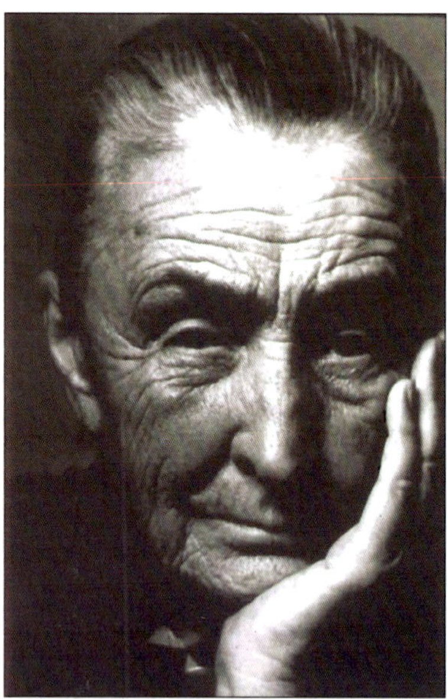

**Figure 3-6.** Relaxed skin tension lines (RSTLs). This photograph of artist Georgia O'Keefe shows relaxed skin tension lines that have developed over many years of living and painting in the Southwestern US.

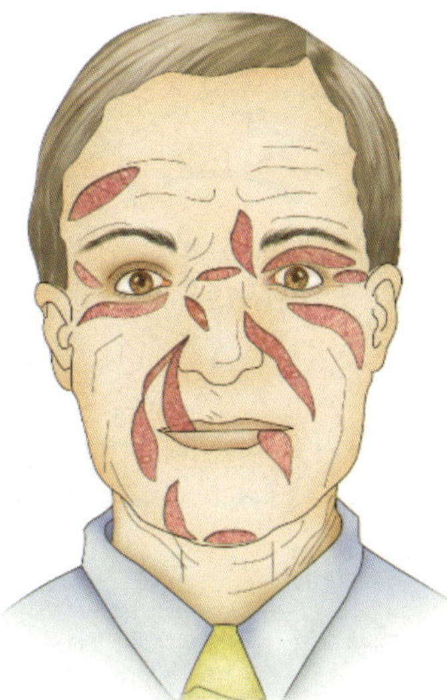

Figure 3-7. Incision placement along relaxed skin tension lines. Placement of incisions along RSTLs minimizes tension and scarring and maximizes cosmesis.

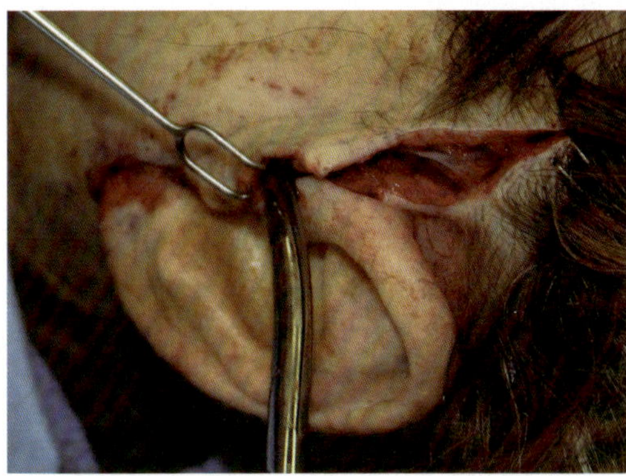

Figure 3-9. Proper Technique for Undermining Soft Tissue. Gentle countertraction from the assistant and traction with a tissue hook or tissue friendly forceps, without grasping the skin edge directly, provides for elevation of the tissues with the least trauma.

are elevated (**Figure 3-9**). Elevation with a 15 or 15c blade will accomplish undermining with the least amount of tissue trauma; however, for larger flaps a facelift scissor is quite effective and efficient. The edge of the flap should be grasped with a tissue hook or in the subcutaneous tissues with a forceps that will provide a secure purchase and minimal trauma such as a Brown–Adson forceps that has multiple teeth in two rows along the edges. Single-toothed forceps tend to tear through the tissue creating more trauma. Grasping the epidermal edge should be avoided if at all possible, as this will affect the final outcome of the scar.

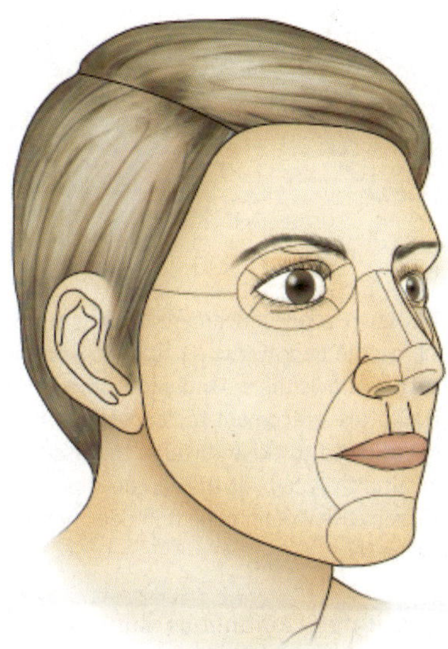

Figure 3-8. Facial esthetic subunits. The subunit principle permits appropriate pre-op planning for reconstruction of facial defects. As much as possible reconstructions should avoid overlap into adjacent subunits or should run along borders between them.

Studies have been performed looking at the amount of undermining necessary to create a tension-free closure. It has been shown that there is no significant advantage to undermining beyond 2 cm from the edge of the wound. Additionally, there have been a number of studies evaluating the advantage of rapid intraoperative tissue expansion as a means of reducing wound-closing tensions. It has been shown that the advantage gained with rapid intraoperative tissue expansion is equivalent to that obtained by undermining and is primarily attributable to biomechanical creep.

## Wound Closure Techniques

All facial wounds involving full-thickness defects should be closed in a layered fashion. In general, this would involve closure of any deep tissues such as muscle or deep fascia followed by closure in the subcutaneous plane and finally a skin or cuticular closure. Prior to closure, it is essential that adequate hemostasis is obtained. This is accomplished

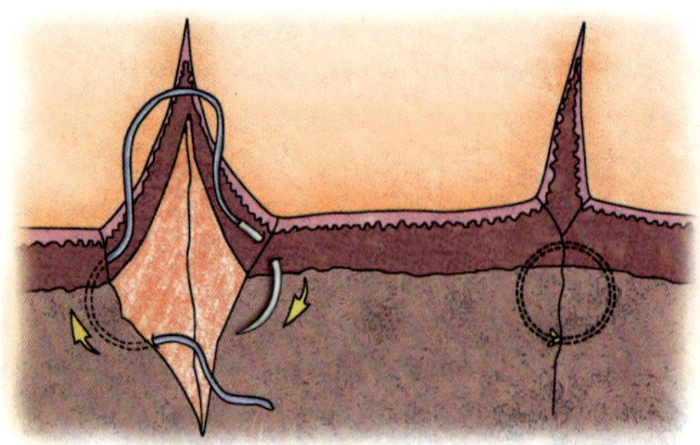

**Figure 3-10.** Buried intradermal suture. By initiating the closure in the deep surface of the wound the knot is buried in the depth of the wound, lessening the risk of suture abscess and extrusion.

with the use of a bipolar cautery or an ophthalmic thermal cautery. The advantage of the ophthalmic thermal cautery is that it is battery powered and convenient for small cases. It is not as efficient as bipolar cautery in achieving hemostasis, however.

Deep sutures should be placed as interrupted sutures whose knots are buried in order to minimize suture extrusion or abscess as the wound heals (**Figure 3-10**). Cuticular closures should be accomplished so that the full curvature of the needle is used to create eversion of the wound edge (**Figure 3-11**).

In addition to the simple suture, seen in Figures 3.5 and 3.6, there are a number of suture techniques that are useful and with which the surgeon should be aware. Mattress suture techniques are useful in distributing tension across a larger area of the wound. In the vertical mattress suture (**Figure 3-12**), the suture is passed several millimeters away from the wound edge in the first pass. A second pass is made in line with the first but closer to the wound edge. This distributes the tension in the vertical plane to the deeper tissues.

In the horizontal mattress suture (**Figure 3-13**), tension is distributed horizontally along the edge of the wound by passing the needle several millimeters away from the wound edge on either side of the wound and then advancing down the wound edge and performing a similar pass with the needle at the same level in the subcutaneous plane. This permits the tension to be distributed up and down the length of the wound, thus taking tension off of the wound edge.

Sutures may be placed as interrupted sutures or as a continuous suture (**Figure 3-14**), also termed

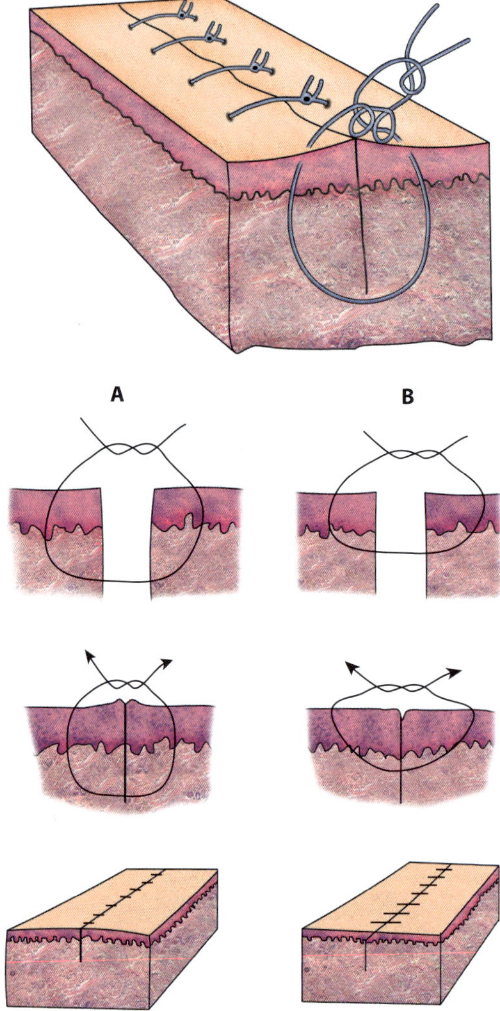


**Figure 3-11.** (A) Proper placement of the suture by allowing the needle to traverse its full arc through the tissues. This allows the wound edges to be slightly everted. (B) Suture placement too superficial because the needle is allowed to skive through the tissues resulting in suture placement that is too superficial and too far from the wound edge and does not evert the edges properly.

a running suture. Continuous sutures may be simple continuous sutures or running locking sutures. Running sutures may be placed as cuticular sutures with an external component or as an intradermal (subcuticular) suture that surfaces only at either end. When a continuous suture is used, care must be taken to avoid pulling the suture too tightly

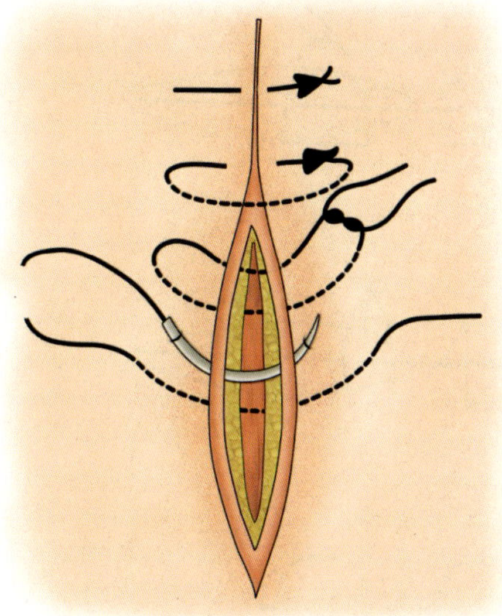

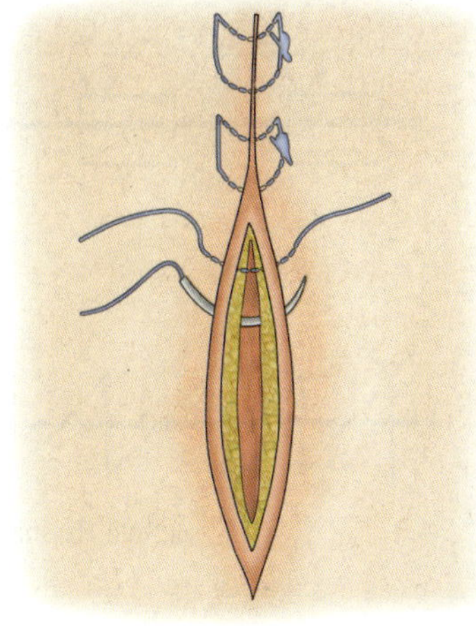

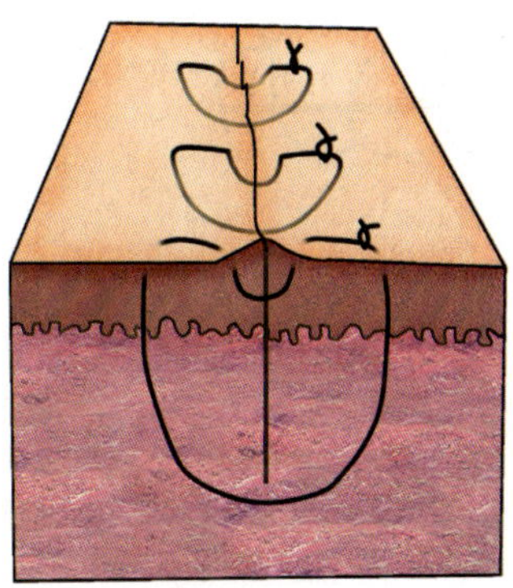


**Figure 3-12.** Vertical mattress suture. The vertical mattress suture allows the closing tension to be shared with deeper tissues in addition to the skin surface.

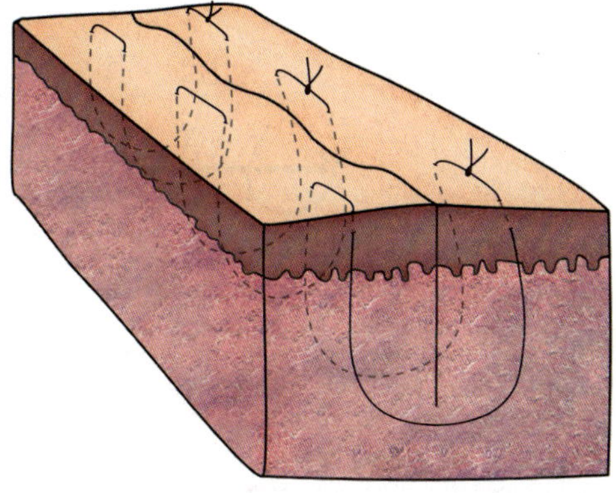


**Figure 3-13.** Horizontal mattress suture. The horizontal mattress suture distributes the wound closing tension over the surface of the wound horizontally.

and creating strangulation of the wound edge and bunching of the incision. This impairs healing and can leave suture track marks on the scar after the sutures are removed.

Except in unusual circumstances, purse-string sutures should be avoided as they create too much strangulation of the tissues. Similarly, three-way sutures that encompass the tip of a flap should be avoided, as they place too much tension on the tip of the flap, which has the least amount of blood supply.

## Suture Selection

The surgeon should be familiar with the various sutures and needles that are available for subcutaneous and cuticular closure. Absorbable sutures are sutures that retain tensile strength for a varying period of time and then are hydrolyzed by the tissue fluids. They are generally used below the surface of the epidermis or for mucosal closures; however, they are useful for epidermal closures in special circumstances where it would be undesirable to remove

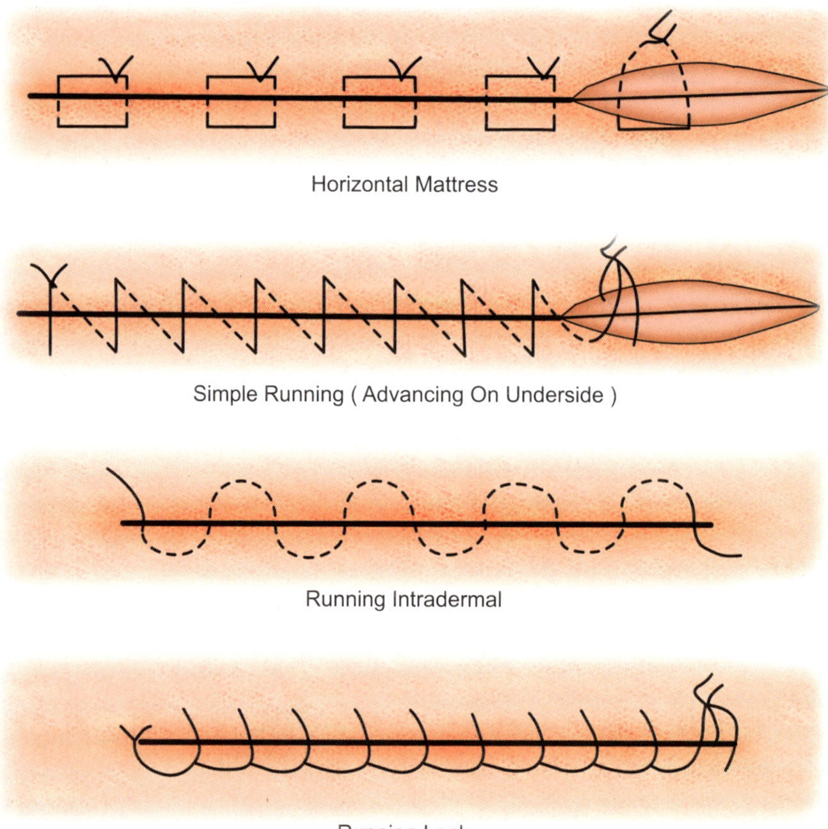


**Figure 3-14.** Various suture techniques. The surgeon should be familiar with a large number of different suturing techniques that offer specific advantages.

sutures at a later time. For example, in the subciliary incision of a lower eyelid blepharoplasty, it is disconcerting to the patient to have these sutures removed in the office, and for this reason a small absorbable suture is typically used. In pediatric cases where removal of permanent sutures would necessitate sedation or general anesthesia, absorbable sutures would be preferable. Because they cause a greater tissue response and more inflammation, absorbable sutures do have the potential to create a less desirable scar. It is for this reason that the author prefers a permanent monofilament suture in most cases for skin closure.

The most important factors to consider when choosing an absorbable suture are its tensile strength, knot-tying characteristics, and tissue reaction (**Figure 3-15**). In general, the deeper and more substantial the tissue, the longer you want the suture to retain its tensile strength and the less concern there is for tissue reaction. Extrusion rates are less for monofilament sutures than for braided ones and are higher the longer the suture is retained and the more superficially it is placed in the wound. The choice of absorbable suture should fit the desired goals of the surgeon and should persist only as long as needed. The size of the suture selected should be as small as possible to get the desired result. As a general rule, 5-0 sutures are used in the subcutaneous plane with occasional 4-0 sutures used for deeper subcutaneous closures and 6-0 sutures for closures that are superficial in the dermis.

Nonabsorbable (permanent) sutures are similarly monofilament and braided in type (**Figure 3-16**). In general, braided sutures should not be used for cuticular closures in the face, head, and neck. Braided sutures are very useful in areas in which the surgeon desires long-term tensile strength and are the author's choice for use in facelifts to suspend the su-

| | Suture | Brand Name | Composition | Tensile Strength(d) | Common Uses |
|---|---|---|---|---|---|
| Gut | Plain | | Animal-derived collagen | 7–10 | Subcutaneous closure minimal support |
| | Chromic | | Plain gut treated with chromium salts to slow absorption | 10–14 | Dermal Subcutaneous Mucosa |
| | Rapidly (fast) absorbing gut | | Plain gut heal treated to accelerate absorption | 5–7 | Skin closure |
| Synthetic | Polyglycolic acid | Dexon | Braided strands of polyglycolic avid | 14–21 | Fascial deep closures |
| | Polyglyconate | Maxon | Monofilament strands of glycolic acid and trimethylene carbonate | 14–21 | Subcutaneous |
| | Polydioxanone | Polydioxanone II | Monofilament polyester of polydioxanone | 14–42 | Dermal subcutaneous |
| | Poligtecaprone 25 | Monocryl | Monofilament copolymer of glycolide and epsilon caprolactone | 7–14 | Dermal subcutaneous |
| | Polyglactin 910 | Vicryl | Braided copolymer of lactide and glycotide | 14–28 | Dermal subcutaneous mucosa |
| | Polyglactin 910 | Vicryl Rapide | Molecular with copolymer of lactice and glycolide | 5–7 days | Superficial skin and mucosa |
| | Polyglactin 910 plus antibacterial | Vicrul Plus | 90% glucolide/10% L-lactide with antibacterial triclosan brad spaectrum | 14–28 days | Dermal subcutaneous |

**Figure 3-15.** Commonly used absorbable sutures.

perficial musculoaponeurotic system (SMAS) layer, for example. Silk sutures are still commonly used for mucosal closures and for closures on the lips because it is soft and will not irritate the oral cavity or lips during chewing.

For facial skin closures, a 6-0 or 7-0 monofilament suture is best. The smallest suture that will accomplish the task is preferable. Occasionally, 5-0 sutures are used in the neck. Because monofilament sutures are very slippery, they are useful when the surgeon needs the suture to be able to slide after the first throw. Five throws of the knot are usually necessary to ensure that a monofilament suture will not unravel over time. Care must be taken to reverse the throws in order to square the knot and lock it sufficiently. Conversely, braided sutures have significant friction with the first throw and will lock after two throws. Usually, three throws are sufficient to prevent knot failure with braided sutures.

## Cutaneous Tissue Adhesives

Once the subcutaneous closure is complete, or in the case of a very superficial wound requiring only a single layer cuticular closure, a skin adhesive may be used to accomplish the cuticular closure. The most commonly used material for this purpose is Dermabond (octylcyanoacrylate), which is quite popular among physicians treating pediatric patients and in ER patients with clean wounds as they obviously do not require a follow-up visit for suture removal. Dermabond is a derivative of superglue (cyanoacrylate) and dries quickly. It should not be used in contaminated wounds or in wounds that are greater than 5 cm in length. Dermabond is left undisturbed and dry until sloughing occurs at 5–7 days. It is not a substitute for suture in a deep wound that requires a layered closure, as it lacks tensile strength to hold such a wound together and does not adequately

| Source | Suture | Brand Name | Composition | Tensile Strength (d) | Common Uses |
|---|---|---|---|---|---|
| Natural fibers | Silk | Silk | Fibrin protein strands spun & braided. Coated with wax silicone | 1 year | Mucosa<br>Dry portion of lips<br>Rarely skin |
| Synethetic fibers | Nylon monofilament | Ethilon<br>*Dermalon* | Nylon 6 or Nylon 6-6 | 5 years | General skin closure |
| | Nylon braided multifilament | Nurolon<br>*Surgilon* | Nylon 6-6 | 80% at 180 days | General deep tissue closure |
| | Polyester braided | Mersilene | Polythylene Terepthalate | The apparent loss of tensile strength over 1 year | Deep tissue closure where long-term retention of tensile strength is needed. |
| | Polyester braided and coated | Ethibond | Polythene terephthalate coated with polybutilate | The apparent loss of tensile strength over 1 year | Deep tissue closure where long-term retention of tensile strength is needed. |
| | Polypropylene | Prolene<br>*Surgilene* | Polypropylene | No apparent loss of tensile strength at 1 year. | Vascular repair<br>Long-term deep tissue closure |

**Figure 3-16.** Commonly used nonabsorbable sutures.

obliterate the dead space because it cannot be used subcutaneously.

## References


1. Maas CS, ed. *Wound Management and Suturing Manual.* American Academy of Facial Plastic and Reconstructive Surgery, Alexandria VA, 2001.
2. Weerda H, ed. *Reconstructive Facial Plastic Surgery: A Problem Solving Manual,* Thieme, New York, 2001.
3. Branham GH, ed. Local skin flaps. *Facial Plast Clin N Am* 4(4), 1996.
4. Ehlert TK, Arnold DE. Local anesthesia for soft-tissue surgery. *Otolaryngol Clin N Am* 23(5), 1990, 831–844.
5. van Rijssel EJ, Brand R, Admiraal C, et al: Tissue reaction and surgical knots: The effect of suture size, knot configuration, and knot volume. *Obstet Gynecol* 1989, 74(1), 64–68.
6. Touma S, Jackson JB. Lidocaine and prilocaine toxicity in a patient receiving treatment for mollusca contagiosa. *J Am Acad Dermatol* 2001, 44(2 Suppl), 399–400.
7. Hahn IH, Hoffman RS, Nelson LS. EMLA-induced methemoglobinemia and systemic topical anesthetic toxicity. *J Emerg Med* 2004, 26(1), 85–88.
8. Henry LR, Pizzini M, Delarso B, Ridge JA. Methemoglobinemia: Early intraoperative detection by clinical observation. *Laryngoscope* 2004, 114(11), 2025–2026.
9. Birchem SK. Benzocaine-induced methemoglobinemia during transesophageal echocardiography. *J Am Osteopath Assoc* 2005, 105(8), 381–384.
10. Papel ID, et al., eds. *Facial Plastic and Reconstructive Surgery,* 2nd ed., Thieme, New York, 2002.
11. de Jong, RH. Tumescent anesthesia: Lidocaine dosing dichotomy. *Int J Cosmet Aesthetic Derm* 2001, 4(1), 3–7.

# 4

# Principles of Flap Design and Preoperative Analysis

Gregory H. Branham, MD, FACS

## Introduction

In this chapter, we discuss the factors to consider in the preoperative analysis of the reconstructive patient, the defect analysis, and the nomenclature of the local flaps and their definitions. This will include a discussion of the types of flaps based on their movement and vascular supply (**Table 4-1**). We also discuss optimal placement of resultant scars and various esthetic subunits of the face.

The major goals of any reconstruction are to preserve function and achieve an esthetically acceptable result. In order to achieve these goals, there are a number of major factors to consider in the preoperative analysis of the reconstructive patient. The factors include vascular supply, available flap choices, location of defect, and other factors such as underlying disease and comorbidities. All of these will impact how difficult it may be for the flap to survive and how well the flap will heal. The facial anatomical subunits that will be involved or affected by the reconstruction, the relaxed skin tension lines in the area, and how incision placement can be optimized are also necessary considerations.

**TABLE 4-1 Classification of Flaps**

| Movement | Vascularity |
|---|---|
| • Advancement-linear sliding movement of adjacent tissue | • Random Pattem-rely on subdermal and subpapillary plexus |
| • Rotation-movement of adjacent tissue around an arc of rotation or pivot point | • Axial Pattem-direct cutaneous arteries within the pedicle of flap |
| • Transposition movement of tissue across an intervening segment of tissue | • Musculocutaneouscontain overlying muscle fascia and skin with vascular pedicle |

Flaps can be classified based on their blood supply or the movement that is displayed during their transfer into the defect.

## Vascular Supply

Intact vasculature is essential to the survival of any flap and knowledge of the facial vascular anatomy is critical. Although we have discussed the microanatomy of the skin in Chapter 1, the major vascular supply to the face will be addressed here.

The face derives its primary blood supply from the branches of the external carotid artery (**Figure 4-1**). The external carotid artery is a branch from the common carotid artery where it branches into the internal and external carotid arteries. The internal carotid artery proceeds through the neck and into the base of the skull without branches, and the external carotid artery provides a number of branches to structures in the neck and face.

The facial artery gives rise to the superior and inferior labial arteries that supply the upper and lower lips as well as a submental branch. Branching from

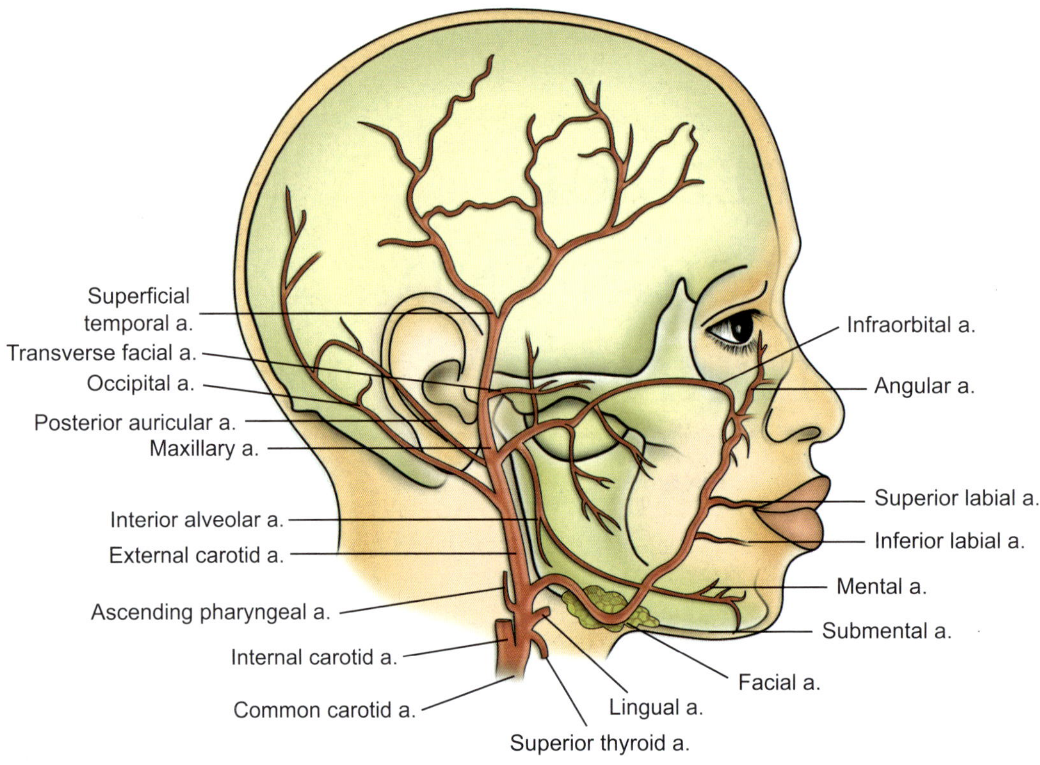


**Figure 4-1.** Vascular anatomy of the face. External carotid artery and its branches.

the superior labial artery is the angular artery that branches upward along the nasofacial groove anastomosing with branches of the infraorbital artery (a branch of the maxillary artery) in the medial canthal region.

The transverse facial artery is the next most superior branch supplying the musculature in the buccal or midfacial region. Superior to this, the external carotid artery then gives off the zygomatico-orbital artery that provides blood supply to the orbicularis oculi and other periocular muscles. One of the two terminal branches of the external carotid artery is the superficial temporal artery, and it branches into the anterior and posterior superficial temporal artery that supplies the frontal region and the parietal region, respectively. Posteriorly, the occipital artery arises from the external carotid artery and supplies the postauricular skin and occipital scalp.

The maxillary artery, the second terminal branch of the external carotid artery, is divided into three portions or divisions. The branches of the first division dive deep to supply the middle-ear structures and the meninges via the middle meningeal artery. In addition, the inferior alveolar artery that supplies the mandible arises from the first division. The second division of the internal maxillary artery supplies the infratemporal fossa musculature such as the medial and lateral pterygoid muscles. The third division enters the pterygopalatine fossa giving rise to several important branches including the infraorbital and sphenopalatine arteries that supply the midface and internal structures of the nose, respectively.

The major vascular supplies to the forehead are the paired supratrochlear and supraorbital arteries. The supraorbital and supratrochlear arteries are branches from the ophthalmic artery, which is a branch from the internal carotid artery.

## Facial Esthetic Units

The face can be divided into facial esthetic units (**see Figure 4-2**). These correspond to areas that are visually distinct and comprise a functional unit of the face. These include the forehead, temporal, periorbital, nasal, cheek, perioral, and chin regions. Whenever possible, construction of a defect should be confined to a single esthetic unit. When a

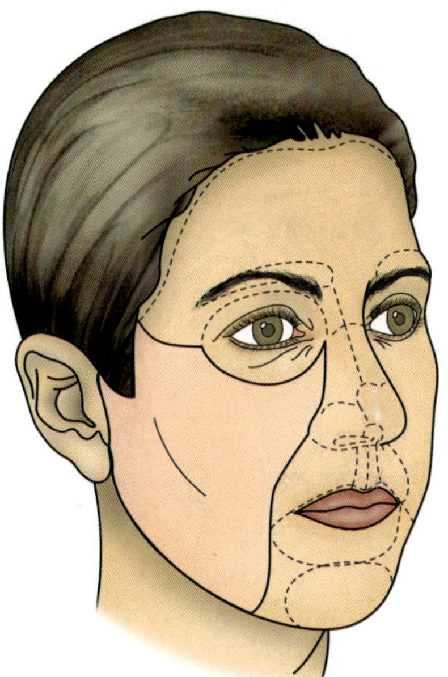

**Figure 4-2.** Facial esthetic subunits represent areas that are visually distinct and functionally unique.

defect crosses two or more esthetic units, every effort should be made to place incisions at the junctions of these esthetic units. Additionally, when a defect involves two or more esthetic units, it may be preferable to reconstruct each of these units in a different manner to create the best cosmetically acceptable and functional result.

Each of these facial esthetic units can be further subdivided into esthetic subunits (**Figure 4-3**). One of the most important examples of this is the nose. The nasal esthetic unit can be divided into the paired nasal sidewall subunits, the nasal dorsal subunit, the nasal tip subunit, the alar lobule subunits, and the columellar subunit. The same general principles apply to facial aesthetic subunits as do the reconstructive principles for the facial aesthetic units. Discussion of aesthetic subunits is undertaken in subsequent specific chapters.

## Relaxed Skin Tension Lines

Another factor to consider in preoperative analysis of facial defects and their reconstruction is the orientation of the defect to the facial relaxed skin tension lines. Relaxed skin tension lines (RSTLs) are those lines that form on the face due to the action of muscles of facial expression on the skin (**Figure 4-4**). These are most evidenced as we age. RSTLs run perpendicular to the action of the muscles of facial expression so that, in the forehead, the RSTLs run in a horizontal plane perpendicular to the orientation of the frontalis muscle. The RSTLs in the perioral aesthetic unit are radially oriented due to the sphincteric circular orientation of the orbicularis oris. The RSTLs in the periorbital region tend to

A

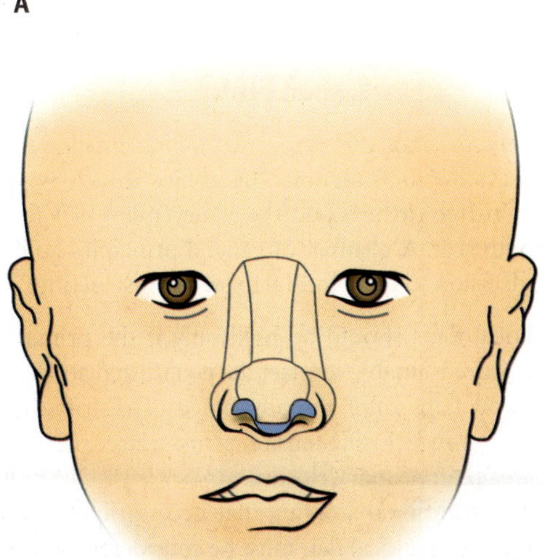

B

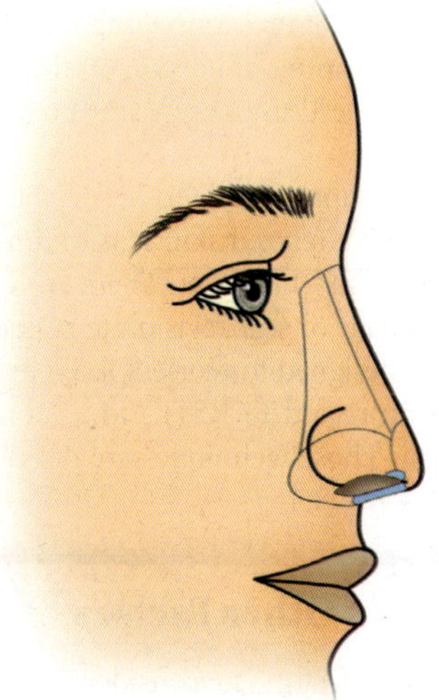

**Figure 4-3.** Facial esthetic units can be further divided into subunits that allow for more detailed and specific operative planning as is depicted here for the nose.

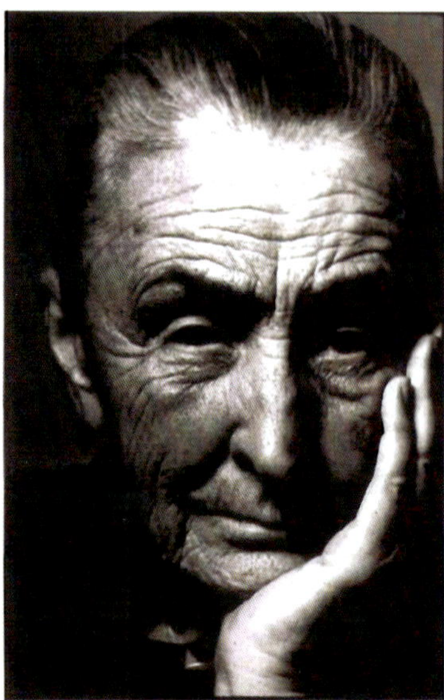

**Figure 4-4.** Relaxed skin tension lines (RSTLs). This photograph of the artist Georgia O'Keeffe shows relaxed skin tension lines that have developed over many years of living and painting in the Southwestern United States.

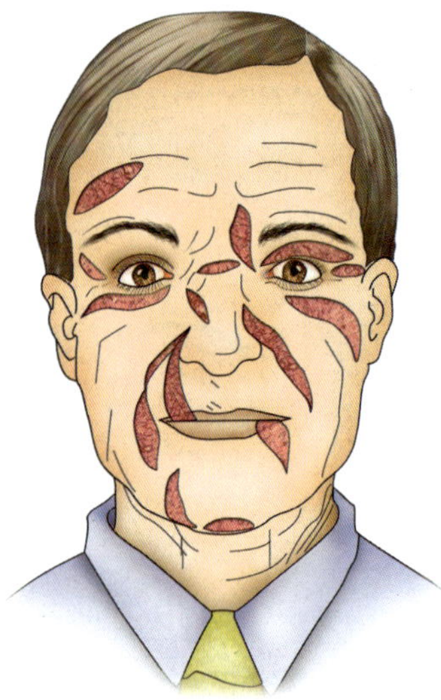

**Figure 4-5.** Incision placement along relaxed skin tension lines. Placement of incisions along RSTLs minimizes tension and scarring and maximizes cosmesis.

be radially oriented at the lateral canthal area due to that same sphincteric muscular action of the orbicularis oculi and tend to be horizontally oriented in the lower eyelid. The RSTLs in the cheek are oriented obliquely perpendicular to the orientation of the zygomaticus major and minor muscles that originate from the body of the body of the zygoma and insert into the skin along the melolabial fold. The orientation of incisions along these RSTLs creates the least amount of tension on the scar, thereby creating the finest, smoothest scar possible (**Figure 4-5**).

When it is not possible to orient the scar or the incision along a relaxed skin tension line, it should be oriented parallel to them. There are a number of scar camouflage or scar revision techniques that are specifically designed to reorient scars that are unfavorable with regard to RSTLs to a more favorable orientation. Those techniques are discussed in this text in Chapter 11.

## Other Factors

Finally, other factors to consider in preoperative analysis include comorbidities and underlying disease such as diabetes, which affects the microvasculature and thus impacts the oxygenation of the tissues as well as predisposing these individuals to postoperative infection. Smoking creates tissue hypoxia by diminishing overall pulmonary function and vasoconstriction by nicotine. Patients on immunosuppressive medications such as steroids or certain chemotherapeutic agents will have their wound healing negatively impacted, and this should be taken into consideration when planning a facial reconstruction.

## Local Flaps

The major goals of any reconstruction include the preservation of function, the ability to achieve a tension-free closure, and the achievement of a flat, smooth scar. A number of general principles guide the decision to use a local flap for reconstruction:

1. Local flaps should be used only if the primary closure is unable to meet the goals listed above.
2. Local flaps offer the advantage of distributing the wound-closing tension across a larger surface area than primary closure.
3. The additional scarring that necessarily attends the use of a local flap must be considered.
4. The option of healing by secondary intention and/or partial healing by secondary intention with secondary skin grafting must also be considered when analyzing a defect for reconstruction.

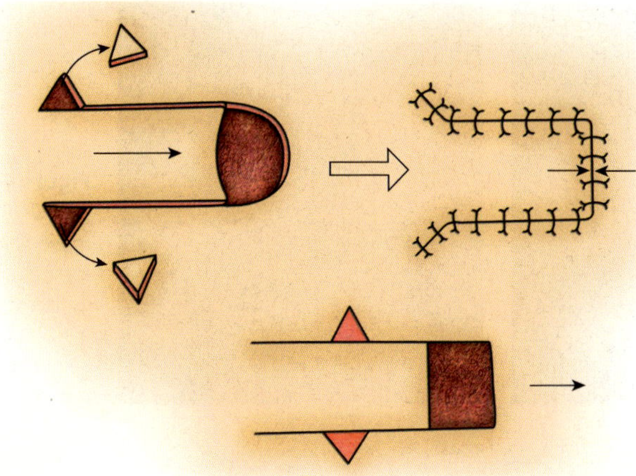

**Figure 4-6.** Advancement flaps. Advancement flaps involve the movement of adjacent tissue in a linear fashion along a straight line.

## Types of Local Flaps

Local flaps may be characterized based on their movement as well as their vascular supply. Most commonly, they are divided based on the type of movement that is characteristic of that flap and include the advancement flap the transposition flap and the rotation flap.

The advancement flap (**Figure 4-6**) is a random pattern flap that involves the movement of adjacent tissue in a linear sliding fashion to accomplish closure of the primary defect. Examples of advancement flaps include V-Y and O-T as well as horizontal advancement flaps.

A rotation flap (**Figure 4-7**) is a random pattern flap that involves the movement of adjacent tissue

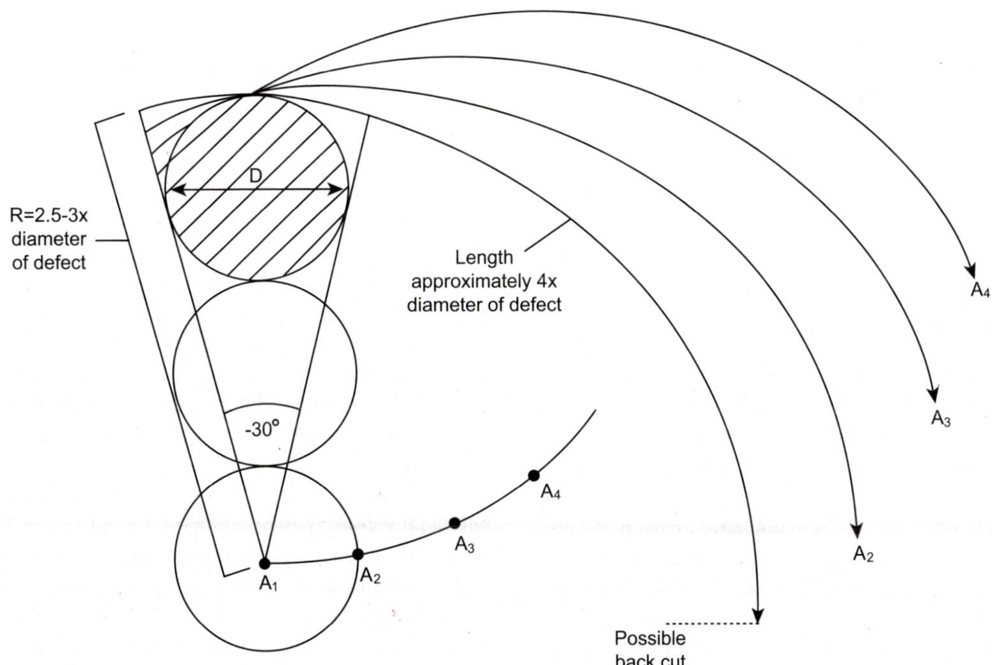


**Figure 4-7.** Rotation flap. A rotation flap involves the movement of tissue around an arc of rotation or pivot point.

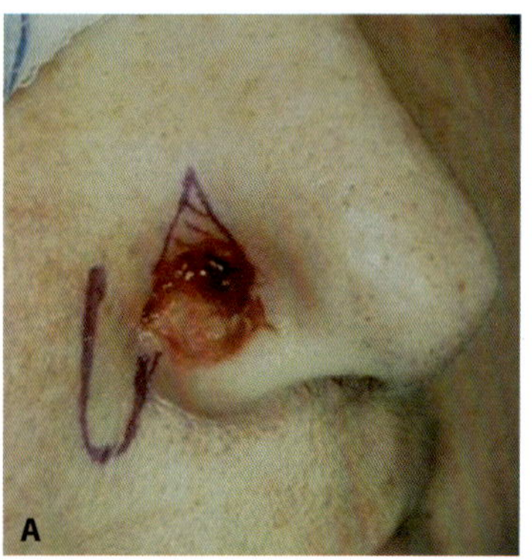


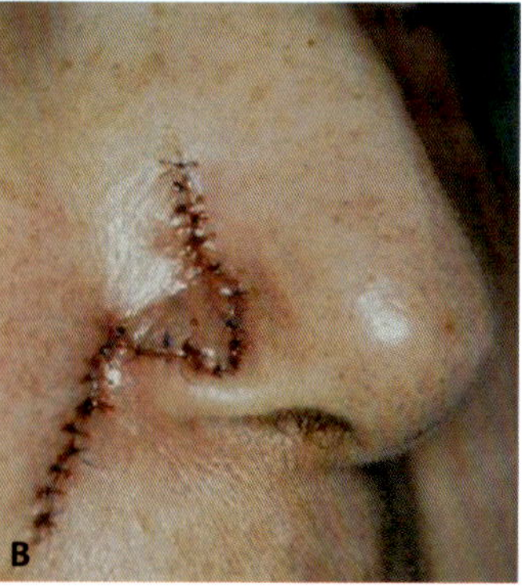


**Figure 4-8.** Transposition flap. (A) This flap involves the movement of tissue across an intervening segment of tissue. This is a superiorly based melolabial flap. (B) Flap has been transposed over the alar lobule and sewn into position.

around an arc of rotation or a pivot point. The sliding glabellar flap is a good example of a rotation flap.

The transposition flap (**Figure 4-8**) is a random pattern flap that involves the movement of tissue across an intervening segment of tissue. Perhaps the most common transposition flap is the superiorly or inferiorly based melolabial flap, which is used in reconstruction of the nasal and perioral subunits.

Local flaps can also be characterized based on their blood supply (**Figure 4-9**). Random pattern flaps (**Figure 4-9A**) are flaps that rely on the musculocutaneous perforating branches for their blood supply and the anastomotic connections to the subdermal and subpapillary plexuses. The flaps are elevated at the subcutaneous level, and the musculocutaneous perforating vessels are divided with only the most proximal ones remaining intact to supply the microcirculation of the subdermal and subpapillary plexuses. Survival of the random pattern flap is dependent on the capillary filling pressure at the distal end of the flap.

Axial pattern skin flaps are flaps that are based on direct cutaneous arteries that are contained within the pedicle of the flap (**Figure 4-9B**). Survival of the axial pattern flap is dependent on maintaining its intact vascular pedicle. The distal end of the skin paddle of an axial pattern flap is also random in its vascular supply, as the terminal branch ends as a musculocutaneous perforating vessel.

Musculocutaneous flaps (**Figure 4-9C**) contain the muscle, fascia, and the overlying cutaneous paddle of skin. In musculocutaneous flaps, it is helpful to anchor the skin paddle to prevent shearing of the perforating vessels between the skin paddle and the deeper tissues. If this occurs, then a portion of the skin paddle becomes random distal to the sheared perforating vessels, negating some of the advantage of the flap.

## Advancement Flaps

The horizontal advancement flap is classically designed with a length-to-width ratio of approximately 2:1. However, as we noted in Chapter 1, adherence to this principle does not guarantee flap survival, as the real indicator of distal flap survival is sufficient capillary flow (**Figure 4-10**). This requires the wound tension to be below the capillary filling pressure at the distal end of the flap. The typical advancement flap is a rectangular flap with two parallel sides that slide forward to fill the defect (**Figure 4-11**). It will always involve creating a standing cone deformity that will need to be addressed. The advantage of the advancement flap is that it is quick and simple to design and execute.

The major disadvantage of this flap is that maximal wound closing tension is at the distal end of the flap, and as these are random pattern flaps this creates a significant risk for distal flap necrosis. One way to lessen that tension is to reconstruct the defect with bilateral advancement flaps (**Figure 4-12**). This involves two opposing advancement flaps that are designed to each close half of the defect by meeting in the middle. In theory, this decreases the closing tension by 50% for each individual advancement flap. The traditional use of the horizontal advancement flap either singly or bilaterally is in the forehead where the RSTLs are horizontally oriented.

The advancement flap is not confined to two parallel lines and may be configured in any number of various ways to accommodate esthetic units or RSTLs (**Figure 4-13**). Other examples of nonlinear advancement flaps include the O-to-Y and the O-to-T closures. These two closures represent an alternative to the rotation flaps to close circular defects such as in the scalp.

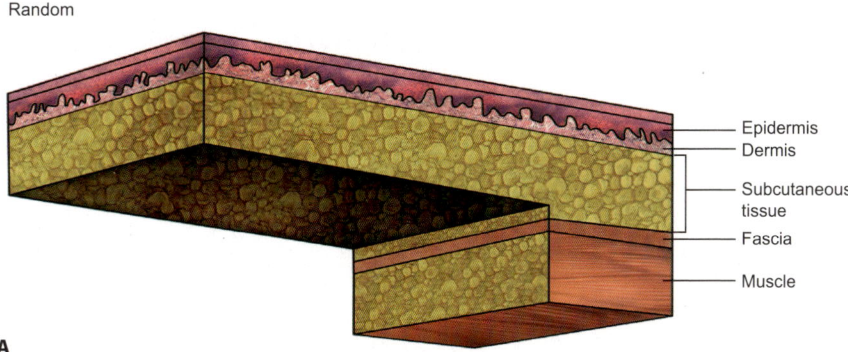


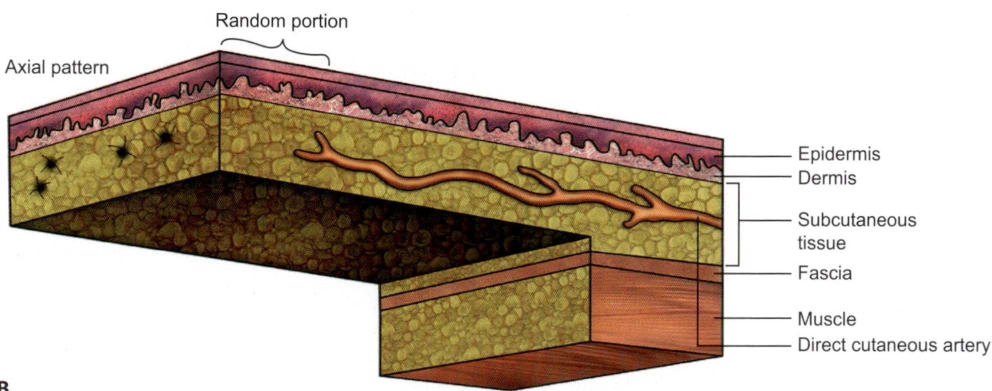


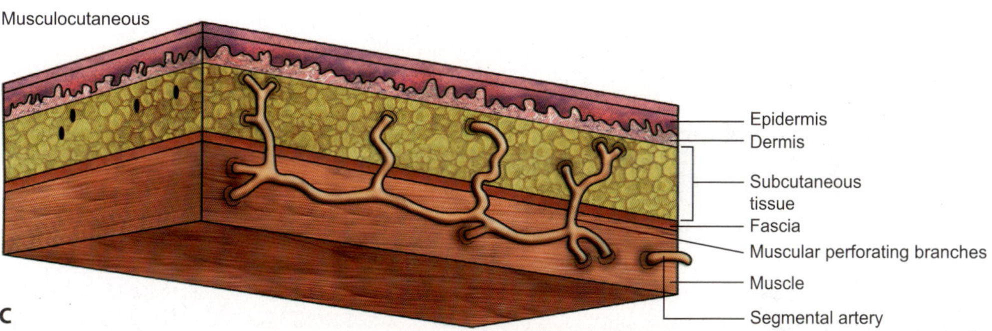


**Figure 4-9.** Classification of local flaps based on vascular anatomy. (A) A random pattern flap relies on the musculocutaneous perforating branches for its blood supply. (B) An axial pattern flap relies on direct cutaneous perforating arteries from a named segmental muscular artery. (C) A musculocutaneous flap derives its blood supply directly from a named segmental artery.

The O-to-Y closure is appropriate in areas where there is an equal degree of skin elasticity on all sides of the defect and where a stellate scar would be acceptable. The defect is divided into three equal parts (**Figure 4-14**). The ideal final scar configuration is determined and outlined (**Figure 4-14B**). Wide undermining is accomplished, and the maximal advancement occurs at the midportion of each flap to the center of the wound where the maximal wound-closing tension occurs (**Figure 4-14C**). Although a three-way suture is tempting to pull all three of the points together, they should be avoided because they tend to be strangulating to the tips of the flaps that are already under maximal tension.

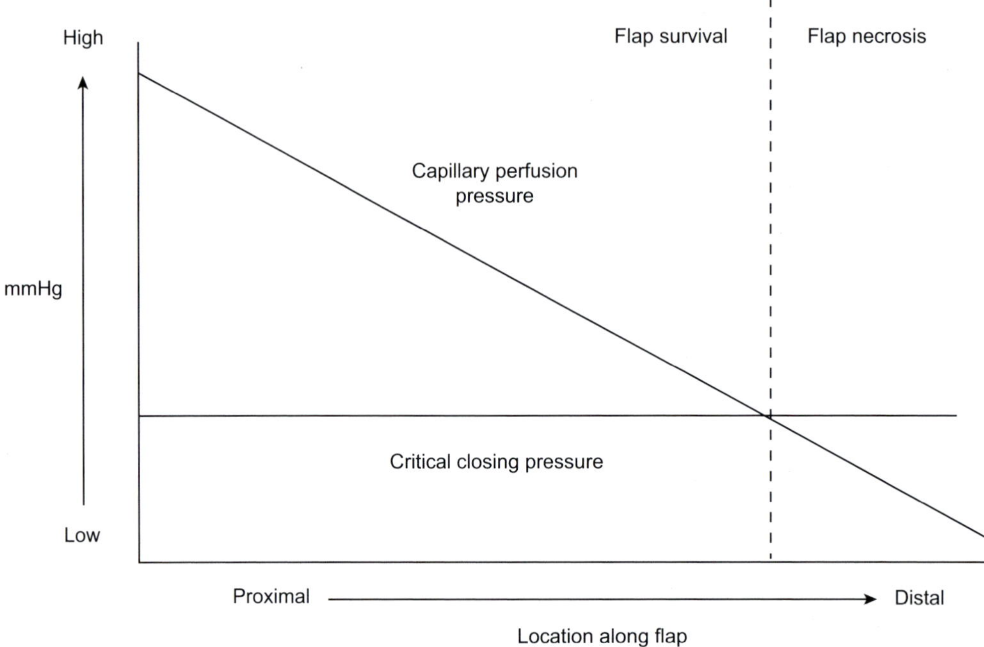


**Figure 4-10.** Relationship of capillary perfusion pressure to flap necrosis. Flap necrosis occurs when the capillary perfusion pressure is exceeded by the closing pressure of the vessel. This does not correlate to a specific length–width ratio.

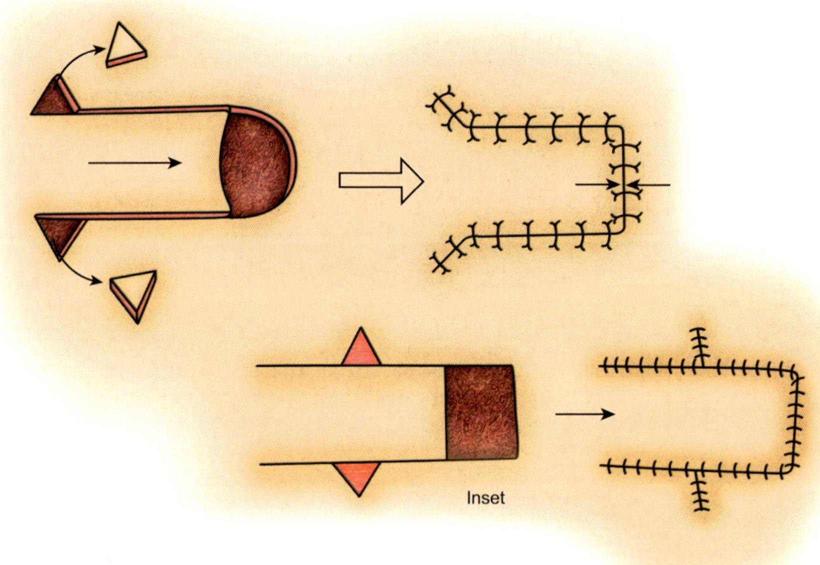


**Figure 4-11.** Horizontal advancement flap. The horizontal advancement flap has its greatest tension at the distal end of the flap. Burrow's triangles are usually resected at the base of the flap but can be excised anywhere along the edge. See insert.

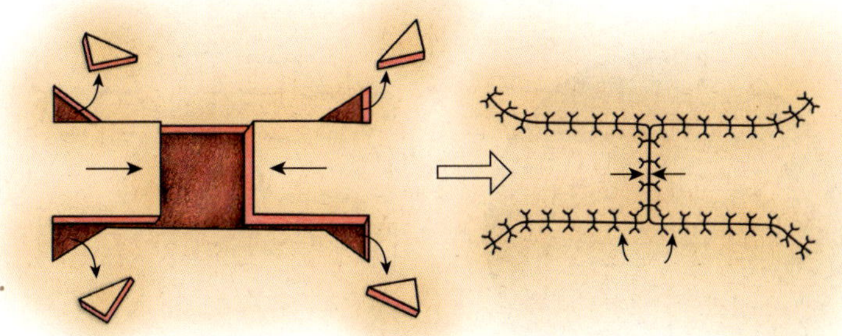

**Figure 4-12.** Bilateral advancement flap. Closure of a defect with opposing bilateral advancement flaps decreases tension at the distal end of each flap.

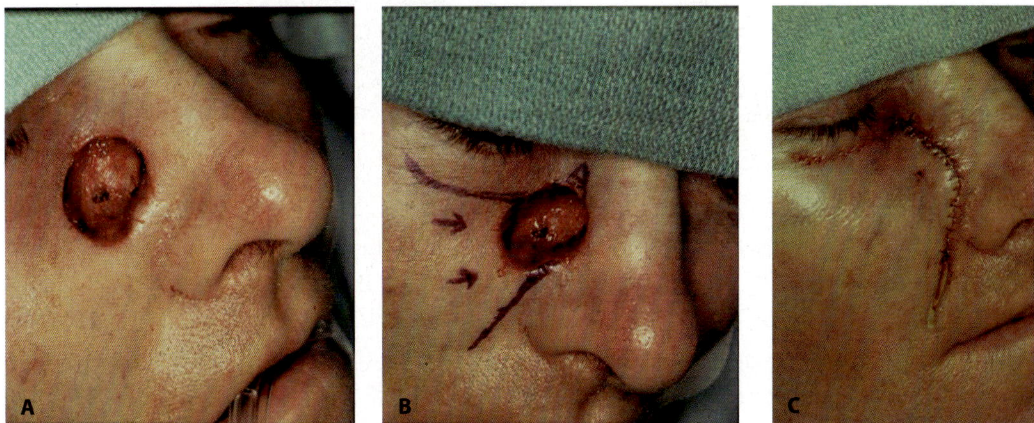


**Figure 4-13.** Cheek advancement flap. Most advancement flaps do not follow straight lines and should be designed to follow the borders of subunits and along RSTLs.

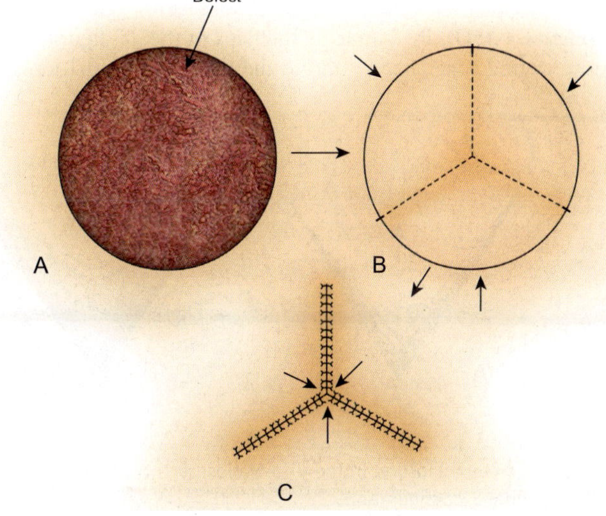


**Figure 4-14.** O to Y closure. An O-to-Y closure involves an equal sharing of the closure between three equally spread advancement flaps. The ideal scar configuration is outlined (B). Equal advancement of each of the flaps to the center of the wound results in the Y configuration of the scar (C). Maximal wound closing tension is at the center of the scar.

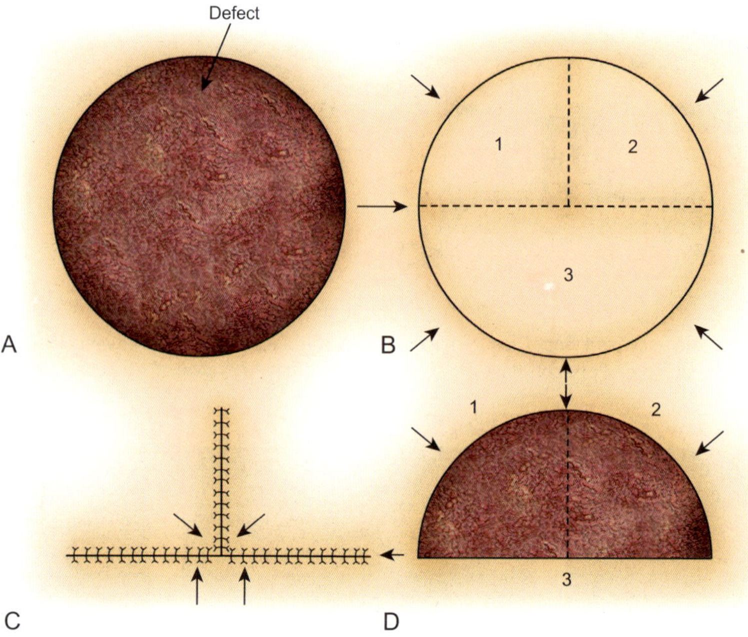


**Figure 4-15.** O-to-T closure. The inferior half of the defect has greater adjacent skin elasticity than the superior half. Half of the closure is accomplished by inferior flap 3 and the superior half by 1 and 2 equally.

The O-to-T closure is very similar to the O-to-Y closure; however, it is best suited to defects where one half of the wound borders an area that has significantly more skin elasticity than the other half (**Figure 4-15**) . This allows half of the wound to be closed with one flap converting it from an arc to a straight line, which corresponds to the horizontal bar of the T (**Figure 4-15C**). The vertical scar is formed by advancing the other half of the wound edge as two equal flaps similar to the O-to-Y closure (**Figure 4-15D**). By advancing the flaps to the opposite wound edge (1 to 2) and to the horizontal flap (3), a vertical line is created, completing the O-to-T closure.

The V-to-Y and Y-to-V advancement flaps represent special advancement flaps that are particularly useful in scar revision and defect repair when the defect is adjacent to a structure such as the eyebrow that needs to be raised or lowered. In the V-to-Y (**Figure 4-16**) closure, a triangular flap is elevated and pushed away from its apex. The resultant defect at the apex is closed primarily to create a Y configuration. In the Y-to-V (**Figure 4-17**) closure, an incision is made that corresponds to the inferior or

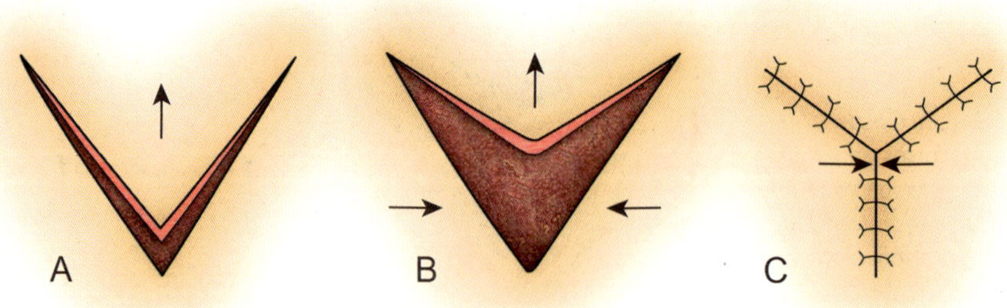


**Figure 4-16.** V- to-Y closure. In the V-to-Y closure, a triangular flap is elevated and pushed away from its apex creating the final Y configuration.

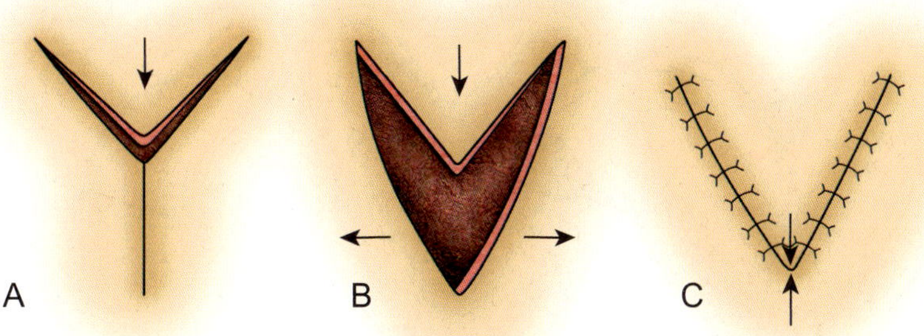


**Figure 4-17.** Y-to-V closure. In the Y-to-V closure, an incision is made that corresponds to the inferior or vertical limb of the Y. This is then opened and the apex of the triangular flap is advanced into the incision creating the V configuration.

vertical limb of the Y. This is then opened and the apex of the triangular flap is advanced into the incision, creating the V configuration.

The advancement flap invariably involves the creation of standing cone deformities at the base of the flap. Care should be taken never to excise these standing cone deformities or Burrow's triangles without first securing the flap in position. Burrow's triangles should be excised from the base of the flap and never into the base of the flap, as this will compromise the perfusion by narrowing the base of the flap. Excision of Burrow's triangles should fall within RSTLs as much as possible.

An alternative to the standard Burrow's triangle excision is the inverted Burrow's triangle described by Baker (**Figure 4-18**).

## Rotation Flap

The rotation flap involves the movement of tissue around an arc. In general, it will also involve advancement of tissue and, for this reason; some surgeons prefer to use the term "rotational-advancement flap." The author's preference is to define the flap based on its primary movement. Thus, a rotational flap is one whose primary movement is that of pivoting or rotating around an arc of rotation. Although there may be some advancement involved, these flaps can generally be considered rotation flaps. The shape, size, and configuration of the rotation flap are infinite and should be based on the defect including the size and location of the defect and the RSTLs. The standard rotation flap is a design with an arc of rotation of approximately 90° (**Figure 4-19**). This is accomplished by placing the pivot point at a distance of 2–2.5 times the diameter of the defect. The line from the edge of the defect to the pivot point then becomes the radius for the rotation flap. This allows a flap length or arc of rotation (from the edge of the defect to the base of the rotation flap) of approximately four times the diameter of the defect. This configuration will

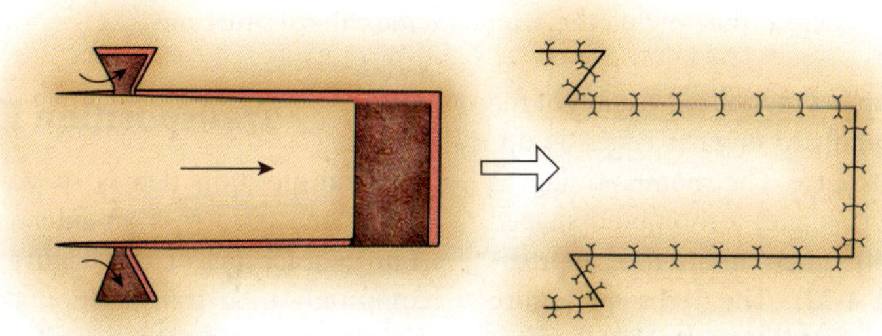

**Figure 4-18.** Inverted Burrow's triangle excision. Can be excised in an inverted fashion an alternative to the standard Burrow's triangle excision. A small triangular flap is rotated into the defect to accomplish advancement of the flap and removal of the standing cone deformity.

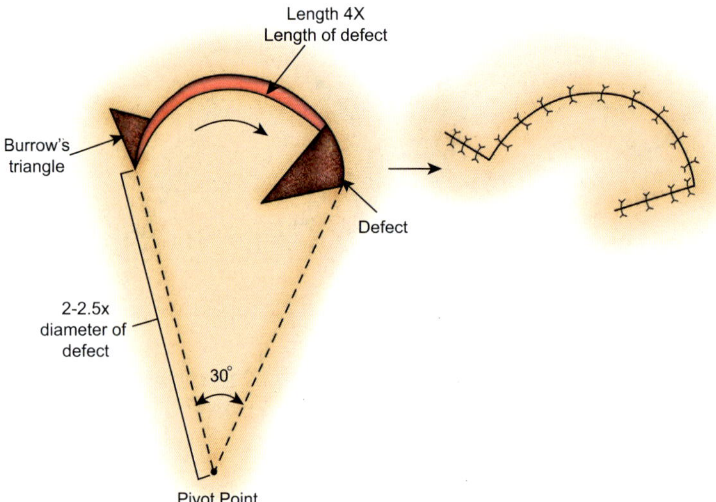


**Figure 4-19.** Classic rotation flap. The pivot point is at a distance 2–2.5 times the diameter of the defect. The line from the edge of the defect to the pivot point then becomes the radius for the rotation flap. This allows a flap length or arc of rotation (from the edge of the defect to the base of the rotation flap) of approximately 4 times the diameter of the defect. This configuration will achieve an approximate 30° rotation to allow the defect to be closed. An arc of rotation greater than 30° will usually necessitate excision of a standing cone deformity (Burrow's triangle).

achieve an approximate 30° rotation to allow the defect to be closed. A shorter radius will increase the angle of rotation and this requires looser tissues to accommodate this degree of rotation. Of necessity, the rotation flap also creates a larger standing cone deformity.

A classic example of a rotation flap is the large and versatile cervicofacial rotation flap that is very useful in reconstructing large cheek defects (**Figure 4-20A–D**). As with the advancement flap, the rotation flap can be paired with an opposing flap that allows recruitment of tissue from opposite sides of the defect, lessening tension on the individual flaps and allowing closure of defects that might otherwise not be (**Figure 4-21**).

The rhomboid flap is a specialized version of the rotation flap that has sharp angular edges as opposed to a curvilinear edge. The rhomboid flap, as described by Limberg, rotates a rhomboid-shaped flap into a defect with an arc rotation of approximately 60° (**Figure 4-22**). The Webster (**Figure 4-23A**) and Dufourmental (**Figure 4-23B**) flaps are variations of the rhomboid flap. They require less tissue rotation, as they rely on tissue advancement from adjacent tissue to complete the reconstruction, also known as secondary movement.

It should be noted that although these flaps are described in the classic manner, their execution in the clinical situation does not require such strict adherence to the geometry and angular edges. When one examines the RSTLs of the face and neck, there are few areas that can accommodate such sharp angles. For example, the rhomboid flap with its sharp points and defined angles is rarely executed with such precision but instead is modified to accommodate the location and nature of the defect, often with softer rounded edges instead of points. However, it is important to understand the basic concepts of these flaps that then allows for modification in specific clinical situations.

## Transposition Flaps

The transposition flap is so named because the flap is moved across an intervening segment of skin to reach the defect (**Figure 4-24**). The most commonly used transposition flap is the nasolabial flap or, more aptly named, the melolabial flap as it is derived from tissue from the cheek and the donor scar lies in the melolabial fold and along the nasofacial junction (**see Figure 4-25A,B**). The melolabial flap should not be taken from nasal tissues.

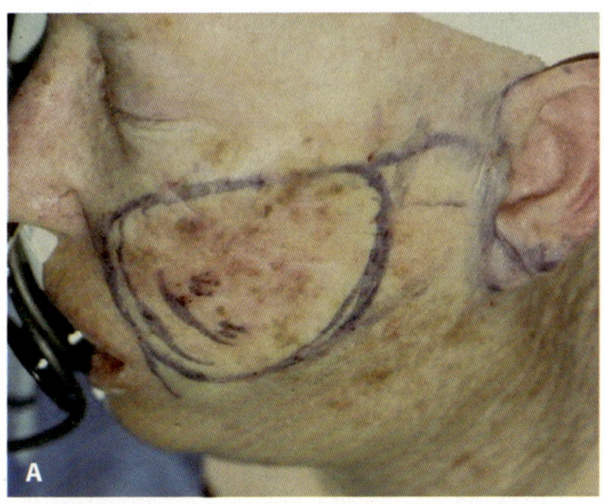


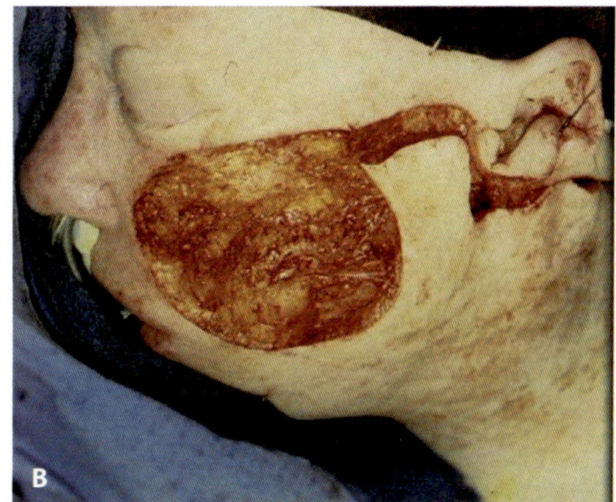


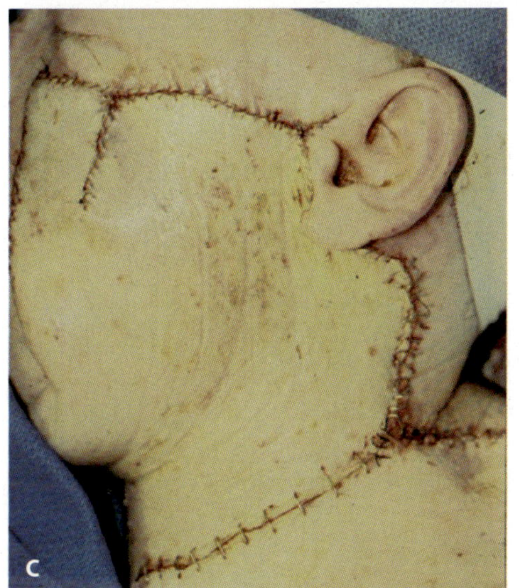


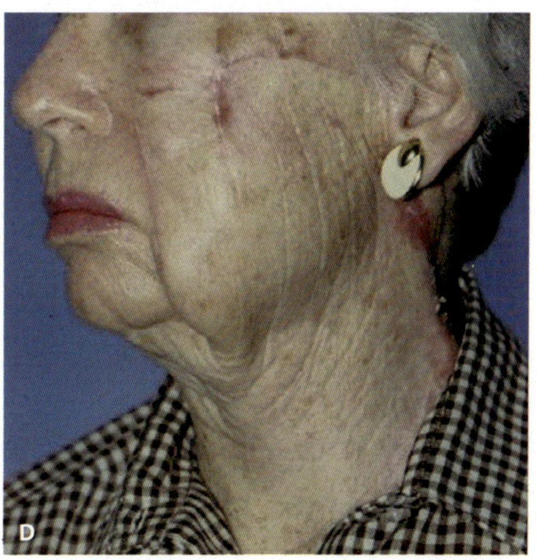


**Figure 4-20.** Large cervicofacial rotation flap for closure of a large cheek defect. (A) This patient has a melanoma that required excision of a large amount of skin with a superficial parotidectomy. Excision of the skin is outlined as is the flap. (B) Excision is completed and cervicofacial rotation flap is elevated. The skin between the ear and the defect is incorporated into the reconstruction and the remainder of the flap is postauricular. Neck skin is advanced and rotated into position necessitating a vertical scar on the anterior cheek. (C) Flap is rotated and sutured into position. Vertical lines on the flap represent previously horizontal relaxed skin tension lines in the neck reflecting a 90° rotation. (D) Healed flap with a prominent standing cone deformity at the jowl area. This was not excised at the time of the reconstruction, as it would have required cutting across the base of the flap. Despite its size, this flap is a random pattern flap and as such should not be placed under tension. The standing cone deformity can be excised once the flap has healed fully.

The melolabial flap is especially useful in nasal and perioral reconstruction. It can be developed as a superiorly based flap that is used primarily for nasal sidewall reconstruction or as an inferiorly based flap that is useful for upper and lower lip and some nasal alar reconstruction. It derives its blood supply from branches of the angular artery, which arises from the superior labial artery. Generally, the angular artery is not incorporated into the flap as a true pedicled flap, and so it is a well-vascularized axial pattern flap based on direct cutaneous branches from the angular artery. Because of this, it is very robust and can be thinned significantly to reconstruct the more shallow nasal sidewall defects or turned on itself to recreate the nasal ala and reconstruct both internal and external nasal defects.

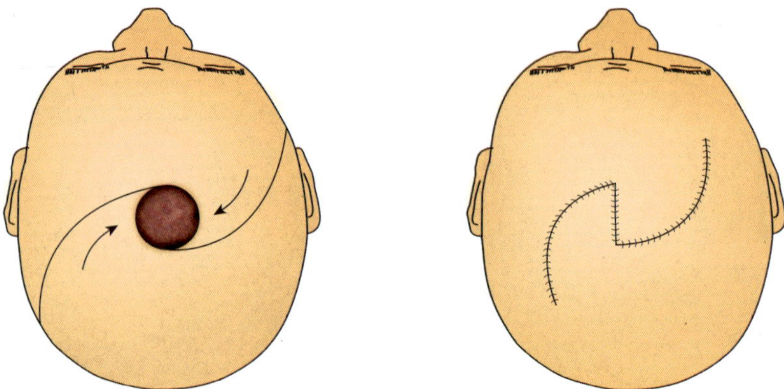

**Figure 4-21.** Bilateral rotation flap. The bilateral rotation flap (yin/yang) flap is helpful in large defects to balance the tension on the distal end of the flaps, as it reduces tension by 50% over a single large rotation flap.

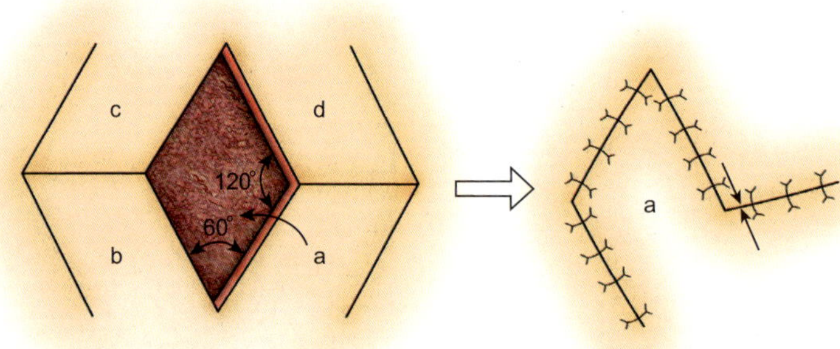


**Figure 4-22.** Rhomboid flap. The original design by Limberg allows for four different potential flaps.

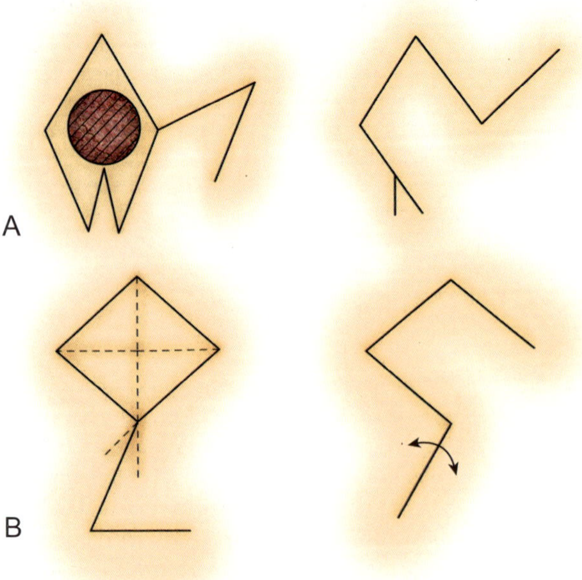


**Figure 4-23.** Webster and Dufourmental flaps. Webster (A) and Dufourmental (B) variations of the classic rhomboid flap require less tissue rotation because they rely on both rotation and tissue advancement to accomplish closure.

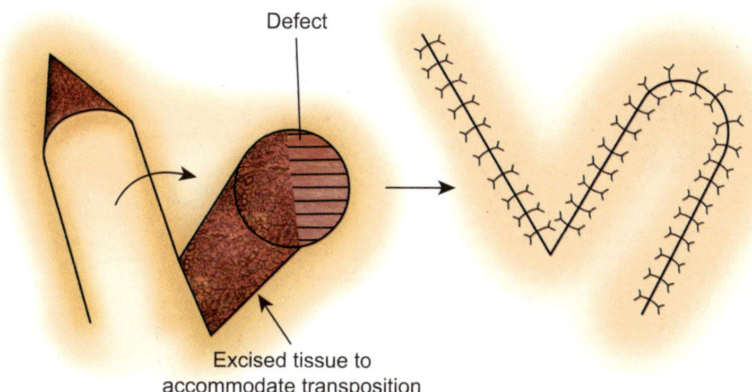


**Figure 4-24.** Transposition flap. The transposition flap moves across an intervening segment (red area) of tissue to reach defect.

The tubed or pedicled interpolation flap (**Figure 4-26**) is a specialized transposition flap in which the tissue travels over an intervening segment of tissue. With tubed or pedicled interpolation flaps, the pedicle must be divided at a later time when the recipient site is able to supply the needed vascularity. A 2–3 week delay is generally adequate for patients with normal healing. After the delay, the pedicle is divided and discarded and the remainder of the flap is tailored and sutured into place.

With an intact pedicle that is based on the supratrochlear vessels, the paramedian forehead flap is a true musculocutaneous flap, as it is transposed with its muscle and vascular pedicle (**Figure 4-27A**). Again, like most flaps used in facial reconstruction, its distal segment becomes a random pattern due to the thinning of the flap to accommodate specialized reconstructive needs, however. It is the workhorse flap for large nasal reconstructions, able to completely resurface the exterior nose. In most instances, it is an interpolation flap as well, as the pedicle crosses over intact glabellar tissue to reach the defect. The pedicle is divided and the remainder of the flap is inset into the defect at three weeks (**Figure 4-27B**).

In the case of the island flap (**Figure 4-28**), the pedicle does not need to be divided at a later time because the epithelium is removed from the portion of the pedicle that is buried. However, the buried pedicle does create bulk and must have an adequate

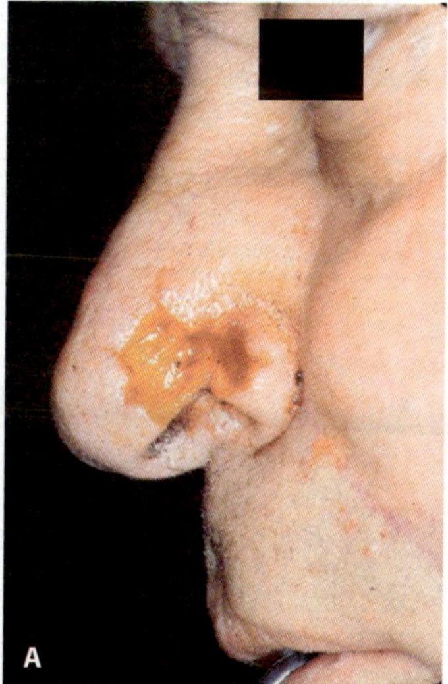


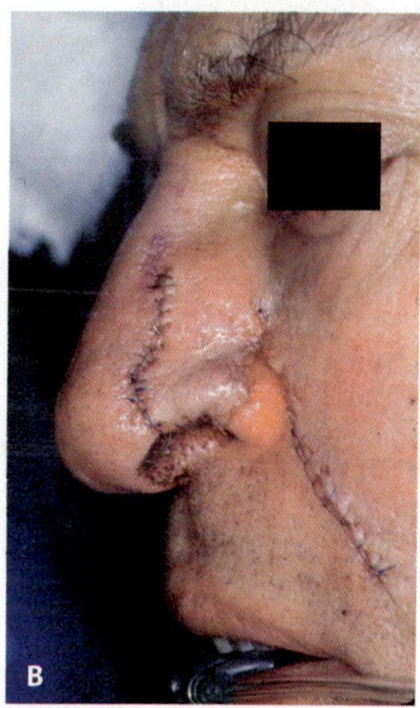


**Figure 4-25.** Melolabial flap nasal reconstruction. (A) The melolabial flap is a very versatile and hearty flap for nasal reconstruction. Nasal defect extends into the nasal cavity requiring internal and external reconstruction. (B) A superiorly based melolabial flap has been used as a "turn-in" flap to reconstruct the internal and external deformities demonstrating its versatility.

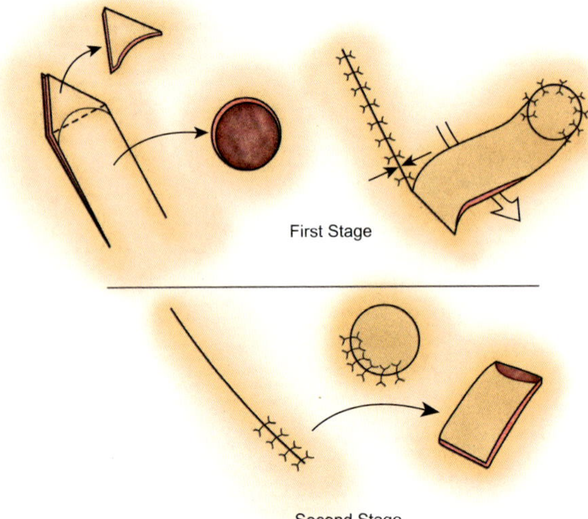


**Figure 4-26.** Interpolation flap (tubed or pedicled). The interpolation flap spans a segment of normal tissue and requires a second stage to divide the pedicle and inset the remainder of the flap after a delay of 2–3 weeks.

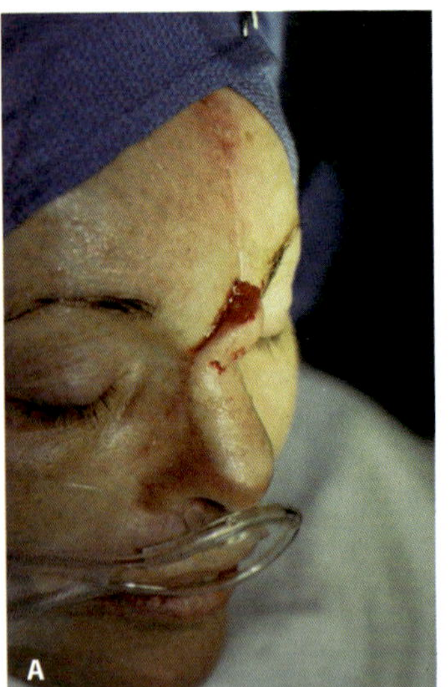


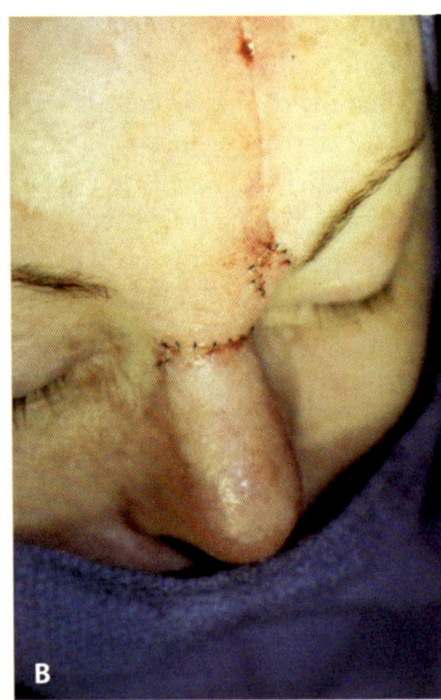


**Figure 4-27.** Paramedian forehead flap. (A) Paramedian forehead flap with intact pedicle prior to division at 3 weeks. (B) Paramedian forehead flap with pedicle divided and flap inset into superior margin of defect.

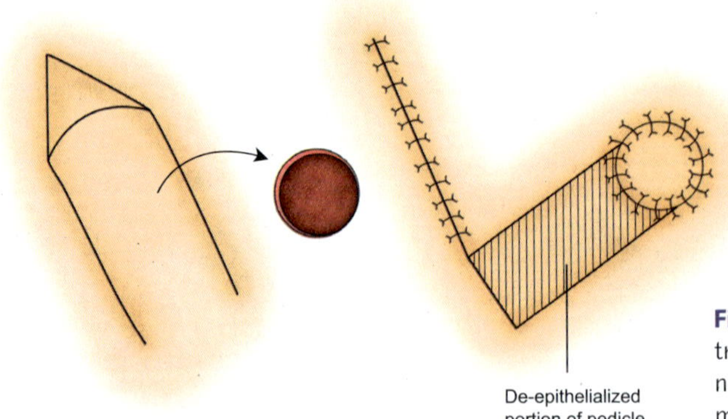


**Figure 4-28.** Island flap. The Island flap is transposed under an intervening segment of normal skin. Because the pedicle is buried, it must be de-epithelialized before it is inset.

pocket so that it does not become strangulated by the intervening normal tissue. The transposition flap is particularly useful when moving a flap of tissue from one facial subunit to reconstruct another, allowing the donor defect to be closed at their junction. The transposition flap in its many forms is perhaps the most common way to reconstruct defects and has very few constraints relative to geometry. Because of this, it can take many different forms and sizes as needed.

A specialized transposition flap is Z-plasty, which can be used to lengthen scars or to close defects (**Figure 4-29A**). It is a double transposition flap that involves the movement of two flaps into the position occupied by the other. In doing so, the scar is lengthened and reoriented. The amount that a scar is lengthened is proportional to the angle at which the flaps arise from the central or common incision (**Figure 4-29B**). The amount of lengthening is proportional to the angle between the central member and the flaps. An angle of 30° yields a scar that is 25% longer, a 45° angle yields a 50% longer scar, and a 60° angle yields a 75% increase in scar length.

The bilobed flap is a unique transposition flap that closes the original defect (primary defect) with a flap (primary flap) that is adjacent to the defect and

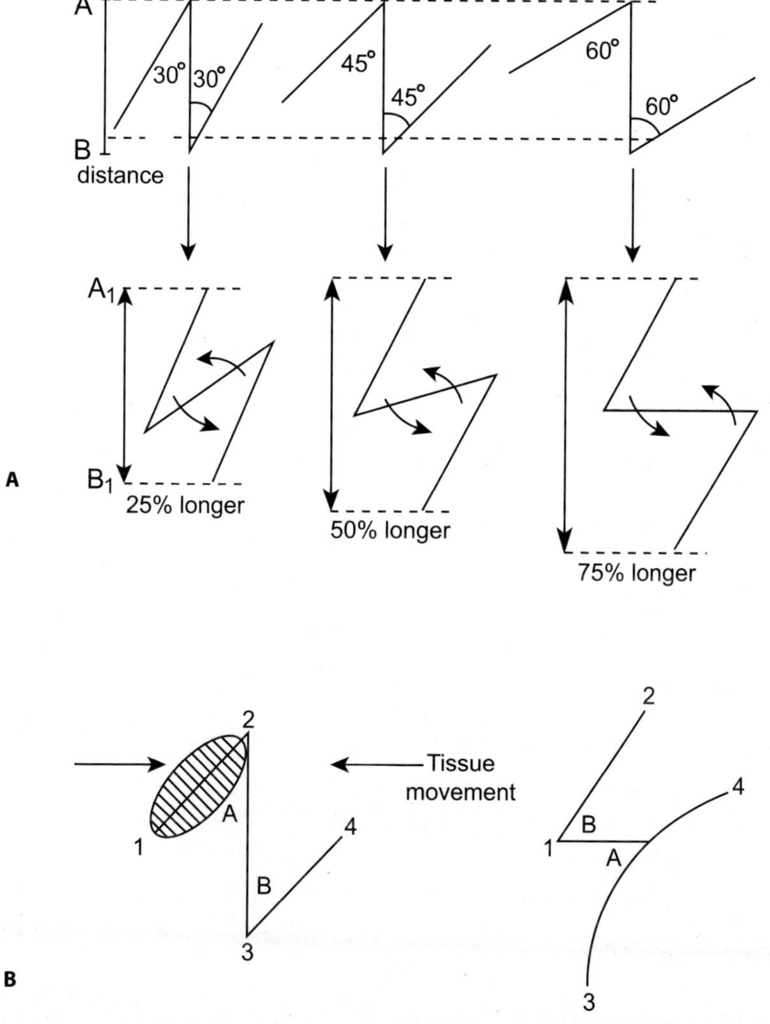


**Figure 4-29.** Z-plasty flap (A) and Z-plasty. (A) The Z-plasty can be used as a double transposition flap to close defects and reorient the scars as depicted here. (B) The Z-plasty is an excellent technique to lengthen scars and reorient them. This is ideal for contracted linear scars that are binding, impairing function. It is also ideal to reorient scars to a more favorable plane.

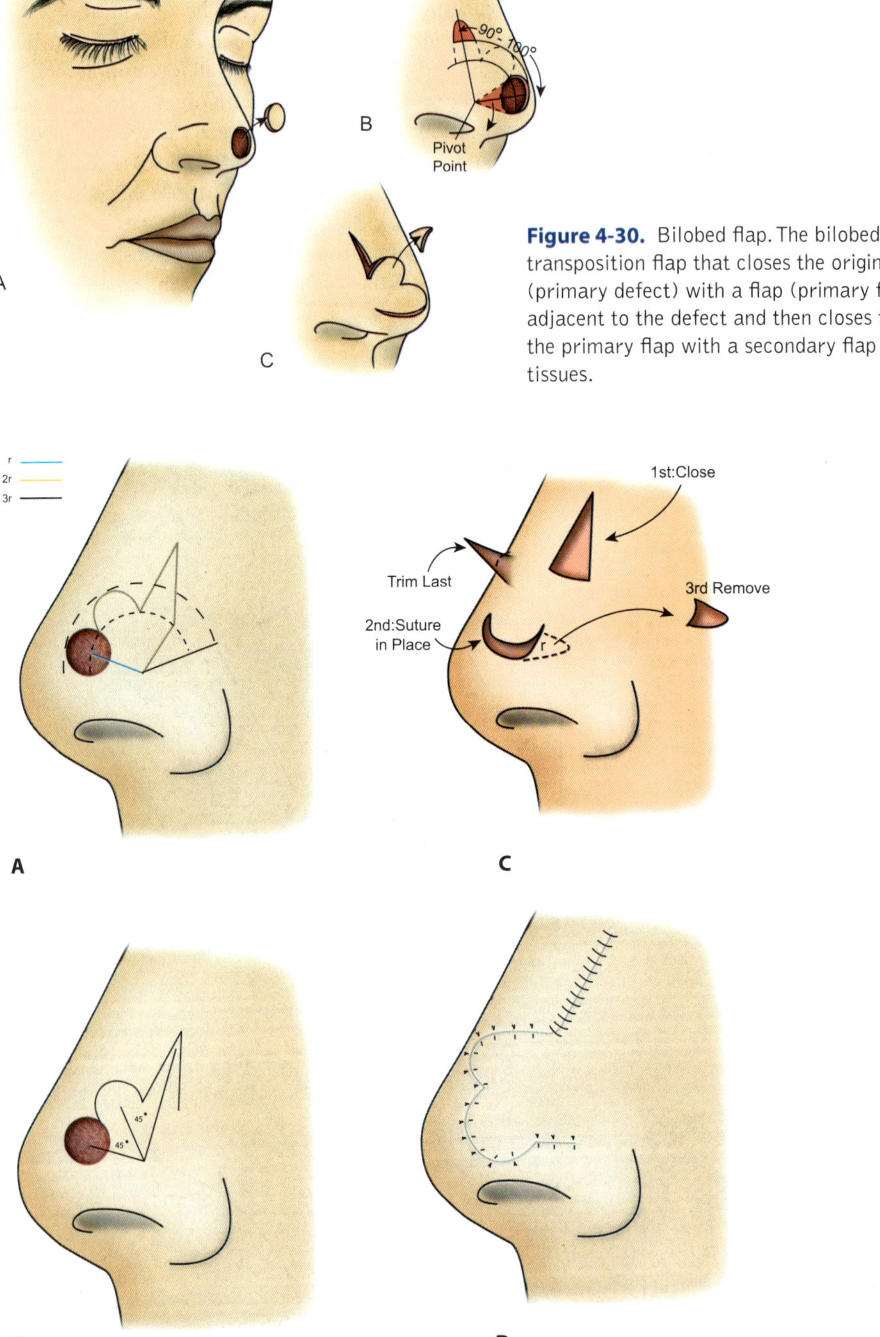


**Figure 4-30.** Bilobed flap. The bilobed flap is a unique transposition flap that closes the original defect (primary defect) with a flap (primary flap) that is adjacent to the defect and then closes the defect from the primary flap with a secondary flap from adjacent tissues.

**Figure 4-31.** Technique for bilobed flap. The bilobed flap is typically rotated around an arc of 90 degrees from the axis of the secondary flap to the radius of the defect. The primary flap is oriented at 45 degrees to the defect and is the same size as the defect, although this can be smaller depending on surrounding skin elasticity. The secondary flap is typically 50% of the size of the defect and is closed primarily. The success of this flap requires extensive undermining and attention to detail in its planning. It is very useful in nasal and facial reconstruction.

then closes the defect from the primary flap with a secondary flap from adjacent tissues. The axes of the defect and primary and secondary flaps are oriented at 90° from each other (**Figure 4-30**). However, this flap like many others has many possible variations and can be adapted to fit many locations and needs. This flap is particularly useful for smaller nasal defects (**Figure 4-31**). Like most other flaps, its success depends heavily on wide undermining to allow the flaps to be transposed into position with as little tension as possible.

A major concern in using the transposition flap is avoiding tension on the flap. If the flap is not wide enough or long enough and undue tension is exerted on the flap, then its viability is compromised. This can occur at any point along the length of the flap and is especially harmful if the base is compromised. In this situation, the surgeon should rely on secondary movement of adjacent tissue that is created by undermining the edges of the primary defect. Proper planning is essential to avoid this complication. This preoperative planning should include ensuring that the donor site scar lies within RSTLs.

In this chapter we introduced the types of flaps that are useful in facial reconstruction and discussed the preoperative planning and analysis that is necessary to have a successful reconstruction. Specific applications of these techniques will be discussed in subsequent chapters as they relate to each specific esthetic unit.

## References


1. Branham, GH, ed. Local skin flaps. *Facial Plast. Clin. NA* 4(4), 1996.
2. Hochman, M, ed. Conceptual considerations in head and neck reconstruction. *Otolaryngol. Clin. NA* 30(4), 1997.
3. Papel, I, et al., eds. *Facial Plastic and Reconstructive Surgery,* 2nd ed., Thieme, New York, 2002.
4. Park, SS, ed. Local cutaneous flaps. *Facial Plast Clin N Am* 13(2), 2005.
5. Thomas, JR, ed. Facial plastic surgery. *Otolaryngol. Clin. N Am* 23(5), 1990.
6. Weerda, H, ed. *Reconstructive Facial Plastic Surgery: A Problem-Solving Manual,* Thieme, New York, 2001.
7. Baker, SR. Local Flaps in Facial Reconstructive. Philadelphia: Elsevier 2007.
8. Sclafaui, AP. Fozo, M. Rhombic Flaps Emedicine. Feb 12, 2009.

5

# Skin Grafts

Gregory H. Branham, MD, FACS

## Introduction

In facial reconstruction, both full thickness and split thickness skin grafts are useful and should be considered as an alternative when planning the closure of a facial defect. It is safe to say, however, that primary closure and local flaps represent a better alternative for most facial defects. In this chapter, we review the types of skin grafts and their current uses.

A skin graft is an area of skin that has been removed from a remote donor site and transplanted to the recipient site or defect. As such, it is completely removed from its blood supply and special considerations regarding its healing become apparent. Skin grafts may be taken as a full-thickness graft that encompasses the complete layer of the dermis and epidermis and is harvested at the subcutaneous plane. Split thickness grafts consist of the epidermis and an incomplete layer of dermis. Depending on the depth at which the graft is taken, it can be considered a thin, intermediate or thick split thickness skin graft (**Figure 5-1**)

## Planning and Preoperative Analysis

Prior to placement of a skin graft, careful analysis of the defect should be undertaken to determine whether a skin graft would be the best reconstructive option. Factors that are essential to consider include a vascularized recipient site, patient comorbidities, and margins clear of tumor, among others (**Table 5-1**).

The best sites for skin grafting in general are those that are flat, shallow, and non-hair bearing. Convex or concave surfaces represent additional challenges but are amenable to skin grafting. The decision to use a split thickness skin graft versus a full thickness graft should be made using the following principles:

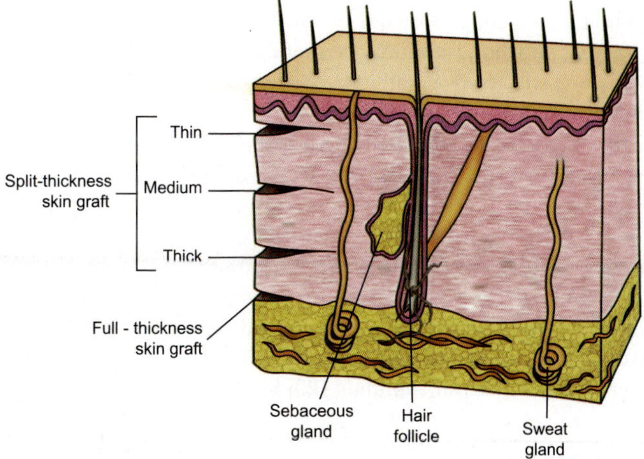


**Figure 5-1.** Skin grafts. Split thickness grafts vary in thickness from thin to thick depending how deep into the dermis they extend. A full thickness graft extends through the dermis into the subcutaneous tissues.

**TABLE 5-1 Factors to Consider in Choosing a Skin Graft**

| |
|---|
| Presence of vital tissue in the recipient site. |
| Inability to easily reconstruct the defect with primary closure or a local flap. |
| Is the reconstruction temporary or definitive? |
| Is the defect sufficiently shallow to be adequately reconstructed with a skin graft? |
| Other comorbidities that would be relative contraindications to skin grafting such as smoking or impaired healing by diabetes or immunosuppression. |
| Are the margins free of tumor in the case of malignancies? |
| Presence of vital tissue in the recipient site. |

1. A full thickness skin graft should be used if at all possible as it will yield a superior cosmetic result, except in specific cases where a thin graft is preferable such as when resurfacing the ear.
2. The use of a full thickness graft is limited by the size of the defect and should usually be confined to defects of 2 cm or less.
3. Full thickness skin graft donor sites are more cosmetically acceptable.
4. Availability of an acceptable donor site for tissue characteristics such as color, texture, and ability to hide the donor site.
5. Full thickness grafts exhibit less contracture than split thickness grafts.

## Recipient Site

The recipient site must have healthy, vital tissue in order to supply adequate nutrition to the skin graft as it heals into place. Skin grafts should not be placed over the bare surfaces of bone, cartilage, or tendons, as they cannot adequately support the graft. Bone with an overlying periosteum or cartilage with an overlying perichondrium may be grafted. Similarly, paratenon will accept a graft if there is adequate immobility during the healing phase.

For the graft to survive, it must adhere to the recipient bed. Therefore, hemostasis is essential to ensure that the graft does not "float" off of the surface. Care should be taken to cauterize judiciously, however, so that excessive char is avoided in the recipient bed. Excessive granulation tissue may need to be debrided if present in an older wound. In some instances, granulation tissue is desirable to bring a deeper defect up to surrounding skin level prior to skin grafting, and, if it not excessive, will permit a skin graft to adhere.

Areas most amenable to reconstruction with skin grafts include the temporal region, the forehead, and the ear. They should be avoided on the nose, cheek, and chin. Grafts can be used successfully in the periorbital region to replace the thin upper and lower eyelid skin but should not extend outside of the bony orbital rim and beyond the orbital esthetic unit, as they become quite noticeable and unsightly.

When reconstructing the temporal region or forehead, it is helpful to allow the wound to develop a bed of granulation tissue that will bring the wound up to the level of the surrounding skin prior to skin grafting. Although this can be annoying to the patient who may wish to have a quick reconstruction, the results are well worth the wait, and the patient should be encouraged to give it time. During this time, significant scar contracture will take place also and will result in the need for a smaller skin graft. Again, when resurfacing the ear with a skin graft, it is essential to have an intact perichondrium on which to place the graft.

## Donor Sites for Split Thickness Grafts

Split thickness grafts can be harvested from any location. They leave a significant scar that is characterized by dyschromia (either hypo- or hyperpigmentation) once healed, and this must be taken into account when harvesting the graft. A color match is not usually as much of a concern with split thickness grafts as is hiding the donor site. The upper thigh, buttocks, and trunk are good sites that will provide the best opportunity to be hidden. The donor site should be free of any suspicious lesions. Grafts from hair-bearing areas should be made sufficiently thin to prevent transplantation of hair follicles. A typical split thickness skin graft of 0.012–0.020 does not contain follicles.

## Harvesting Split Thickness Grafts

Split thickness grafts are generally taken from the lateral or medial thigh with the use of a gas-powered or electric dermatome (**Figure 5-2**). The author generally prefers a split thickness graft 0.015 inches thick, as this works well for most situations. If a thinner graft is taken, it is easy to perforate and can be more difficult to handle. A thicker graft can delay healing at the donor site and create more scarring if it extends beyond the midreticular dermis.

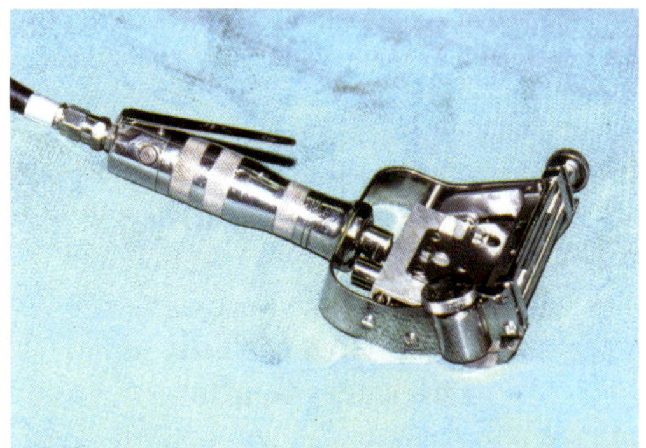

**Figure 5-2.** Dermatome for split thickness grafts. A gas or electric powered dermatome is commonly used to harvest split thickness skin grafts. The one shown here is a typical gas powered dermatome. The width of graft can be selected by choosing a template that fits over the blade. The depth of the cut or thickness of the graft is controlled with a dial on the dermatome. This should always be double checked by gently passing a #15 blade through the gap. It should pass between the blade and the dermatome with no additional gap.

Prior to harvesting the graft, the dermatome should be checked by the surgeon to ensure proper settings. As an additional check on the calibration of the dermatome, a standard #15 surgical blade should just fit in the space between the dermatome and the blade and is roughly 0.015 inches thick. The dermatome has a single blade that is attached to the dermatome and secured with screws. Care should be taken when setting up the dermatome and attaching the blade, as it is very sharp. The dermatome can be set up to take different width grafts by placing one of several different width cover plates over the blade. These usually come in 2-, 4-, and 6-inch widths.

When harvesting the graft, the skin should be lubricated with sterile light mineral oil and spread with a tongue blade (**Figure 5-3A–E**). Firm but gentle pressure should be constantly applied to the skin as the dermatome is activated. It should not be lifted from the skin to check the thickness unless you suspect a major problem, as this will perforate the graft. If the need should arise to check the graft, the dermatome should be deactivated by releasing the handle and allowing the blade to stop prior to checking. It is desirable to check the graft without lifting the blade. As the graft is being harvested, it is preferable to gently lift the graft as it comes through the dermatome to prevent injury to the graft. Once the appropriate length of graft material has been

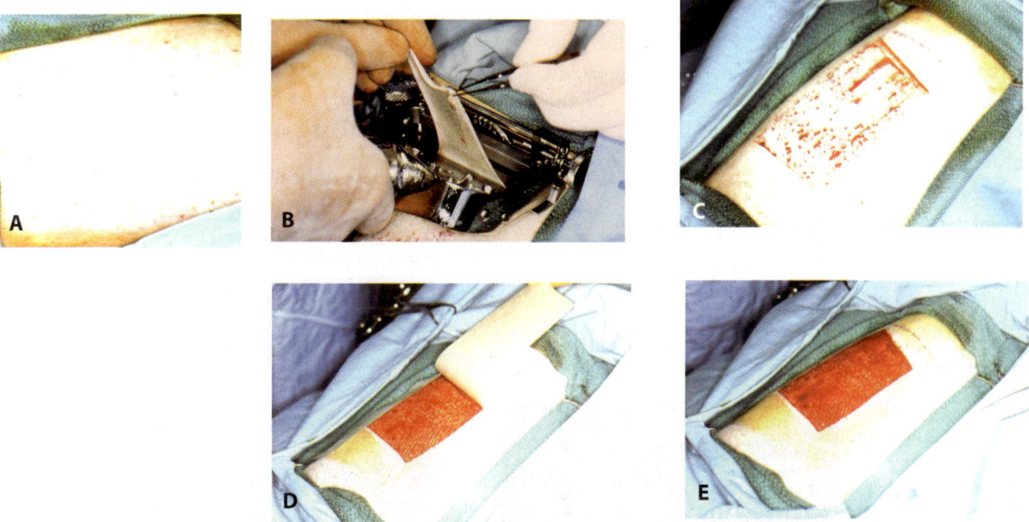


**Figure 5-3.** (A) The lateral thigh is prepared for a split thickness skin graft on the patient depicted in Figure 5.4. (B) The dermatome is used to harvest a split thickness skin graft 0.015 inch thick. The graft is supported and gently lifted as it is being harvested. (C) Punctate bleeding seen immediately after the skin graft is harvested. Gentle pressure with gauze will usually control this bleeding. If not, topical epinephrine at a concentration of 1:50,000 will accomplish hemostasis. (D) A transparent occlusive dressing such as Opsite or Tegaderm is used to cover the donor site. (E) The donor site dressing is complete. Use of an occlusive dressing is recommended for 7 days. This allows the wound to heal in a moist environment and prevents the wound from rubbing against clothing.

harvested, the dermatome is deactivated and the skin is trimmed from the dermatome with a #15 blade. Once the graft is removed, pressure is applied to the donor site to control the punctate bleeding that is present. A solution of topical epinephrine (1:50,000) can be applied to the wound to assist control of bleeding. Once this is accomplished, the donor site is dressed with a transparent occlusive dressing such as Opsite or Tegaderm.

## Placement of the Skin Graft

Split thickness skin grafts should be trimmed to the appropriate size of the defect and anchored to the edge of the defect. Absorbable sutures work well for this and do not have to be removed. This prevents shearing of the graft from the wound edge when the bolster is removed. For larger grafts, it is useful to make several "pie crust" incisions inside the graft. This will allow any accumulating blood or seroma to be cleared and prevent the graft from floating off the recipient bed. Small absorbable sutures placed through these pie crust incisions will anchor the graft to the recipient bed as well. Although these do not take the place of a bolster, they serve as additional security against shearing forces as the graft heals.

Finally, a bolster is placed and anchored into postion with nonabsorbable sutures at the edge of the wound (**Figure 5-4A,B**). Bolster tie-down sutures should be placed on opposite sides of the wound so that opposing sutures can be tied over the bolster. If the defect is small, the bolster is formed from a ball of Xeroform gauze. If the bolster needs to be larger, then the Xeroform is filled with antibiotic ointment-coated cotton balls. The Xeroform is then folded over the cotton balls to complete the bolster.

Full thickness grafts in general should be bolstered as well. Bolsters are generally left in place for 5–7 days to allow the graft to adhere to the recipient bed.

## Donor Sites for Full Thickness Grafts

With full thickness grafts, the donor site should be chosen so that the scar is minimized and the color and texture match is maximized (**Figure 5-5**). The junction of esthetic units and natural borders such as hairlines make good choices for sites to hide scars. As with any other incision, it should follow relaxed skin tension lines and must be closed in a careful, layered closure as any other wound.

Donor sites for any skin graft should be of good quality and free of any suspicious skin lesions. They should have the same tissue color and sebaceous qualities as the recipient site as much as possible. For example, when grafting to an area that has received a lot of actinic exposure like the nose, one should not harvest supraclavicular skin, as this skin has had little exposure to the sun and has very few adnexal structures and glands. A better match for this would be the melolabial fold or preauricular skin.

## Healing of Skin Grafts

The initial phase of healing of the graft to the wound begins immediately. Because there is no blood sup-

A

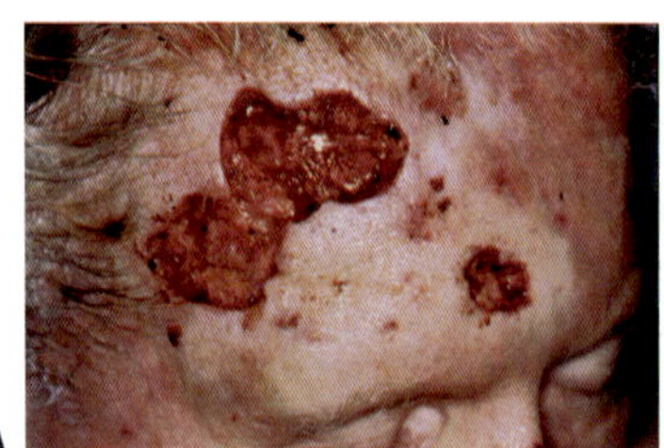

B

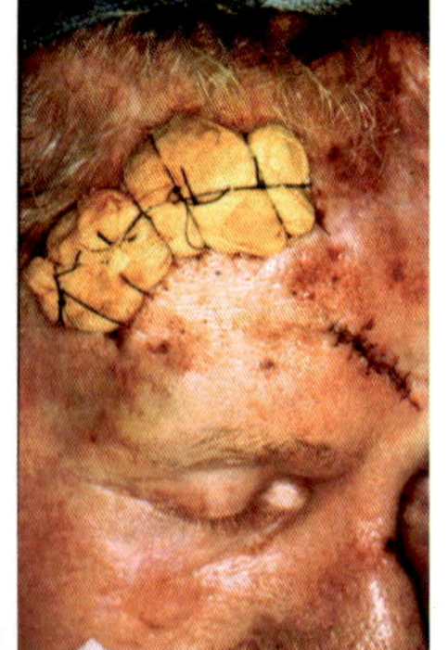

**Figure 5-4.** (A) Forehead defects from multiple skin cancers. Patient has extensive actinic exposure and multiple malignant and premalignant lesions present. In this instance, a skin graft is the most appropriate reconstruction. (B) Reconstruction of multiple forehead defects. A small central defect is closed primarily and the large defect is reconstructed with a split thickness skin graft. The Xeroform bolster is secured with a tie over the sutures.

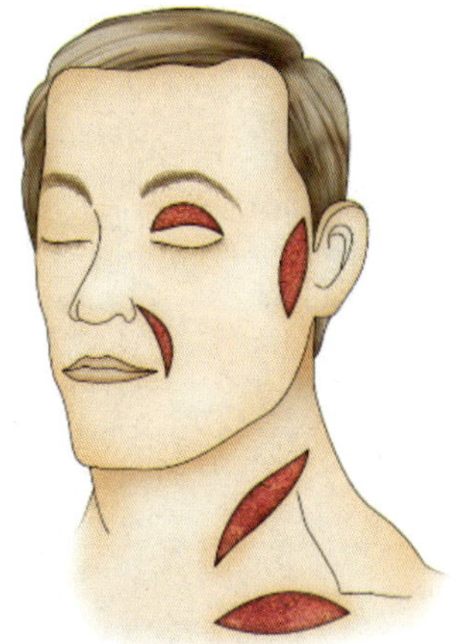

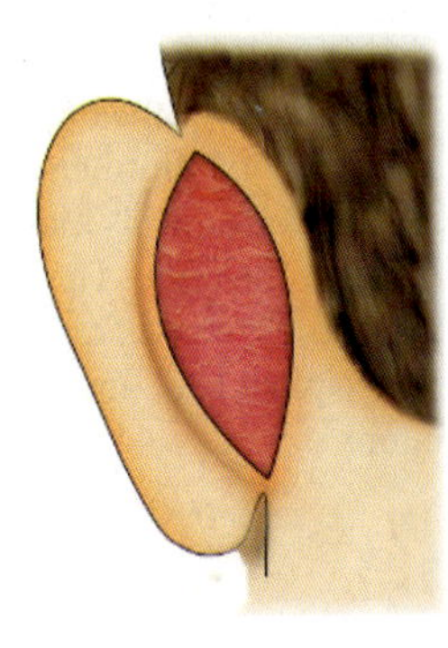

**Figure 5-5.** Full thickness graft donor site. Skin grafts should be taken from areas that will provide a good color and texture match but in areas that will hide scars such as junction of esthetic units and along RSTLs.

ply to the graft at this point, the graft must absorb plasma from the wound by capillary action through a process known as plasmatic imbibition. This process is responsible for nourishment of the graft for the first 48 hours. At this point, the thinner grafts are able to absorb more nutrients and are more likely to survive. There is essentially a race between the ability of the graft to become vascularized and the death of the graft cells from lack of adequate nourishment. During this avascular phase, the graft is pale due to the absence of erythrocytes in the graft.

A network of fibrin is laid down between the graft and the recipient bed, and it is through this matrix that vascular buds develop and work their way into the graft tissue. When this occurs the graft takes on a mottled appearance due to its patchy vascularity. Existing vascular channels within the graft are used to revascularize the graft through a process called inosculation. It is this combination of new vascular buds connecting with existing and newly formed channels that ensures revascularization of the graft. At approximately day 4–5 these anastomotic channels become operational and blood begins to flow into the graft. The flow of blood into the graft exerts a negative feedback loop to inhibit further neovascularization.

In split thickness grafts, no viable adnexal structures (sebaceous glands, hair follicles, etc.) are transplanted and therefore are not present in the healed defect. In the case of a full thickness graft and some thick partial thickness grafts, adnexal structures are present and contribute to a more normal appearance of reconstruction.

Innervation of the transplanted tissue by sensory nerve endings from the recipient bed takes place over time. For full thickness grafts, this process is slower but more complete. As the wound heals, the grafts are subject to scar contracture. In general, the thicker the graft the less scar contracture that occurs and is usually complete by 12 months.

Skin grafts fail for a number of reasons including technical factors, host factors, such as smoking and comorbidities, and others **(Table 5-2)**. Attention to these factors prior to placement will lead to a more satisfactory result or perhaps to the choice of a different reconstructive option.

## Postoperative Care

The skin graft must be immobilized to ensure proper adherence and healing. This is typically done with sutures around the perimeter of the graft as well as a number of tacking sutures between the graft and the recipient surface. In some cases, a bolster that relies on tape can be used in lieu of sutures; however, the author prefers to suture the bolster into place and remove the bolster at 1 week.

The patient is instructed to coat the bolster with antibiotic ointment in an occlusive fashion "like

**TABLE 5-2 Causes of Skin Graft Failure**

| |
|---|
| Recipient bed failure (avascular bed, bone, paratenon, prior radiation) |
| Infection |
| Trauma/shearing of graft from bed |
| Hematoma/seroma under graft |
| Underlying comorbidities (diabetes, malnutrition) |
| Smoking |
| Technical errors in placement (poor contouring, graft upside down) |

icing on a cake" in order to prevent both the bolster and the skin graft from desiccation and infection. Special care should be taken not to get the bolster wet, especially if the bolster is made from Xeroform and antibiotic ointment–coated cotton balls. Once wet, the cotton balls loose their bulk and become a nidus for infection. The bolster should not be hit or bumped, as this will cause shearing of the graft from the recipient bed, one of the leading causes of graft failure.

## References

1. Branham GH, ed.Local skin flaps. *Facial Plast Clin N Am* 4(4), 1996.
2. Branham GH, Thomas JR: Skin grafts. *Otolaryngol Clin N Am* 1990 23(5), 889–897.
3. Park SS, ed. Local cutaneous flaps. *Facial Plast Clin N Am* 2005, 13(2).
4. Thomas JR, Holt GR, eds. *Facial Scars: Incision, Revision, and Camouflage*. Mosby, St. Louis, 1989.
5. Thomas JR. Advanced Therapy in Facial Plastic and Reconstructive Surgery. St Louis; Mosby 2010.

6

# Nasal Reconstruction

Gregory H. Branham, MD, FACS and
Arash Moradzadeh, MD

## Introduction

In this chapter, we review relevant nasal anatomy and discuss reconstruction of the soft tissues of the nose including defect analysis, choice of reconstructive technique, and specific reconstructive techniques most commonly used for nasal reconstruction.

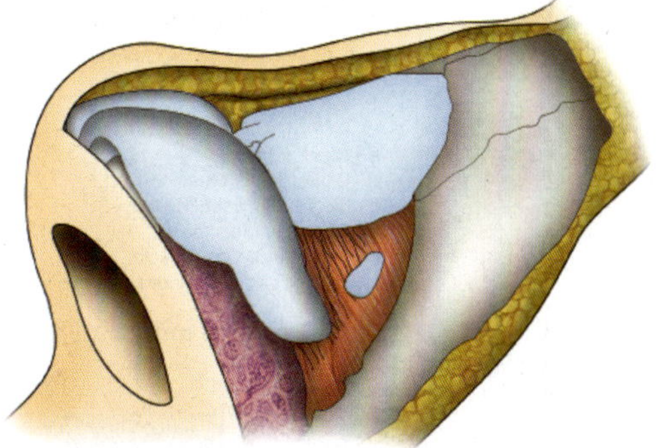

**Figure 6-1.** Skin soft tissue envelope of the nose. The skin varies in thickness largely due to varying amounts of subcutaneous fat. The S/STE is tightly adherent over the lower lateral cartilages in the tip and has abundant sebaceous glands.

## Nasal Anatomy

Along with a thorough understanding of the subunit principle in nasal reconstruction, it is also essential that the surgeon have a firm grasp of the underlying anatomy responsible for this unique topography. The nose is covered with a skin/soft tissue envelope (S/STE) that varies in thickness and sebaceous qualities depending on its location on the nose (**Figure 6-1**). The more cephalic portions of the nose from the nasion down to the supratip region are covered with a relatively thin and loosely adherent S/STE. Similarly, the nasal sidewalls are also covered with thin skin that gradually thickens as the alar groove is reached caudally. The S/STE consists of several layers, with the deepest being the perichondrium or periosteum followed by loose areolar tissue, a deep vascular fatty layer, a fibromuscular layer, a layer of subcutaneous fat, and finally a layer of dermis and epidermis. The tip and columellar and alar subunits are covered by a tightly adherent S/STE that is thick and glandular or sebaceous in quality except for that overlying the columella, which is quite thin and adheres to the medial crura.

The fibromuscular layer, which is continuous with the facial superficial musculoaponeurotic system (SMAS) layer, laterally contains the musculature of the nose (**Figure 6-2**), which consists of the procerus located in the nasion and inserts into the forehead skin that pulls down and creates horizontal lines at the nasion. The nasalis muscle is paired and fans out over the upper lateral cartilage and joins in the midline to form a muscular covering that stabilizes the otherwise floppy middle vault during deep inspiration. The second component of the nasalis muscle is the dilator naris, which extends over the lower lateral cartilages and serves to flare the nostrils during deep or rapid inspiration. The depressor septi is a small muscle that extends superiorly from the orbicularis oris with which it is interdigitated and serves to depress the nasal tip, especially during smiling.

The vascular supply of the nose arises from branches of both the external and internal carotid arteries (**Figure 6-3**). The lateral wall of the nose is supplied by the angular artery that travels along the

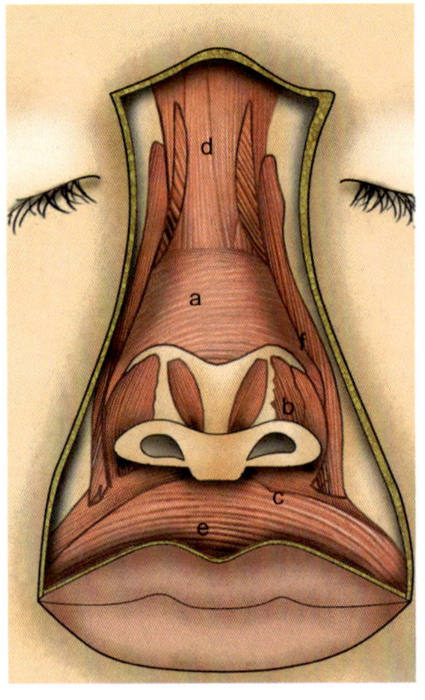


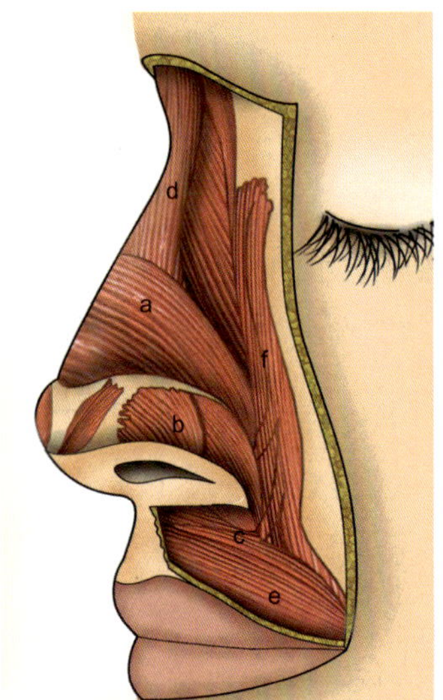


a - Nasalis Muscle
b - Dilator Naris Muscle
c - Depressor Septi Muscle
d - Procerus Muscle
e - Orbicularis Oris muscle
f - Levator Labii Superioris Muscle

**Figure 6-2.** Nasal musculature.

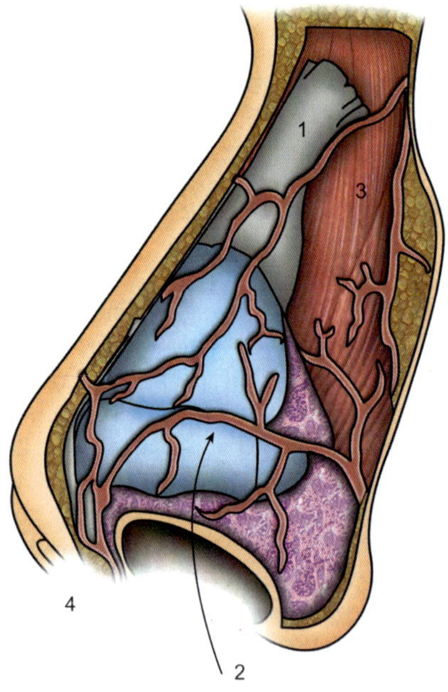


1 - Dorasal Nasal Arteny
2 - Lateral Nasal Artery
3 - Angular Vessels
4 - Columellar Artery

**Figure 6-3.** Vascular anatomy of the nose.

nasal-facial groove and gives off the lateral nasal artery, which supplies the lower lateral portions of the nose and anastomoses with descending branches of the dorsal nasal artery, a branch of the ophthalmic artery. The anterior ethmoidal artery terminates in an external branch that pierces the lateral nasal wall at the junction of the nasal bones and the upper lateral cartilages and supplies the more medial aspect of the sidewall, dorsum, and superior aspect of the nasal tip. The inferior portion of the nasal tip and all of the columella are supplied by an ascending septal and/or separate columellar branch from the superior labial artery.

The nasal skeleton is comprised of two paired nasal bones that comprise the upper one third of the nose (**Figure 6-4**). They are fused in the midline and join with the frontal bone at the nasion and laterally are fused with the ascending process of the maxilla. Attached to the caudal end of the nasal bones are the upper lateral cartilages that comprise the major framework for the middle nasal vault. The paired lower lateral cartilages are responsible for the shape and support of the nasal ala and the tip. They are related to the upper lateral cartilage in a complicated and highly variable manner in a region known as the scroll area. This area correlates with the alar

a - Upper Lateral Cartilage
b - Lower Lateral Cartilage
c - Sesamoid Cartilages (highly variable or absent)
d - Ascending Process Of Maxilla
e - Nasal Bone

**Figure 6-4.** Bony and cartilaginous skeleton of the nose.

groove area and the external nasal valve. The upper lateral cartilages and lower lateral cartilages are connected with a fibrous ligament that may also contain a floating sesamoid cartilage.

Innervation of the nose laterally is from branches of the infraorbital nerve or the second division of the trigeminal nerve ($V_2$). Medially and caudally, the innervation is derived from the external nasal branch of the anterior ethmoidal nerve. The most superior aspects of the nose and glabella are supplied by branches of the supraorbital and supratrochlear nerves.

## Nasal Defect Analysis

In Chapter 4, the topographical anatomical concept of esthetic units of the face was introduced. Within each esthetic unit such as the nose there are subunits that exist and must be considered when planning a nasal reconstruction. The nose can be divided into the nasal dorsum, paired nasal sidewalls, nasal tip, alar subunits, and columella (**Figure 6-5**). Planning a reconstruction with these boundaries in mind will lead to a superior overall result. For instance, it is best not to cross subunits if possible, as this blurs the distinction between the subunits making the repair more obvious. If incisions can be placed along the boundaries of the subunits, the repair is more likely to go unnoticed. If the defect encompasses a large portion of a subunit, it is generally better to remove the remainder of the subunit and replace that entire subunit. Similarly, if a defect encompasses more than one subunit then consideration should be given to reconstructing the subunits separately or reestablishing the distinction between the subunits with further surgical refinements. An example of this would be to re-create the alar groove after reconstruction with a superiorly based melolabial flap.

The nose is a complex structure with multiple complex functions. The nature of the defect and the subsequent reconstruction, of necessity, will impact the functions of the nose. The mucosal lining requires a different reconstructive plan than the skin/soft tissue envelope of the nose. Similarly, loss of structural components such as cartilage or bone must also be considered when planning a reconstruction. The local flaps discussed herein are primarily used to restore the skin/soft tissue envelope of the nose but are occasionally "turned in" to restore the skin of the vestibule of the nose.

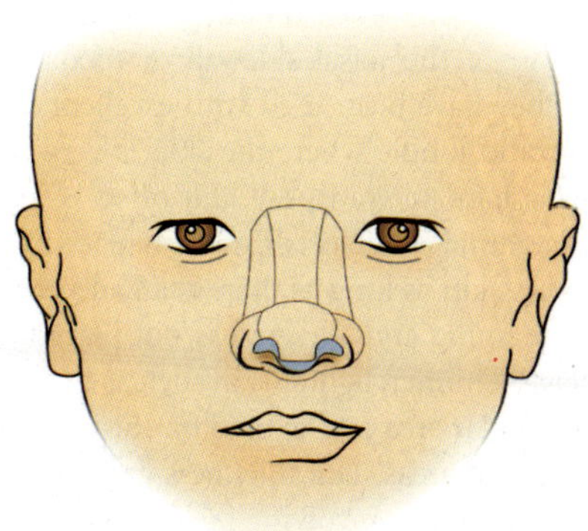


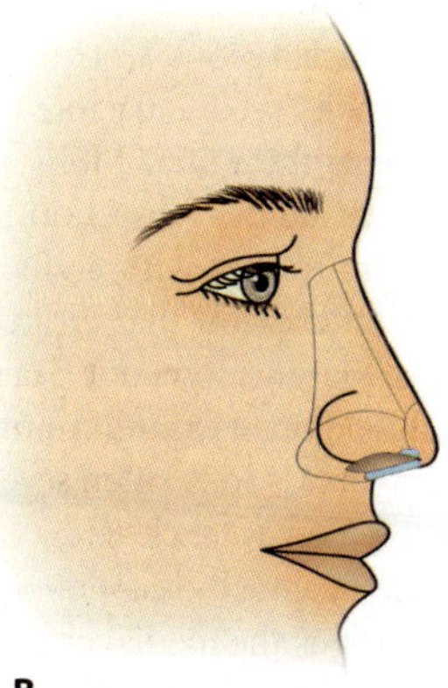


**Figure 6-5.** Nasal subunits. The nose can be divided into a tip, dorsal, collumellar, and paired sidewall and alar lobule subunits.

## Nasal Defect Preparation

When faced with a defect that is fresh, there is little preparation of the wound for repair. However, in many cases, such as those involving Mohs surgical excision, it is not possible to repair the defect on the same day as the excision. In these instances, the wound should be freshened to remove any fibrinous exudate that accumulates in the bed of the wound. Similarly, the edges of the wound should be freshened and any beveling or unevenness should be trimmed to give a defect of uniform thickness with clean, fresh edges.

## Choice of Reconstructive Technique

The prime consideration in the decision of which nasal reconstructive technique to use is the size and location of the defect. This is why the subunit principle is so important to understand and apply in these cases. We will discuss the most commonly used techniques for each subunit and when to use them. The patient's health and desires regarding the reconstruction must be considered as well. Explanation of the reasonable alternatives including healing by secondary intention should always be discussed with the patient so that they can make a proper informed decision. Some patients will opt for a lesser esthetic result in favor of convenience and comfort. These choices of the patient should be respected and not taken personally.

## Alternatives to Local Flaps

Healing by secondary intention can yield surprisingly good results in certain areas. Much of this is known from the early work of Dr. Frederic Mohs and other early Mohs surgeons who routinely allowed wounds to heal by secondary intention. This was necessary because the initial Mohs technique did not use a fresh tissue frozen section technique and the wounds were treated with a zinc chloride fixative paste prior to excision that created significant tissue necrosis. Margins were not cleared at one sitting and patients had open wounds until the margins were cleared. Wounds were often several weeks to months old before they were cleared.

The best areas for healing by secondary intention are concave areas such as the medial canthal area or areas that have a firm base such as the forehead or upper nasal sidewall. This prevents the wound from contracting and creating distortion of the surrounding tissues as it heals. When this method is used, it is imperative that the patient understand that the wound must be kept clean and free from exudate or eschar and should be kept moist with a coating of petrolatum or antibiotic ointment. Water-based antibiotic creams should be avoided, as they are not occlusive and contribute to the buildup of debris in the wound bed. It is often helpful to allow a wound to heal partially by secondary intention even if the intent is to skin graft. In doing so, the depth of the wound is filled preventing the depression that accompanies immediate skin grafting and improving the esthetics of the reconstruction.

Primary closure has limited use in nasal reconstruction unless the defect is small and is in an area with loose skin such as the sidewall or dorsum. This technique is most commonly employed in elderly patients who have significant laxity of the skin. Closure as always should be along relaxed skin tension lines. Areas such as the nasal tip cannot be closed primarily without significant distortion.

Skin grafts are discussed in detail in Chapter 5; however, some comments specific to their use in nasal reconstruction are in order. Split thickness skin grafts should be avoided in the nose, particularly as an immediate reconstructive option. Because they lack adnexal structures associated with full thickness skin or flaps, split thickness skin grafts are thin and will yield an unacceptable result. When split thickness skin grafts are placed on a wound bed that has allowed to granulate up to the level of the surrounding epidermis, the result can be improved but will still remain suboptimal.

Best results with full thickness grafts are obtained when they are used in shallow defects that encompass the entire subunit. Full thickness grafts yield best results when they are used to replace the thin skin of the nasal sidewall or medial canthal area. They have been used with excellent results in the infratip lobule where the skin is very thin and a flap is hard to transpose and often is too thick. Small columellar defects can be replaced with full thickness skin as long as there is an adequate tissue bed remaining and the graft is not placed on bare cartilage. Thinner, lighter skin such as that from the postauricular area can be used for these nonactinically exposed areas. Full thickness grafts should not be used in defects involving the alar margin, as they will contract without a framework underneath to counteract the graft contracture. This results in unacceptable cosmetic and functional results.

## Total Nasal Defects

Nasal defects that involve the entire S/STE of the nose or involve substantial portions of many subunits are best reconstructed by removing the remnants of these subunits and replacing them in their entirety. Defects that extend outside the boundaries of the lateral nasal sidewall should be reconstructed using cheek advancement flaps. These flaps should be anchored into position so that they do not retract and distort the nasal/facial boundary or create tension on the flap used for nasal reconstruction. Reconstruction used for the nasal defect should be used for that purpose only even though it may be tempting to pull the cheek onto the nose or extend the forehead flap out onto the cheek defect.

The paramedian forehead flap represents the best source of tissue in sufficient quantity to complete this type of reconstruction. This flap is a true pedicled flap that is based on the supratrochlear vessels (**Figure 6-6**). If these are compromised or

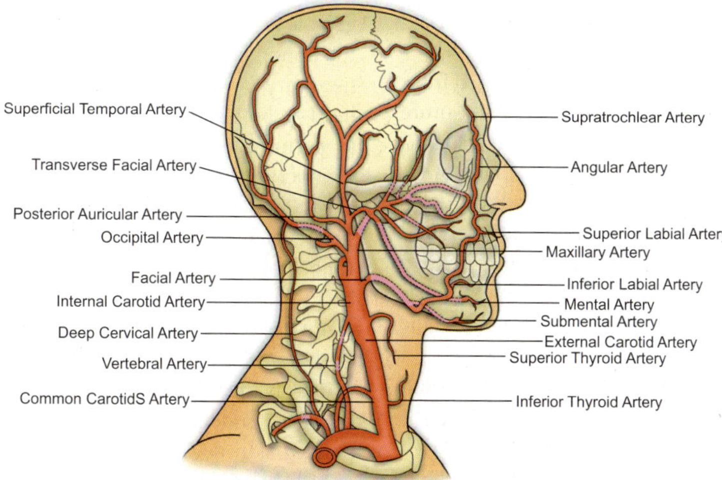


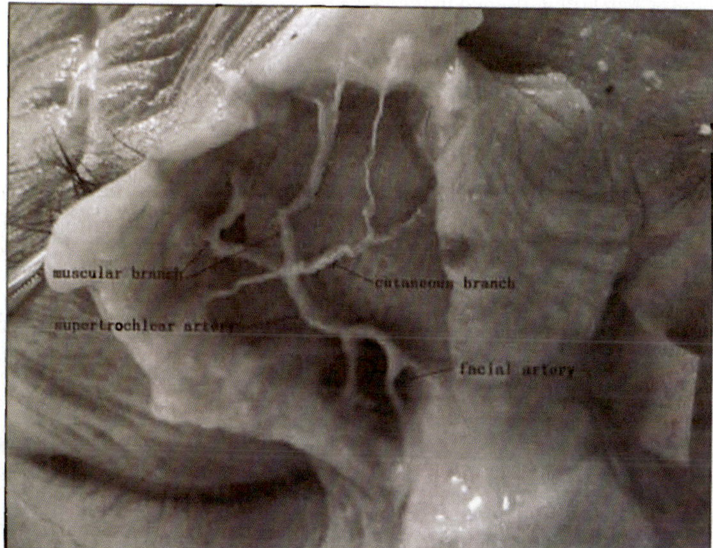


**Figure 6-6.** The supratrochlear artery is the blood supply to the paramedian forehead flap. It is capable of providing a large amount of tissue for nasal reconstructions. If the supratrochlear artery is compromised, a flap can be developed from the supraorbital vessels.

absent, a flap can be based on the supraorbital vessels, but it is harder to rotate into position due to its distance from the root of the nose, thus requiring a longer pedicle and interfering with the upper eyelid and vision on that side. The paramedian forehead flap should be designed to arise from the side contralateral to the defect. This permits easier rotation of the flap into the defect. If the defect is symmetric, then either pedicle can be used for the flap. The vascular pedicle exits at the medial aspect of the brow and is usually just superior to the trochlea, which is palpable just inside the superior orbital rim. The supratrochlear artery should be doppled with a pencil Doppler to map out its exact location and marked with a marking pen.

An exact template of the defect is fashioned from foil or other suitable sterile material. Foil suture packages work well for this as does presterilized aluminum foil. Once the template is made, the distance from the rotation point of the flap at the medial brow is measured by fixing the point of rotation and using 4 × 4 gauze to determine the length of the flap that is necessary. The template is then held in position with the gauze and a final check is made of the measurements.

Having ensured that the template is the right size and configuration and that the flap length is appropriate, the flap can be elevated (**Figure 6-7**). The superior aspect of the flap will require tapering to a fusiform or elliptical shape to promote closure of the donor site. The flap is undermined in the subgaleal plane down to approximately 2 cm above the superior orbital rim. At this point, an incision is made in the periosteum and the flap is elevated in this plane to preserve the neurovascular bundle. Proximal to the defect template of the flap, the pedicle may be tapered, taking care not to radically skeletonize the pedicle and compromise venous outflow or arterial integrity. Some tapering is necessary to permit proper rotation of the flap into the defect. If the skin in the region of the pedicle is too wide it can torque and compromise the circulation. As a general rule, 2 cm of skin should be left associated with the pedicle to prevent this.

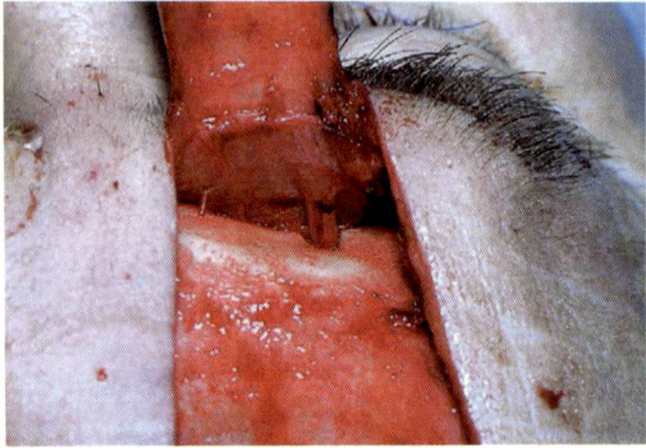

**Figure 6-7.** The flap is elevated in the subgaleal plane taking care to leave the periosteum intact. This is important if the forehead defect cannot be closed and is allowed to heal by secondary intention. The distal end of the flap can be thinned but should only be thinned over the area needed to inset into the defect.

Once the flap has been elevated and the surgeon is assured that it can be rotated into position, the donor site can be closed (**Figure 6-8A–E**). It is necessary to widely undermine the remaining forehead on both sides of the flap in the subgaleal plane to permit closure. A strong suture of 3-0 or 4-0 Monocryl is useful for subcutaneous closure. Skin closure is achieved with a 5-0 or 6-0 monofilament suture such as nylon or Prolene. If the donor site cannot be closed primarily at its widest point, it is best to allow this to heal by secondary intention. It is not necessary to place tissue expanders preoperatively in anticipation of a defect that will not close primarily. In no instance should a tissue expander be placed under the area of the proposed flap, as expanded skin develops into a capsule and becomes less pliable and yields an inferior outcome.

The flap can be thinned appropriately to the thickness of the defect. This thinning should take place only over the template portion of the flap that is to be inset into the defect. It is not necessary to thin the subcutaneous tissues at the proximal end of the pedicle and, in fact, it is to be avoided to prevent compromise of the vascularity. If it is necessary to extend the flap into the hairline for the reconstruction, any hair-bearing skin can be thinned and the follicles removed from the deep surface. Electrolysis or laser hair removal can be used to remove any residual hair following division and inset of the flap. The flap is anchored at key points with 5-0 Monocryl or other monofilament absorbable suture and the skin is sutured with a 6-0 Prolene or nylon. Interrupted sutures are preferable for the inset of the flap. A continuous suture can be used to close the donor site according to surgeon preference.

The exposed portion of the pedicle is dressed with Xeroform gauze that is also coated with a thick coat of antibiotic ointment. The Xeroform is wrapped around the pedicle, taking care not to strangulate it. No other dressings are necessary

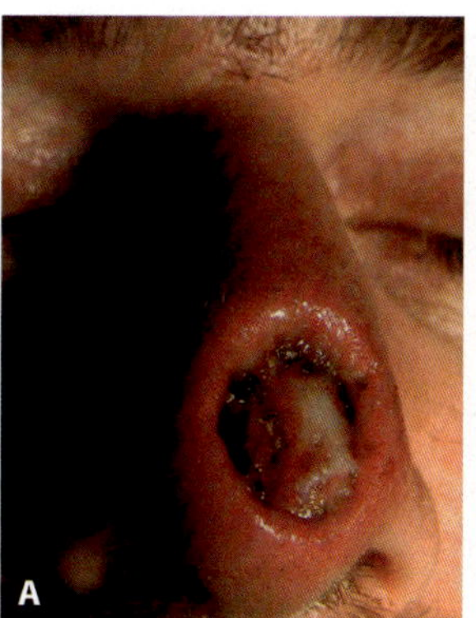


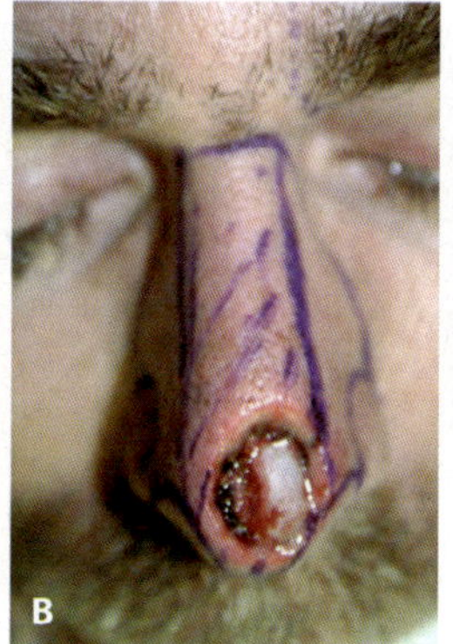


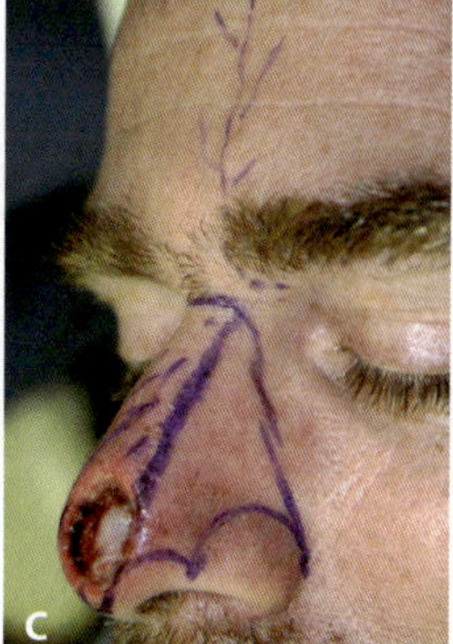


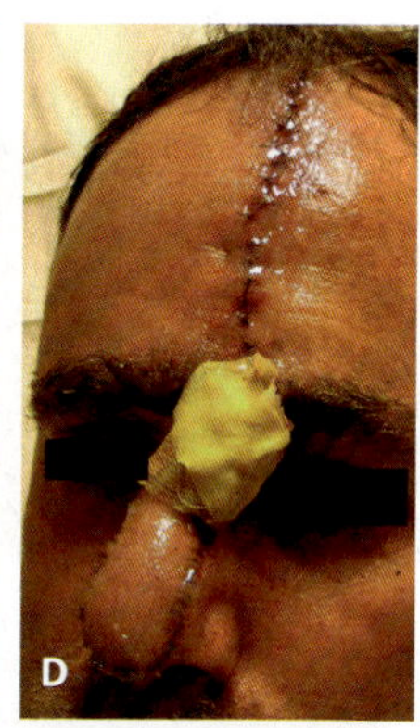


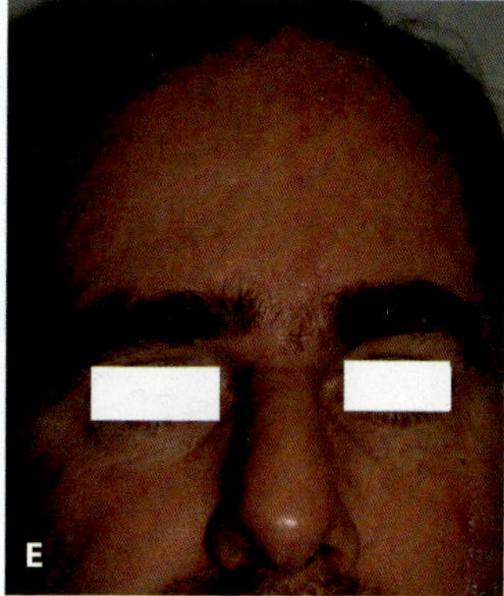


**Figure 6-8.** Paramedian forehead flap for closure of a combined dorsal and tip Defect. (A) Defect prior to the reconstruction planning. (B) Frontal and Lateral view of defect and nasal subunits outlined. (C) The left supratrochlear artery has been doppled to out line its course on the forehead. (D) The tip and dorsal subunits have been resected and the left paramedian forehead flap has been inset into the defect. A xeroform guaze has been used to cover the pedjcle as the flap heals. (E) Final 3 month result of forehead donor scar and nasal reconstruction.

except for an occasional eye pad to catch any oozing from the pedicle into the medial canthal region. In no instance should a dressing be placed over the pedicle that might compress it. Judicious bipolar cautery of any bleeding at the exposed edge of the pedicle is acceptable, but care should be taken not to be too aggressive with the hemostasis. It is not uncommon for these flaps to ooze for the first 6–8 hours postoperatively. The Xeroform should be left intact until the first dressing change at 1 week. Eye pads can be changed on an as needed basis.

The patient is seen postoperatively at 1 week for suture removal and the first dressing change. Patients are taught to replace the Xeroform daily, and the second stage of the procedure—the division of the pedicle and inset of the flap—is scheduled. The pedicle is divided at 3 weeks with assurance that the flap has established its new vascular supply from the native nasal tissues. A tourniquet test is helpful to assure the surgeon that the pedicle can be safely divided. This is performed by occluding the artery with a vessel loop or a rubber band. It is common for the flap to blanch slightly, but if it exhibits capillary refill, it is safe to divide. The author has never had a flap fail after dividing the pedicle at 3 weeks. This portion of the procedure can be easily performed with local anesthesia or, if preferred, under a mild intravenous sedation. No attempt should be made to return any portion of the excess pedicle skin. The defect resulting from the removal of the excess pedicle skin can be closed along relaxed skin tension lines in a curvilinear fashion at the medial end of the brow. Care should be taken to thin this area as well, as the tissues tend to contract and "ball up" and will not lay flat and smooth unless thinned.

The dorsal subunit is often reconstructed with the nasal tip subunit, particularly for large defects, as the cosmetic result is much better when these two units are reconstructed together with one flap. When the forehead flap is extended over the nasal tip, the scars are hidden along the alar/tip junction and in the shadow of the tip of the nose. When the forehead flap is terminated at the tip/supratip junction, a lengthy horizontal scar results that is more noticeable than the scar associated with a tip/dorsum combined reconstruction (**Figures 6-9A–H**).

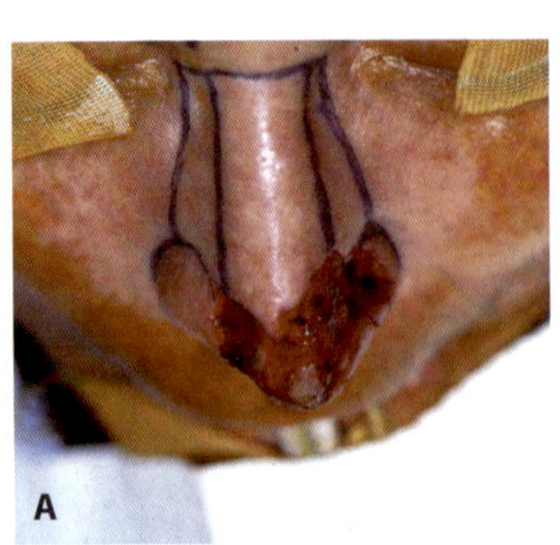
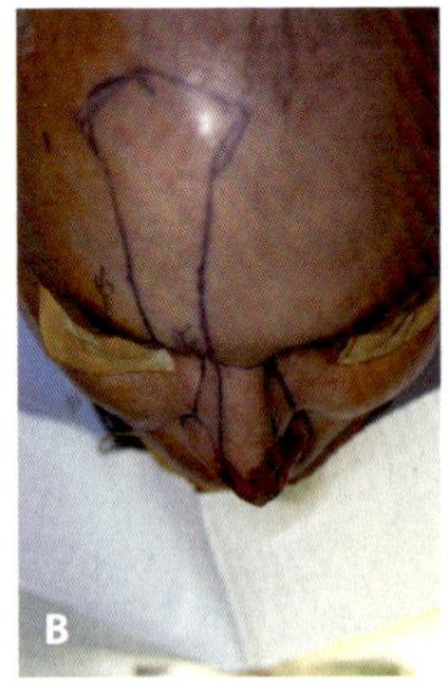
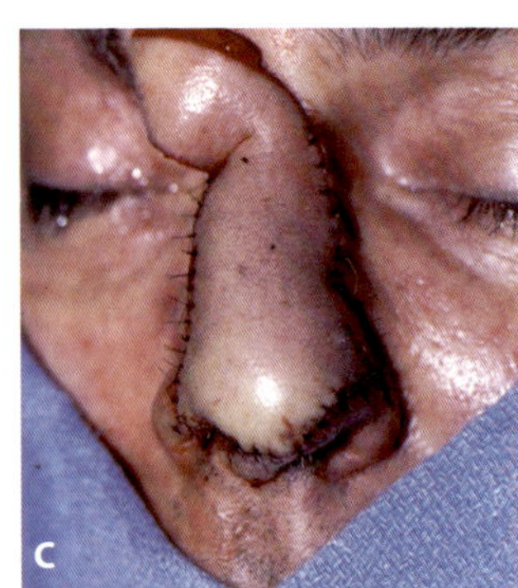
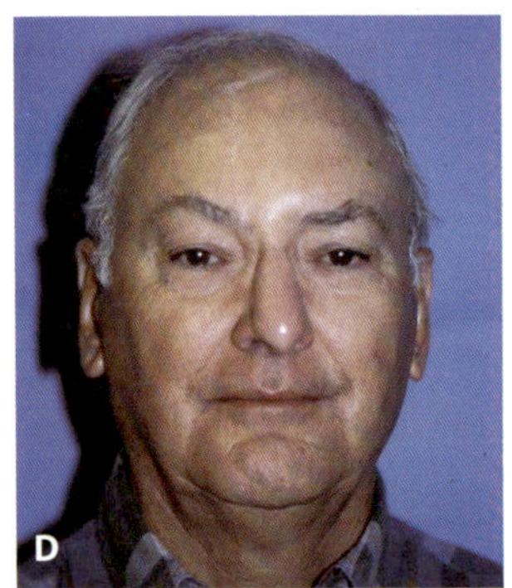
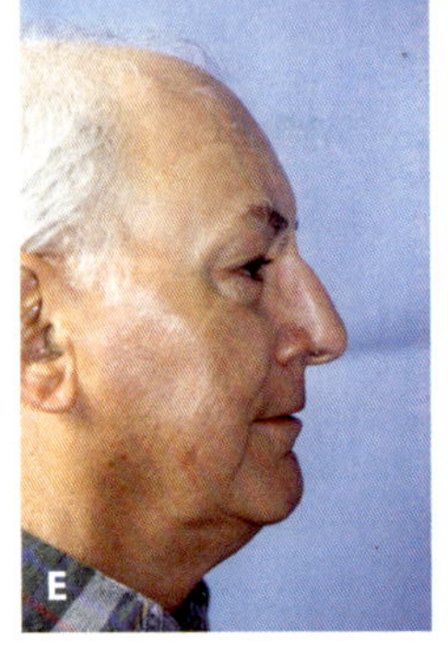
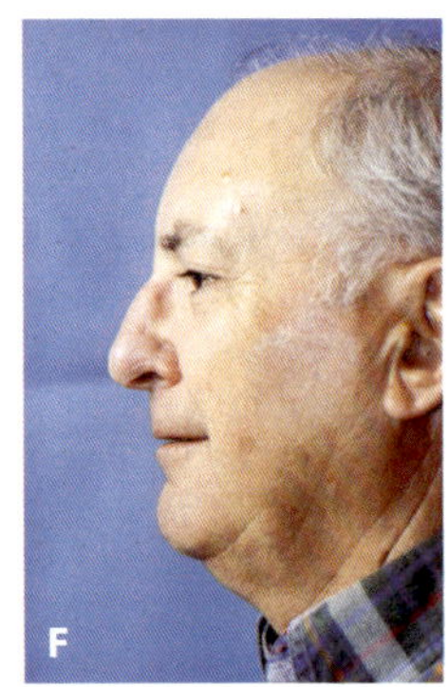
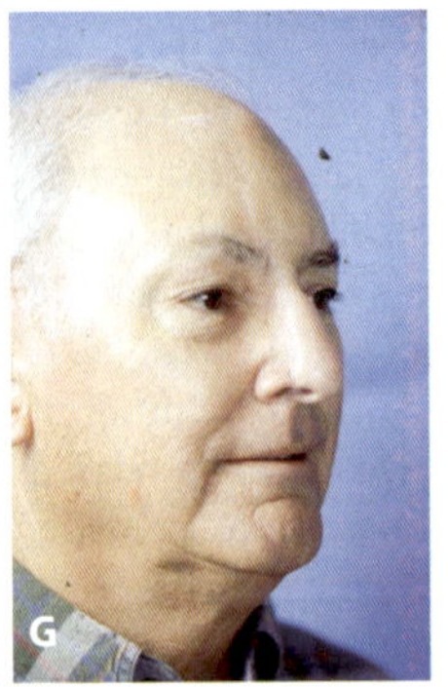
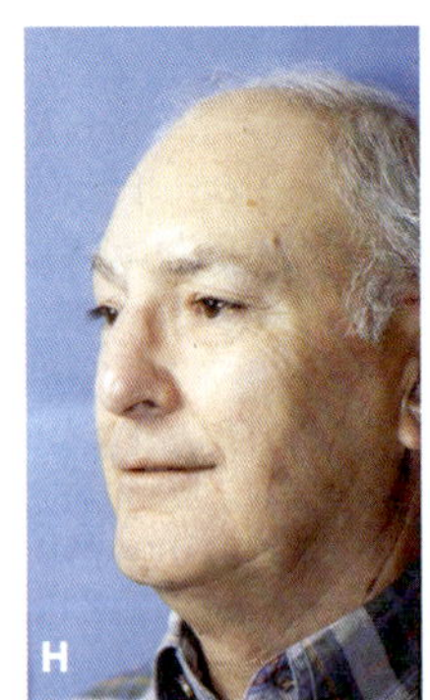

**Figure 6-9.** Paramedian Forehead. Flap reconstruction of nasal tip defect (A) A large tip defect that involves both alar subunits and encroaches on the dorsal subunit. (B) A right paramedian forehead flap has been outlined and measured. The vascular pedicle is outlined by Doppler. The supraorbital pedicle is also outlined. For cosmesis, the dorsal subunit is planned for resection as a part of the reconstruction. (C) Flap has been elevated and the donor site closed primarily with wide undermining of the entire forehead in the subgaleal plane. (D) Frontal view of healed flap (E) Right lateral view of healed flap. (F) Left lateral view of healed flap. (G) Right oblique view of healed flap. (H) Left oblique view of healed flap

## Nasal Dorsum Reconstruction

The nasal dorsal subunit is frequently involved with cutaneous malignancies, most commonly basal cell carcinoma, owing to its prominence and constant exposure to the sun. Although adherence to the subunit principle is critical, some small defects can be reconstructed without excising the entire dorsal subunit. If more than half of the subunit is involved in the defect, however, consideration should be given to excising the remainder and reconstructing the entire dorsum. When reconstructing a small defect, care should be taken to plan the incisions to lie along relaxed skin tension lines and within or along the affected subunit. The most commonly used flap for reconstruction of the entire dorsal subunit is the paramedian forehead flap as previously discussed.

## Subtotal Dorsal Defects

For defects that are smaller and do not necessitate removal of the entire dorsal subunit, there are a number of options available. The bilobed flap is particularly useful for both dorsal nasal defects and lateral nasal wall defects. If planned and executed properly, the incisions can be placed along the junction of the nasal sidewall and dorsum and the flap well camouflaged. The bilobed flap is particularly useful in the lower dorsum and tip where the skin is thicker and more sebaceous in quality. By rotating adjacent similar tissue into the primary defect and recruiting more lax sidewall tissue for the secondary flap, the defect can be reconstructed nicely (**Figure 6-10A–D**).

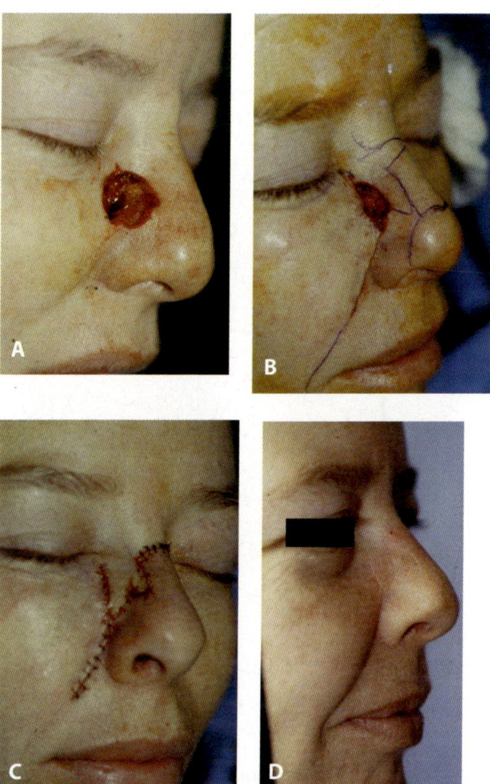


**Figure 6-10.** Combined defect of cheek and nasal sidewall. (A) This defect spans the nasofacial junction and has both cheek and nasal sidewall components. These should be reconstructed using different techniques. (B) Nasal subunits have been outlined and the cheek portion of the defect has been reconstructed using a cheek advancement of the esthetic units. A bilobed flap is outlined using the subunit principle. (C) The nasal reconstruction is completed by rotation the bilobed flap into place. The primary flap is oriented to stay within the sidewall subunit. The secondary flap in this case was taken from the nasion and is transversely oriented to yield the best donor site scar. (D) One year post-operative result demonstrated the importance of adhering to the subunit principle when platming local flaps.

The typical bilobed flap is designed with a total of 90 degrees of rotation around the axis of rotation for the primary and secondary flaps (**Figure 6-11**). The primary flap is oriented at 45 degrees from and tangential to the primary defect. It is classically described as being the same size as the primary defect, but with some undermining of the edges, the primary flap can often be slightly smaller. This is not true in the tip where the skin is tightly adherent and the primary flap should equal the size of the defect. The secondary flap is typically half the size of the secondary defect created by the primary flap. Again, it is typically oriented at 45 degrees from the primary flap but need not be in all cases. In areas where skin is more lax, such as the nasal sidewall, a different angle or orientation that will allow better scar placement is possible. In all cases the adjacent tissues should be undermined to permit optimal rotation of the flaps into position and to minimize standing cone deformities.

In all reconstructions, it is helpful to close the donor sites prior to completing the inset of the flap. Similarly, one should refrain from excising Burrow's triangles in a preformed fashion until the reconstruction is nearly complete and the flaps have been inset. This prevents over resection of tissue based on a plan that was conceived preoperatively and may have changed during the reconstruction as the surgeon experiences the movement of the tissues. As the bilobed flap is a random pattern flap, care must be taken not to back-cut the base of the flap when elevating the flap or excising standing cone deformities.

## Nasal Sidewall

The nasal sidewall is the easiest of the subunits to reconstruct. The tissue here is thin and loosely adherent to the skeletal framework unlike the tip and lower dorsum. Small defects can be closed primarily with adequate undermining and scars oriented along the nasal/facial or dorsal/sidewall junctions. The workhorse flap for reconstruction of lateral nasal defects is the melolabial flap. This flap is generally considered to be a random pattern flap that can be based superiorly (**Figure 6-12**) or inferiorly (**Figure 6-13**) and is most commonly used as a superiorly based flap. There are a number of arterial perforators that arise from the adjacent musculature in addition to direct branches from the angular artery (**Figure 6-14**). This rich dual blood supply allows the flap to be based superiorly or inferiorly. The decision

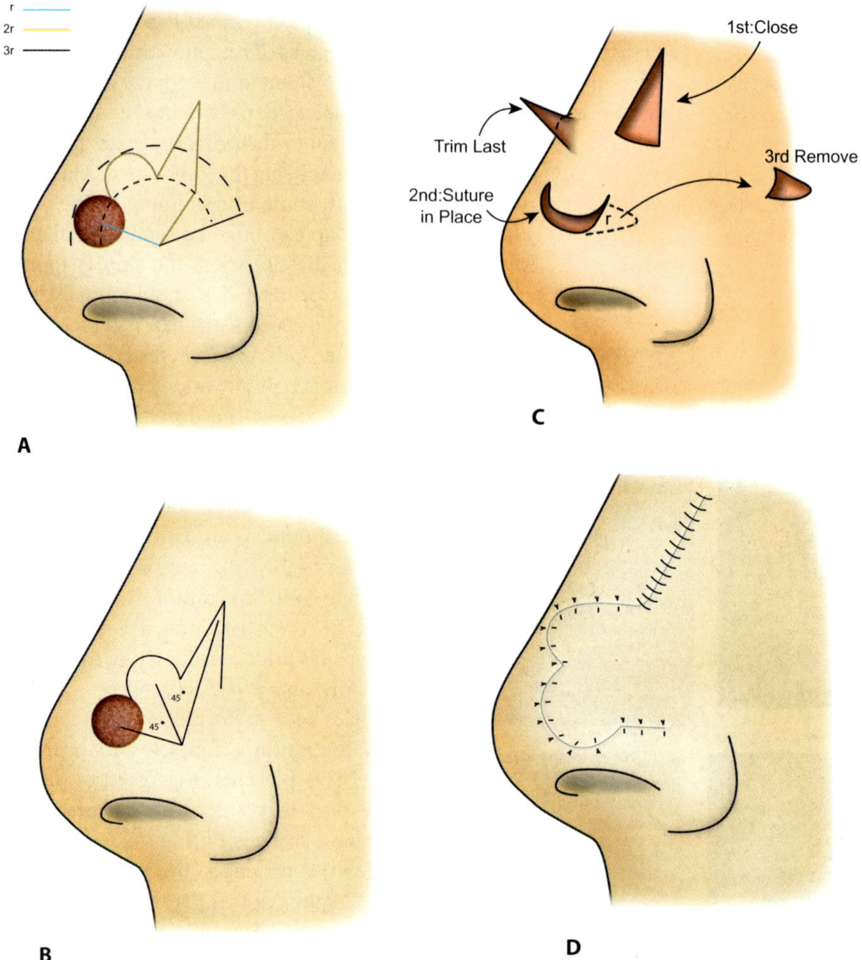


**Figure 6-11.** Bilobed flap. The bilobed flap is an excellent tool for small to medium nasal defects of the sidewall and tip.

of which one to use is determined by the location of the defect. Small superior defects can be closed with either a superiorly based flap or an inferiorly based flap. Large defects are best reconstructed with a superiorly based flap. The major disadvantage of the inferiorly based flap is that it crosses over the alar groove and can obliterate it if used for inferior defects. This necessitates a secondary procedure to take down a portion of the flap if it is pedicled or to recreate the alar groove. Using a superiorly based flap avoids these secondary procedures. The major disadvantage of the superiorly based flap is that the distal end of the flap is in a dependent position and is prone to chronic swelling and lymphedema. This can be minimized by thinning the flap aggressively when insetting it. Care must be taken to properly align the skin edges so that the scar is smooth and flat. Triamcinolone acetonide (Kenalog) 10 mg/ml is also helpful in treating the chronic thickening.

In designing the melolabial flap it is critical that the tissue is recruited lateral to the melolabial fold. In no instance should the flap be centered over the melolabial fold as is shown in some texts. This can lead to distortion of the lip and perioral area, thus violating a key principle in soft tissue reconstruction. A large flap both in length and width can be obtained from the cheek tissues and closed along the fold with an excellent result. Patients should be warned that the cheek mound will be less full on the donor side, but this represents a small price com-

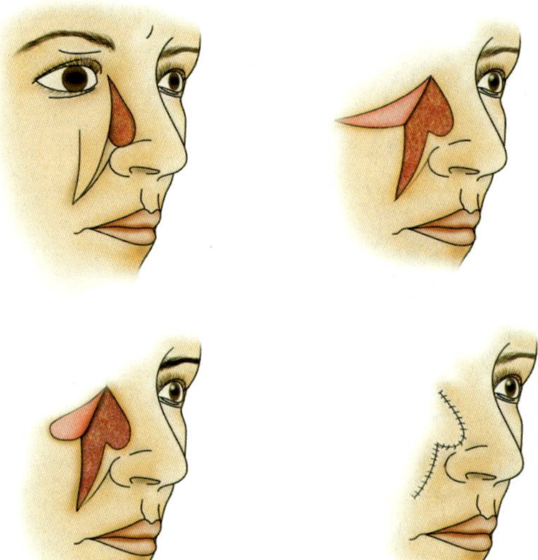

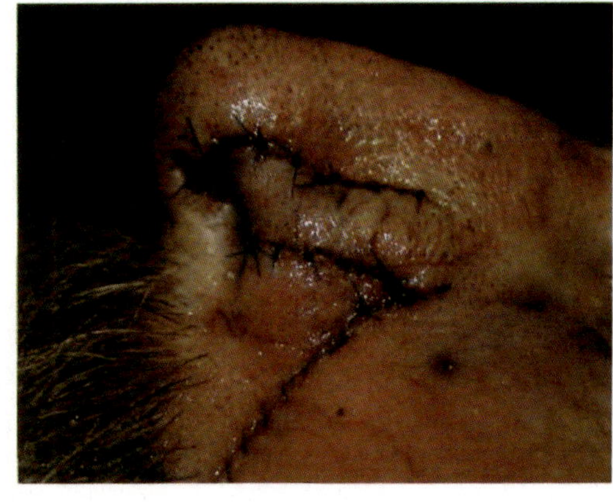

**Figure 6-12.** Superiorly based melolabial flap.

pared to the volume of tissue that is available for reconstruction. Care should be taken when elevating the flap to avoid injury to the underlying angular artery and the underlying musculature.

Another useful flap for the reconstruction of lateral nasal wall defects is the dorsal nasal flap. It has also been termed the sliding glabellar flap and the Reiger flap **(Figure 6-15)**. This flap takes advantage of the V-to-Y advancement concept in the glabellar region and allows this excess tissue to be advanced or slid down the nose along the nasal-facial junction to close lateral defects. It is based on the angular artery and its many branches onto the nose. It is essential that the incision for this flap be made along the nasofacial junction and that extensive undermining of the skin/soft tissue envelope of nearly the entire nose be made to allow this flap to lie smoothly **(Figure 6-16A,B)**. A standing cone deformity is encountered at the root of the nose and should be excised in a horizontal fashion at this junction. This flap is not ideal for reconstructing medial canthal defects, although it has been described for this purpose. The skin is too thick and bulky to recreate the thin skin of the medial canthus. Reconstruction of this region is addressed in Chapter 10 entitled "Orbital/Periorbital Reconstruction."

As mentioned earlier, full thickness skin grafts can be used on the nasal sidewall if necessary and will provide an adequate but not optimal result.

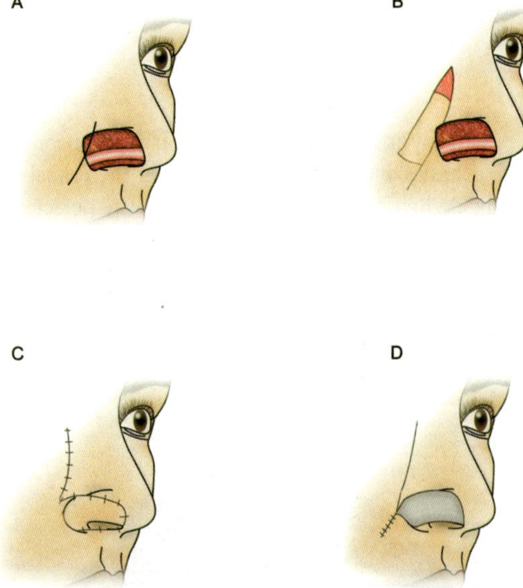


**Figure 6-13.** Inferiorly based melolabial flap. The inferiorly based melolabial flap can be used for defects along the alar rim (A). Based along the melolabial fold, the pedicle is inferior to the defect (B) and once transposed obliterates the alar-facial groove (C). This necessitates a second stage procedure to divide the pedicle and recreate the alar-facial groove (D).

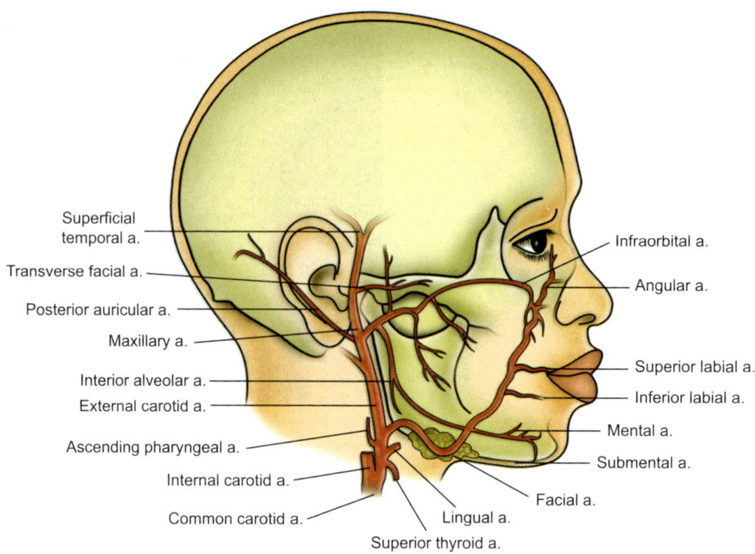


**Figure 6-14.** Vascular anatomy of the melolabial flap numerous perforating arteries from adjacent muscles provide additional blood supply to the skin in this area in addition to the direct branches of the angular artery. This allows the flap to be based either superiorly or inferiorly.

## Nasal Tip

As previously mentioned, this subunit is often reconstructed as a larger reconstruction of the dorsal subunit. When faced with an isolated tip defect, rarely does it encompass the entire tip subunit. However, it is best reconstructed as a subunit whenever possible. It is unusual to be able to close this area primarily as the skin is tightly adherent to the underlying cartilages and is thick and nonpliable. One should avoid the temptation to place skin grafts in this area, as they rarely yield an acceptable result. The skin has such unique qualities that adjacent skin of similar quality and thickness represents the best method of reconstruction. If skin grafts are to be used on the tip, they should encompass the entire subunit and should be tailored to the exact thickness of the defect. Skin that is significantly lighter should also be avoided, and the best option for a skin graft donor site for the nasal tip is the melolabial fold

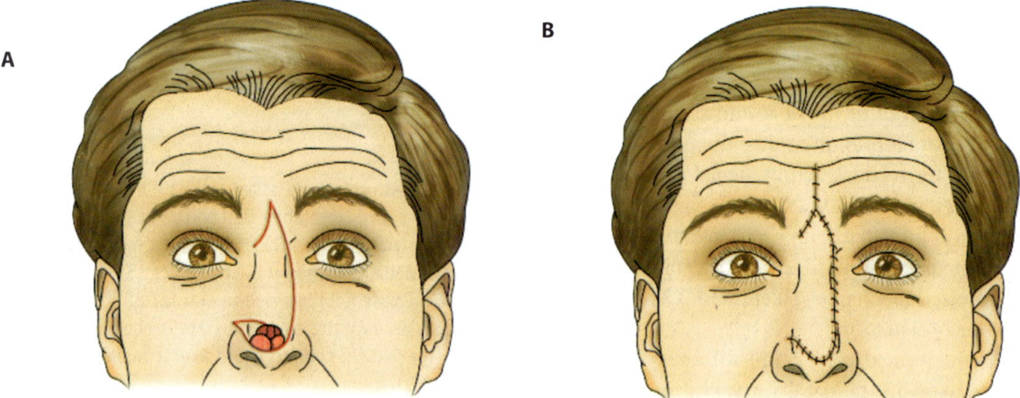


**Figure 6-15.** Dorsal nasal flap. The dorsal nasal flap is most useful for lateral defects although in selected patients it can be used to reconstruct tip defects.

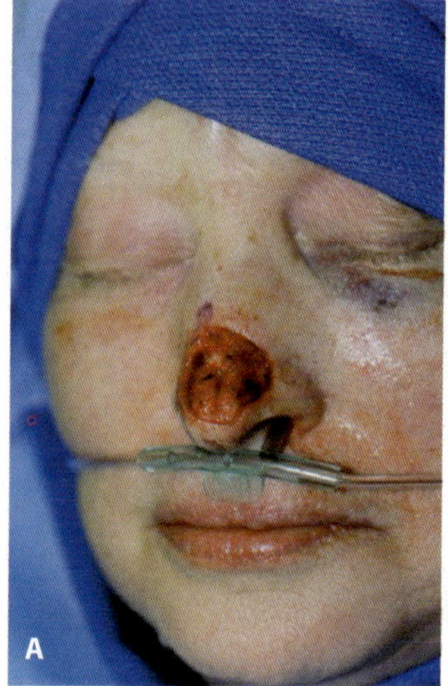


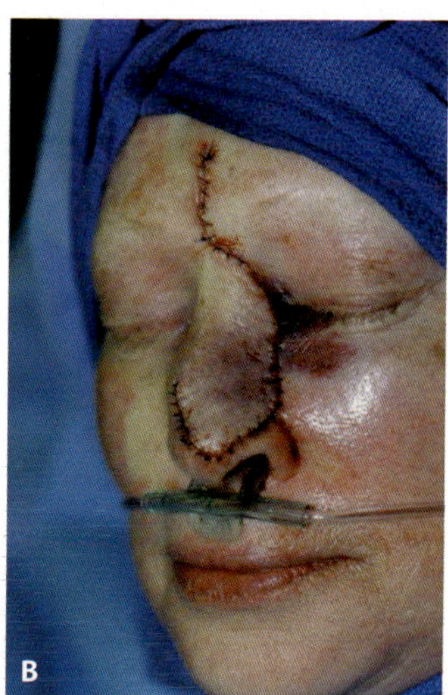


**Figure 6-16.** Dorsal nasal flap. (A) Large nasal tip and dorsal subunit defect. (B) Dorsal nasal flap has been used to reconstruct this defect. It's sucess depends on wide undermining of the entire dorsum and sidewalls of the nose.

area. The skin here is thick and sebaceous and has similar actinic exposure as the nasal tip. Donor sites with less actinic exposure such as the postauricular or supraclavicular skin should be avoided.

For small nasal tip defects, the bilobed flap is a good choice, as it recruits adjacent skin for the primary defect and allows the secondary reconstruction to be hidden laterally. The sliding glabellar flap has been used for nasal tip defects as well but is less well suited for central defects as a rule.

The infratip lobule is an exception to the rule regarding skin grafts and a full thickness skin graft in this location will often yield a superior result to a local flap.

## Nasal Ala

The nasal ala represents a unique reconstructive challenge owing to its unique geometric shape. The alar groove is difficult to recreate once obliterated or resected. In addition, alar defects often extend intranasally as full thickness defects that require special consideration. The superiorly based melolabial flap is the best option to re-create this subunit. It is amenable to turning in on itself to reconstruct the full thickness of the ala. Although the alar subunit does not have a cartilaginous framework to support it in its normal condition, such a framework is often required to prevent alar retraction once the ala is reconstructed. Conchal cartilage works well for this purpose and does not create significant donor site morbidity or scar (**Figure 6-17A–D**). A full thickness helical rim has also been described as a composite chondrocutaneous graft reconstruction for this area, but it has not been found to be as useful, and it is prone to failure and resorption. For this reason, the author's preference is a conchal cartilage graft with a turn-in melolabial flap. The major issue with composite graft reconstruction of the ala is the inability of the surrounding skin to provide n adequate blood supply quickly enough to ensure viability. For this reason, when using these chondrocutaneous grafts it is advisable to keep them smaller than 1 cm. Skouge has described a technique that involves insetting the border of the composite graft into the recipient site. This increases the surface area exposure of the graft to the vascular recipient site, increasing its chance of survival. In this technique the cartilage of the composite graft is larger than the cutaneous portion and this is inserted between the layers of the alar skin. This increases surface area and serves to further stabilize the graft from shearing forces.

## Columella

The columella represents the most difficult area to reconstruct despite being the smallest subunit. There is no adjacent tissue that lends itself to an easily rotated or transposed flap, and it is so small that one has a hard time justifying a forehead flap for its reconstruction. Small lip transposition flaps do not work well in my experience and are the most reliable technique for reconstructing large columellar defects into a pedicled melolabial flap that is divided and inset at 3 weeks. Free composite grafts are not generally successful in this are due to its small surface area and lack of contact with surrounding skin from

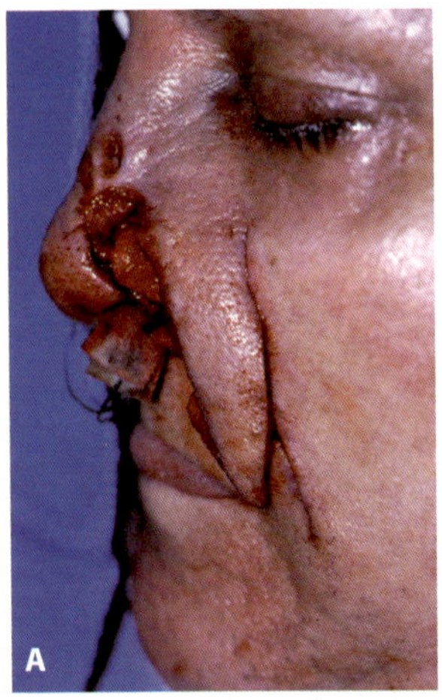


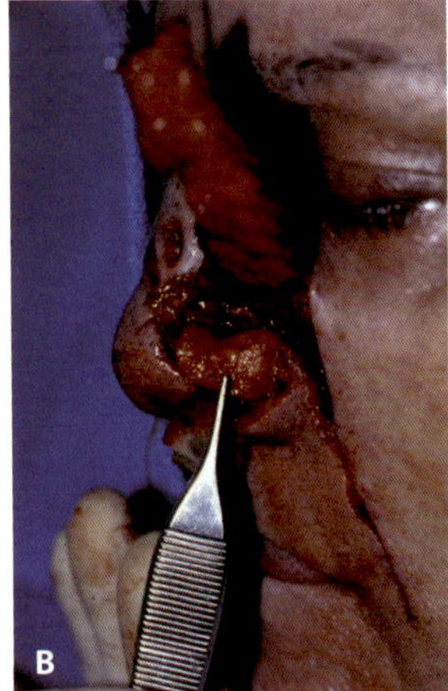


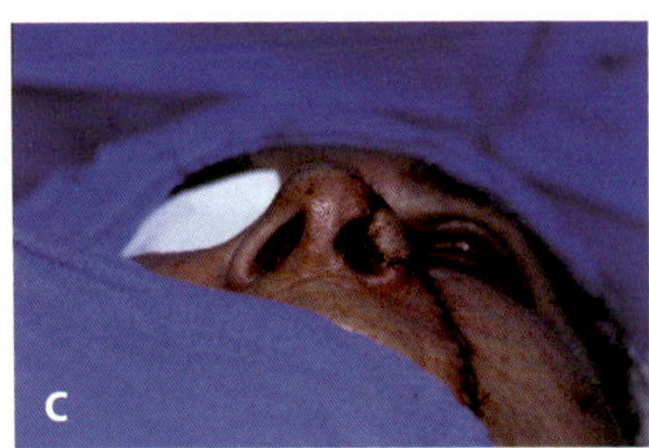


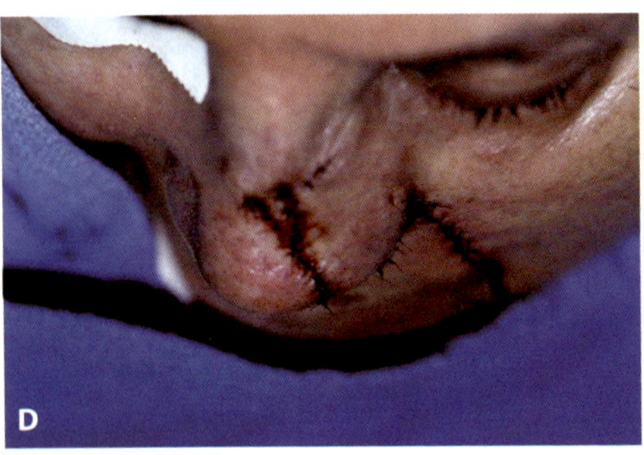


**Figure 6-17.** Alar rim reconstruction. (A) A superiorly based melolabial flap has been elevated for use as a tum in flap for reconstruction of a full thickness alar defect. (B) Conchal cartilage has been harvested and placed at the level of the alar margin. This is necessary to prevent flap retraction even though cartilage does not normally extend to the margin. (C) Basal view demonstrates structural integrity of reconstruction. The conchal cartilage prevents soft tissue collapse into the nasal vault. (D) Superior view demonstrates closure of the donor site and contour restoration of the alar rim. The second scar represents a primary closure of an adjacent Mohs defect.

which to quickly obtain a reliable vascular supply. If adequate vascularized tissue is present and there is no exposed cartilage, full thickness skin grafts can be used for small columellar surface defects.

## Nasal Lining Restoration

Nasal reconstruction was dramatically improved when reconstructive surgeons realized that restoration of lining was critical to surgical outcomes. A well-vascularized lining will support structural grafts and help resist wound contractile forces, ultimately resulting in optimal functional and esthetic outcomes.

Tissue should be replaced with like tissue whenever possible. The internal lining of each nasal subunit has different characteristics, which need to be considered when reconstructing the nasal lining. The ala and soft-tissue triangles are lined by skin, whereas the columella, septum, and nasal sidewalls are lined by nasal mucosa. The nasal mucosa helps humidify inhaled air and moisturize the nasal cavity. Replacing the mucosa with skin can lead to dryness and crusting.

Although a variety of techniques and flaps exist, the ideal tissue for lining reconstruction remains adjacent nasal mucosa. The choice of flap for lining defects is based on size, location of defect and availability of vascularized pliable thin tissue for coverage (**Table 6-1**). Skin grafts, local skin hangover flaps, paramedian forehead flaps, and free flaps are all alternatives to the mucosal flaps. However, they each have limitations such as bulk, rigidity, poor vascularity, or the inability to support cartilaginous grafts. In this chapter we discuss the common flaps and composite grafts used to manage small- to moderate-sized defects of the lower and middle nasal vault. The upper vault rarely requires reconstruction of the lining.

## Auricular Composite Grafts

Auricular composite grafting is a simple, fast method of providing a thin flap with structural support

**TABLE 6-1 Nasal Lining Reconstruction Options**

| *Options* | *Primary Features* | *Defect Location* | *Other Characteristics* |
|---|---|---|---|
| Grafts | | | |
| Full-thickness skin graft | Thin and dry | Multiple | Needs vascular bed; little contraction; cannot use support grafts simultaneously |
| Split-thickness skin graft | Thin and dry | Multiple | Needs vascular bed; variable contraction; cannot use support grafts simultaneously |
| Chondrocutaneous grafts (auricular composite) | Thin and dry | Ala | Needs vascular bed; unpredictable; incomplete take |
| Chondromucosal free grafts | Thin and moist | Ala, tip, lower vault; middle vault | Needs vascular bed; unpredictable; incomplete take |
| Mucosal flaps | | | |
| Bipedicled vestibular | Thin and dry | Ala | Little available tissue |
| Septal mucoperichondrial flap | Thin and moist | | May incorporate cartilage; well vascularized and versatile if axial; may use flap from contralateral airway |
| Septal mucosal (ipsilateral) | Thin and moist | Ala, tip, lower vault | Bilateral flaps possible; lining and structure; may obstruct nasal airway |
| Hinged septal mucosal (contralateral) | Thin and moist | Middle vault | Can be composite; lining and structure; septal perforation |
| Local flaps | | | |
| Nasal turn-in flap (epithelial) | Thick and dry | Ala, tip, lower vault, middle vault | Poor vascularity; needs secondary thinning |
| Nasolabial flap | Thick and dry | Lower vault, middle vault | Bulky; multistage |
| Forehead flap (turn-in) | Thick and dry | Complete lining | Bulky; multistage; robust |
| Composite septal pivotal | Thin and moist | Tip, columella, middle vault | Difficult dissection; septal perforation; bilateral lining |
| Inferior turbinate | Thin and moist | Caudal, occasional, middle vault | Difficult dissection; airway obstruction; avoid septal perforation |

Adapted from Tollefson TT, Kriet DJ, Complex nasal defects: Structure and internal lining. *Facial Plast Surg Clin N Am*, 13 (2005), 333–343.

to small defects of the ala. Small rim defects can be reconstructed with composite grafts harvested from the root of the helix. A composite graft from the conchal bowl is favored for alar lobule defects. Composite grafts are limited by the poor vascular supply to the region. In the authors experience composite grafts are best limited to a maximum of 1.5 cm in size and can only be used reliably for alar rim defects.

## Bipedicle Vestibular Skin Advancement Flap

The bipedicled skin advancement flap can be used to line alar full-thickness defects 1 cm or less in height. An intercartilaginous incision is made and the mucosa is released to facilitate transposition to the alar margin (**Figure 6-18**). Cartilage grafts can be secured to the flap to provide nostril support and to local cutaneous flaps for external coverage. The resulting donor site is then repaired with a thin full-thickness skin graft or other mucosal flap.

## Septal Mucoperichondrial Hinge Flaps: Ipsilateral and Contralateral

The hinge flap is the workhorse of nasal lining flaps. Intranasal lining flaps are thin, supple, and allow for placement of cartilaginous grafts. The limitations of intranasal flaps are morbidity and limited flap dimensions. A flap 4 cm long and 3 cm wide can line the entire lower third and some of the middle vault. Burget and Menik (1985) have shown that the

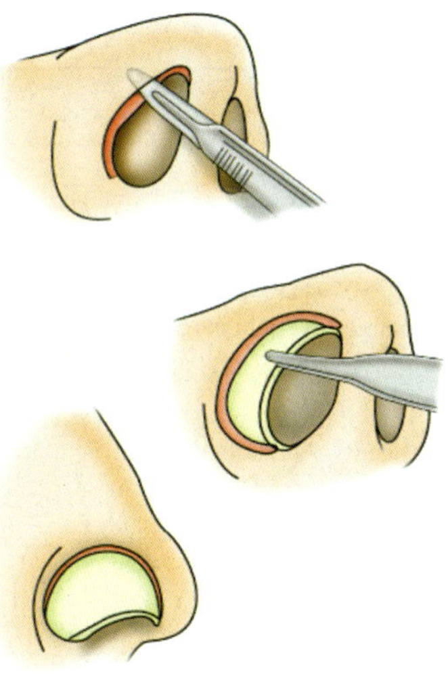

**Figure 6-18.** Bipedicle vestibular skin advancement flap. An intercartilaginous incision allows mucosal release and transposition to the alar margin.

ipsilateral septal flap can be based anteriorly off a narrow pedicle containing the septal branch of the superior labial artery to line defects of the lower vault (**Figure 6-19**).

Alternatively, the hinge flap can be based dorsally off the anterior and posterior ethmoid arteries to line the contralateral sidewall of the nose. The rectangular mucoperichondrial flap should always be designed larger than expected and cartilage grafts should be use to reestablish structure and contour. Good injection of the flap before incisions are made will limit bleeding and help with flap elevation in the subperichondrial plane.

For the ipsilateral flap, the two incisions should start 1 cm posterior to the caudal septal margin and can be extended beyond the bony cartilaginous junction. The inferior horizontal incision can be placed at the floor of the nose, whereas the dorsal incision should be placed 1 cm below the roof of the middle vault (**Figure 6-20A–F**). The exposed bone

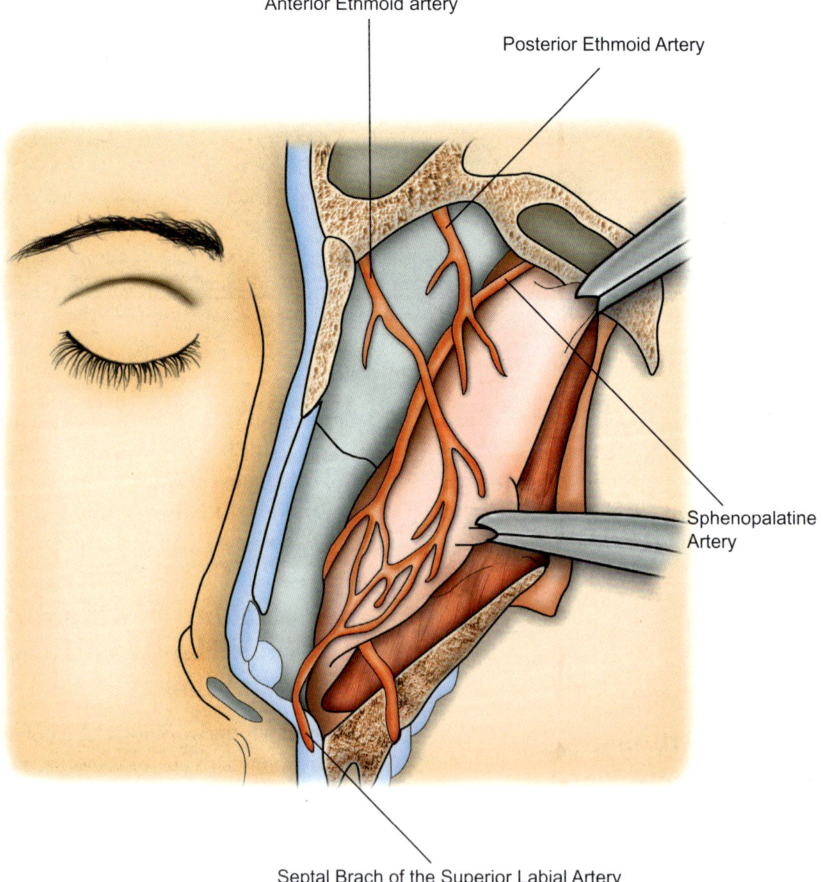


**Figure 6-19.** Blood supply to the septum. The anterioly based ipsilateral septal mucosal flap relies on a narrow pedicle supplied by the superior labial artery.

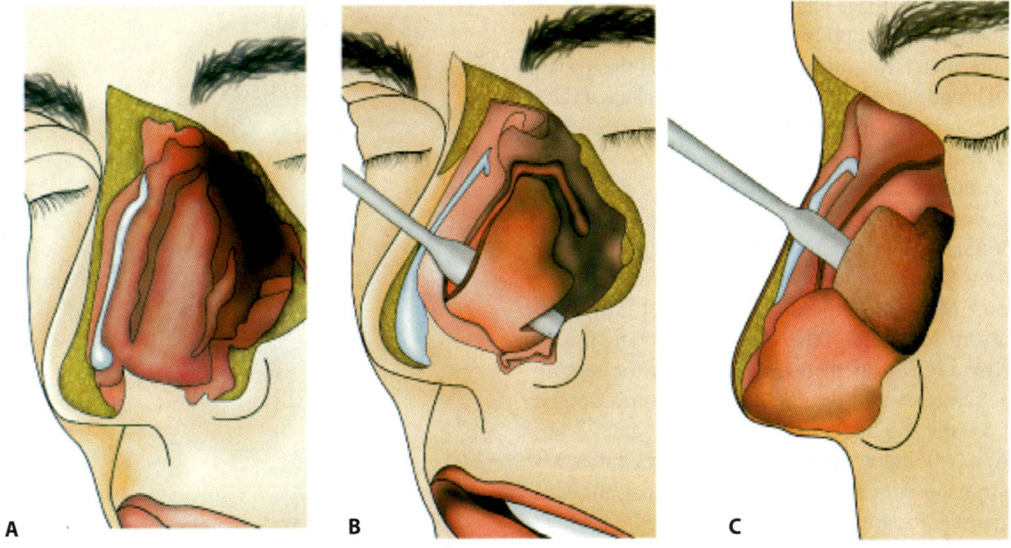


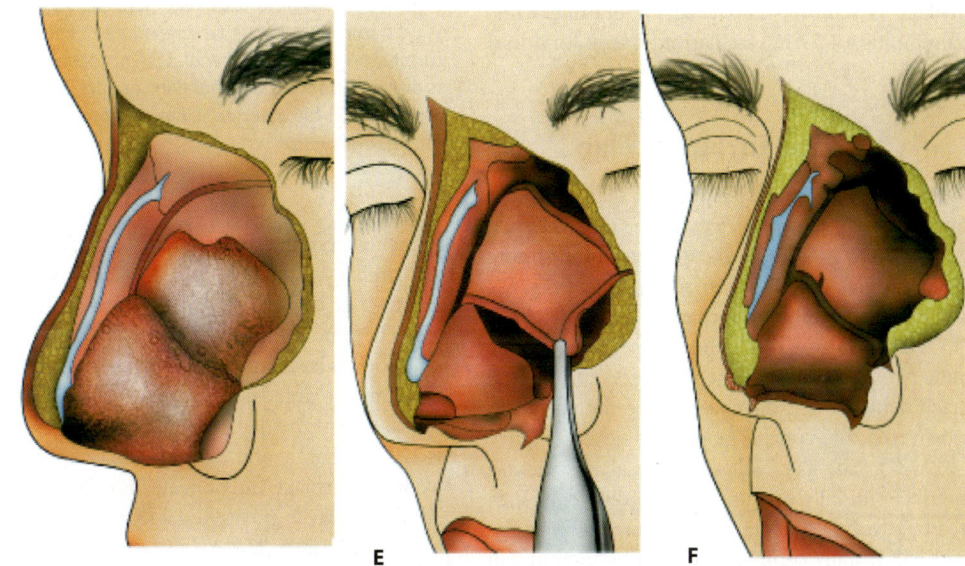


**Figure 6-20.** (A) Markings for the ipsilateral mucoperichondrial hinge flap. The dorsal septal incision is 1cm below the dorsal margin. The inferior incision is at the septal- nasal crest junction. (B) Flap is elevated in the subperichondrial plane. (C) The hinge flap based on the caudal mucoperichondrium is reflected laterally and the septal cartilage is freed from the contralateral muchoperichondrium. A 1.5 cm L-strut of septal cartilage is preserved. (D) The contralateral muchoperichondrium is intact and the septal cartilage has been removed for grafting. (E) The contralateral flap is incised and reflected laterally. (F) Both flaps are sutured in position.

and septal cartilage will remucosalize by secondary intention if the opposing mucoperichondrium remains intact. It is important to note that the ipsilateral hinge flap pedicle may cause internal nasal valve obstruction requiring flap division 3 weeks after reconstruction.

Similar surgical techniques are used to harvest the contralateral dorsally based septal mucoperichondrial hinge flap to line the middle vault of the nose. Anterior and posterior incisions are made from the floor of the nose to within 1 cm of the dorsum to maintain the septal L strut. The mucoperichondrium is then dissected from the septum and released at the floor. The flap is then transposed across the midline and secured in the desired position. A window in the septum may be necessary to transpose the flap if septal cartilage has not been harvested for grafting.

Bilateral hinge flaps based on the superior labial artery can be used to line total nasal tip defects. Each flap lines the hemitip structures, leaving behind a permanent septal perforation. The exposed cartilage is removed and used for grafting while maintaining a 1.5-cm vascularized L strut for dorsal support.

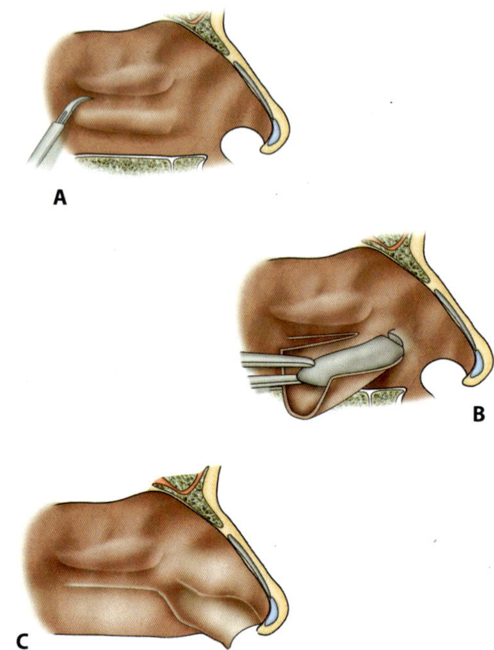


**Figure 6-21.** Inferior turbinate flap. (A) sickle knife is used to release boney attachments of the inferior turbinate from the nasal wall. (B) mucoperiosteum is disected from the conchal bone and the bone is removed. (C) the anterior pedicled flap is then used to line the entire ala.

## Inferior Turbinate Flap

The inferior turbinate is a highly vascular tissue that can be use to line small defects in the nose. The anteriorly based inferior turbinate is useful for lining ipsilateral alar defects when septal mucosa is not available or if multiple approaches are needed. The flap is developed with an anterior pedicle. A sickle knife is used to detach the posterior and central attachments of the turbinate. Once the turbinate is delivered, the conchal bone is removed (**Figure 6-21A–C**). The flap will cause nasal obstruction anteriorly initially because of a standing cone created by pivoting the flap 180 degrees. However, the graft will usually contract and the obstruction will resolve. If needed, the pedicle can be revised after 3 weeks. One of the benefits of the inferior turbinate flap is that it avoids septal perforation.

## Septal Composite Chondromucosal Pivotal Flap

Septal composite pivotal flaps can be use to repair bilateral defects of the nasal tip, columella, and dorsum. The composite flap is based on bilateral septal branches from the superior labial arteries. Incisions are similar to the ipsilateral septal mucosal flap, except they are carried out through all tissue layers. The amount of septum pivoted caudally and anteriorly is based on the size of the defect. The flap is useful for large tip defects. When used to repair dorsal defects the flap is pivoted 45 degrees (**Figure 6-22A, B**). For tip and columella defects, an anterior wedge of cartilage and bone needs to be removed to allow the flap to pivot 90 degrees for proper positioning (**Figure 6-23A–C**).

## Forehead Flap

The nasal lining can be restored by turning in a paramedian forehead flap. Two paramedian forehead flaps can be used to restore the lining and external coverage with cartilage grafts between them for structure. The pedicles of the flaps are usually divided in a staged manner 3 weeks apart from each other. Due to the bulk of these flaps, extensive

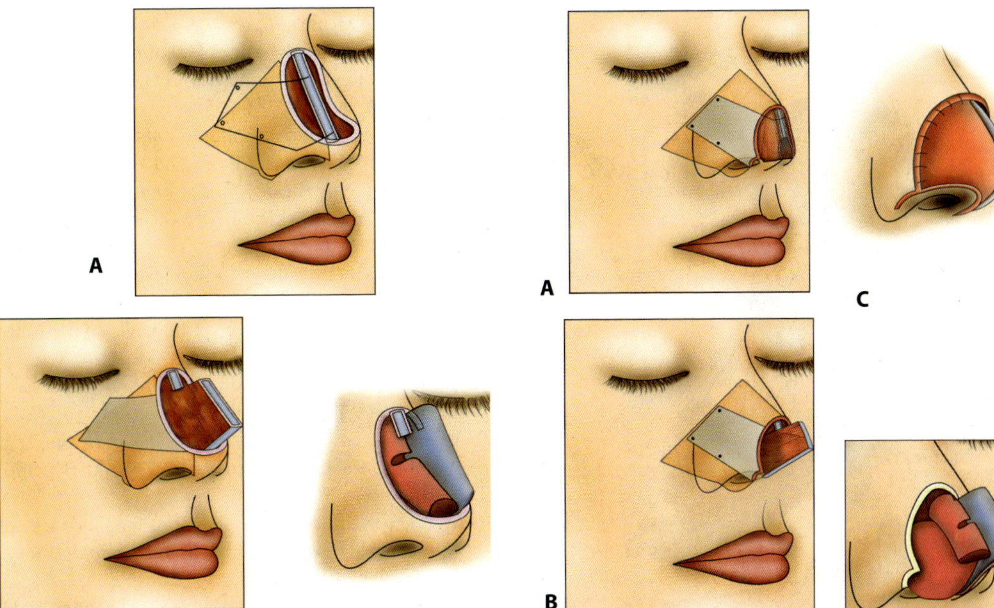


**Figure 6-22.** Septal composite chondromucosal pivotal flap for dorsal defects. (A) The broken line shows the full-thickness incisions made to create the composite flap. (B) The flap is pivoted 45 degrees to repair dorsal defects. After positioning, bilateral muchoperichondrial flaps are reflected laterally to line the nasal vault. The excess septal cartilage and bone are then trimmed.

**Figure 6-23.** Septal composite chondromucosal pivotal flap for tip and columella defects. (A) The broken line shows the full thickness incisions made to create the composite flap. Wedge of cartilage is removed (wedge not show) to allow the flap to be pivoted 90 degrees. (B) The flap is positioned and the mucoperichondrial flaps are reflected laterally to line the nasal tip. (C) Excess septal cartilage is trimmed and the mucoperichondrium is sutured to the border of the defect.

thinning is required to obtain a good result. Menik advocates for a three-stage double paramedian forehead flap for large three-layer defects. The surgical techniques are similar to the harvest described earlier in the chapter.

## Epithelial Turn-in Flap

Based on the principles of subunit reconstruction if greater than 50% of a subunit is involved, the entire subunit should be replaced. An alternative to disposing of this skin is to use it as a turn-in flap. The skin flap can be turned 180 degrees and a cutaneous flap (i.e., forehead flap) is then used to cover the entire external subunit defect after structural grafts are placed. A common use of this technique is for partial defects of the nasal sidewall (**Figure 6-24**).

## Summary

Nasal reconstruction requires careful attention to *skin* coverage, cartilaginous support and mucosal lining. The reconstruction of lining is a very challenging aspect of nasal reconstruction. Without adequate lining nasal reconstruction, efforts will fail as wound contracture continues. With an understanding of anatomy, the subunit principle, and the importance of replacing like tissues with like tissues, reconstructive results can be optimized.

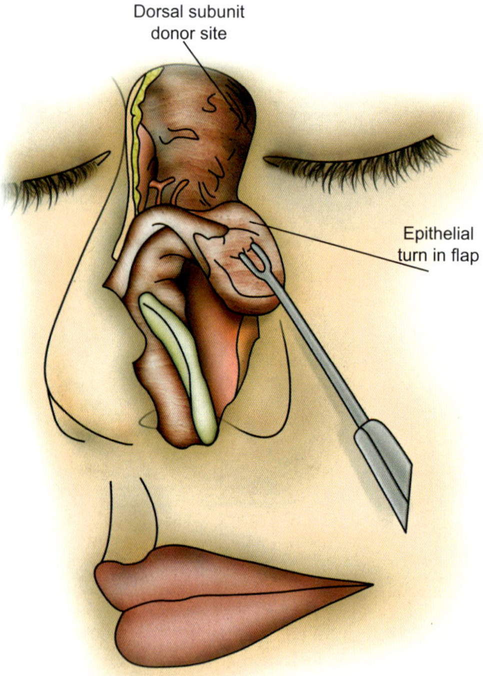


**Figure 6-24.** Partial repair of the nasal side wall using an epithelial turn in flap.

# References


1. Baker SR, Naficy S. *Principles of Nasal Reconstruction*, Mosby, St. Louis, 2002.
2. Branham GH, ed. Local skin flaps. *Facial Plast Clin N Am* 4(4), 1996.
3. Burget GC, Menick FJ. *Aesthetic Reconstruction of the Nose.* Mosby-Year Book Inc., St. Louis, 1994.
4. Jewett BS. Repair of small nasal defects. *Facial Plast Clin N Am* 13, 2005, 283–299.
5. Larrabee W, ed. *Surgical Anatomy of the Face*, 2nd ed. Lippincott Williams & Wilkins Philadelphia, 2004.
6. Papel ID, ed. *Facial Plastic and Reconstructive Surgery*, 2nd ed. Thieme Medical Publishers, Inc., New York, 2002.
7. Park SS, ed. Local cutaneous flaps. *Facial Plast Clin N Am* 13(2), 2005.
8. Skouge JW. *Skin Grafting.* Churchill Livingstone, New York, 1991.
9. Tardy, ME, ed. *Surgical Anatomy of the Nose.* Lippincott Williams & Wilkins Philadelphia, 1990.
10. Weerda H, ed. *Reconstructive Facial Plastic Surgery: A Problem-Solving Manual.* New York, Thieme, 2001.
11. Weisberg NK, Becker DS. Repair of nasal ala defects with conchal bowl composite grafts. *Dermatol. Surg.* 26(11), 2000, 1047–105
12. Cannady SB, Cook TA, Wax MK. The total nasal defect and reconstruction. *Facial Plast Surg Clin* N Am 2009;17, 189–201.
13. Taghiania AH, Pribaz JJ. Complex nasal reconstruction. *Plast Reconstr Surg* 2008;121, 15e–27e.
14. Burget GC, Menick FJ. Nasal support and lining: The marriage of beauty and blood supply. *Plast Reconstr Surg* 1989;84, 189–202.
15. Burget GC, Menick FJ. The subunit principle in nasal reconstruction. *Plast Reconstr Surg* 1985;76, 239–247.
16. Tollefson TT, Kriet DJ. Complex nasal defects: Structure and internal lining. *Facial Plast Surg Clin N Am* 2005;13, 333–343.
17. Menick FJ. The evolution of lining in nasal reconstruction. *Clin Plast Surg* 2009;36, 421–441.

7

# Lip and Perioral Reconstruction

Christina K. Magill, MD and Jill L. Hessler, MD

## Introduction

The lips are a focal point of the face during expression and communication. They also play a vital role in speech and eating. Composed of skin, muscle, and mucosa, the lips lack a rigid underlying ultrastructure, which confers both benefits and challenges for the reconstructive surgeon.

Historically, the reconstruction of the lip has been documented as early as 1000 B.C. in India, with modern techniques emerging from the work by Burrow in the early 1800s, by Dieffenback, Abbe, Sabattini, and Estlander in the later nineteenth century, and most recently by Karpandzic, Hari, and Ohmori in the last 40 years. The frequency of lip involvement from oral malignancies and trauma has mandated the continued evolution of reconstructive techniques.

The fundamental objective for lip reconstruction is the restoration of oral competence. Secondary objectives are the preservation of muscular continuity and sensation, maintainance of the optimal oral aperture circumference, and restoration of the appropriate upper and lower lip proportions. The cosmetic integrity of the lip is an overall goal of lip reconstruction and should be considered in all reconstructive efforts.

## Facial Analysis

The lips themselves are categorized by the tissue comprising them and are often referred to separately as the cutaneous, vermillion, or mucosal lips. There are three esthetic subunits of the upper lip. A central philtral subunit is placed between two lateral hexagonal subunits. The lower lip contains one subunit extending from the vermillion to the mental sulcus and to each oral commissure (**Figure 7-1**).

The upper cutaneous lip is bounded superiorly by the nasal sill and the columella, laterally by the nasolabial grooves, and inferiorly by the vermillion border. The cutaneous upper lip can be further divided into thirds. The philtrum is the middle subunit and appears concave to the middle upper lip by cresting laterally into philtral ridges that extend vertically and inferiorly to the vermillion lip, creating "Cupid's bow." The vermillion tubercle is located

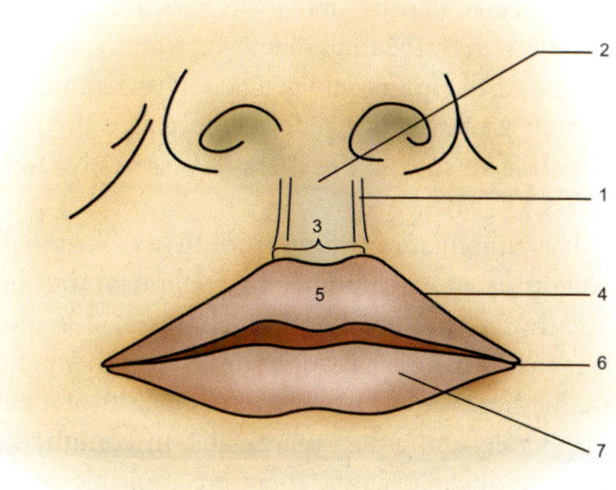


**Figure 7-1.** Topographic anatomy of the lips. 1, Philtral columns. 2, Philtral groove or dimple. 3, Cupid's bow. 4, White roll upper lip. 5, Tubercle. 6, Commissure. 7, Vermilion.

below the depth of the bow. For optimal aesthetic results, great care must be taken in realigning any defect of Cupid's bow, in addition to reapproximating the "white roll." The white roll is the perceptible circumferential outline of the mouth that is found at the cutaneous–vermillion lip junction. From the white roll, one can also imagine radial projections of relaxed skin tension lines that lie perpendicular to the underlying musculature of the orbicularis oris

The modioli are found at the corners of the mouth, and mark the insertion point of lip musculature. The oral commissures demarcate the terminal taper of the vermillion lips and mark the lateral borders of the upper and lower lips. The lower cutaneous lip facial subunit is bounded superiorly by the vermillion lower lip, laterally by the extension of the nasolabial creases, and inferiorly by the mentolabial sulcus. The lower cutaneous lip can be viewed as one subunit and can be reconstructed as such.

The smooth, hairless, stratified squamous epithelium of the vermillion lip is the cosmetic focal point of the mouth, and although there are minor salivary glands on the lip's mucosal surface, the vermillion is devoid of any salivary or eccrine glands. The vermillion lip epithelium is grooved with long vertical dermal papillae carrying a rich network of sensory fibers and capillaries. The dense vascularity and sensory fiber population of the lips are responsible for its red color and discriminate sensitivity. The "red line" is created by the vermillion-mucosal border. When the lips are closed, the upper and lower vermillions come together at the red line junction.

Histologically, the cutaneous lip is composed of epidermis, dermis, and scant subcutaneous tissue, followed by the muscular layer, submucosa, and mucosa of the muscosal lip. These layers should be carefully assessed for lip defects to gauge the need for partial versus full thickness reconstructive techniques.

The musculature of the mouth was originally thought to act with sphincterlike elliptical motions to compress the lip margins. However, it is now clear that the obicularis oris muscle has independent quadrants, and each quadrant consists of a pars peripheralis and a pars marginalis. In conjunction with the obicularis oris, there are multiple paired muscles that create subtle movements of the lips. Superiorly, the zygomaticus major and minor, the levator labii superioris, and the levator labii superioris alaque nasi act as superior tractors. The risorius muscle acts to laterally retract the edges of the mouth, and the depressor labii inferioris and the platysma pars labialis act as inferior tractors. The mentalis muscles are elevators of the lower lip and are mainly responsible for oral competence.

Innervation of the described musculature derives from the buccal, marginal, and cervical branches of the facial nerve. Sensation of the upper lip is provided by the infraorbital nerve and the mental nerve supplies sensation to the lower lip. The facial artery provides the blood supply to the mouth via superior and inferior labial arteries that course between the intraoral mucosa and the orbicularis oris muscle.

## Special Preoperative Considerations

Defects of the lips need to be considered in terms of location, size, and thickness. Primary closures, advancements, and local flap techniques can be determined based on the goals of providing tension-free closure, preserving or restoring oral competence, and maintaining the integrity of the layers of the lip. If patients present with hypesthesia of the upper or lower lip, then imaging may be warranted to evaluate integrity of the infraorbital or mental nerve. Individual patient factors must also be considered when planning a repair. An elderly patient with loose skin can tolerate removal of significantly more tissue than a young person with taut tissues. Similarly, local flaps on a male patient must take into consideration the direction of facial hair growth.

When possible, lip defects should be repaired with tissue within the lip complex for maintenance of oral competence. When this will create significant microstomia, adjacent cheek and chin tissue can be used. Realignment of the vermillion border is paramount to a favorable cosmetic result. A step-off of 1 mm in the vermillion can be recognized at a conversational distance. The vermillion and white roll should be marked prior to reconstruction, as the injection of local anesthetic often distorts the white roll and vermillion border. Techniques to accomplish this include using pinpoint methylene blue or circumventing local infiltration by doing a mental and infraorbital nerve block. Particular attention must also be paid to reapproximate the orbicularis if this muscle is resected. If muscle fibers, particularly those near the free border of the lip, are not meticulously repaired, notching can occur.

Relaxed skin tension lines can also be marked prior to anesthetic infiltration. Facial hair should be trimmed to avoid infection and interference with suture placement. The direction of hair growth in men should also be taken into consideration for flap design.

## Oral/Perioral Defect Analysis

In general, oral and perioral defects can be classified by their location and depth. In general, superficial defects are repaired based on their location and the subunit principles of reconstruction. Full thickness defects are repaired based on the size of the lesion. The approach to each defect must be individualized but mandates a working knowledge of reconstructive techniques and flaps.

## Choice of Reconstructive Technique

### Secondary Intention

As in all reconstructive situations, one must consider healing by secondary intention. This method is best used for small lesions near the alar base or remote from the free margin of the lip. Due to the lack of an underlying rigid framework, lesions near the free border can cause significant retraction and deformity if left to heal by this method.

### Primary Repair

Primary repair is frequently the optimal reconstructive method particularly for defects occupying less than 30% of the long axis of the lip. Incisions should be located in relaxed skin tension lines; Burrow's triangles can extend onto the vermillion if it is necessary to remove bulk from this area. Contour of the vermillion can also be maintained by excising underlying muscle to prevent bulging. A conventional Z-plasty may be performed to lengthen a scar or reduce tension on a repair.

When a Mohs resection is not performed, a full thickness wedge resection repaired with primary closure is good for small, deep lesions. A V-shaped or triangular incision is made around the defect, with the base of the V aligned with the vermillion border and the 30-degree apex of the triangle extending into the cutaneous lip. Variations of this excision include pentagonal or shield incisions, and an M-plasty can also be added to the apex of the wedge excision to avoid extending the incision into an adjacent cosmetic subunit.

Primary closure of lower lip lesions can be done with a cosmetically favorable result, barring extension of the excision outside of the lower lip cosmetic subunit. Incisions that traverse the mentolabial crease may necessitate alternate techniques for closure. Additionally, if a lateral lip lesion is excised where the vermillion lip tapers, primary repair is difficult secondary to vermillion lip width discrepancy. This problem can be corrected by excising a Burrow's triangle from the medial side of the vermillion wound. Alternatively, a diagonal incision can be designed to facilitate maximal surface area and reposition the cut vermillion edges, leaving a maximal vermillion lip at the lateral edge.

Suture choice in primary lip reconstruction is based on layered closure. A small-caliber 5-0 or 6-0 suture should be used. The mucosa is closed with an absorbable suture, such as chromic or Vicryl. The muscle layer is closed with an absorbable suture, such as Vicryl, or a longer-lasting braided polyglycolic acid, or polydioxanon (PDS). Careful attention to the closure of the oribularis oris facilitates not only a functional sphincter mechanism but also an optimal cosmetic repair. The vermillion-cutaneous lip junction should be meticulously reapproximated with an epidermal vertical mattress suture for proper wound eversion. If minimal tension occurs, the dermis and subcutaneous tissues are then closed with a low reactivity absorbable suture such as Monocryl. Finally, a 5-0 or 6-0 Prolene suture is used to close the cutaneous lip with eversion of wound edges to minimize visible scarring.

## Defect considerations

### Partial-Thickness Defects of the Upper Lip

Basal cell carcinoma accounts for most lesions of the upper lip and is usually limited to the perioral skin without involvement of the red lip or vermillion. As this area of the face has limited skin redundancy and sparse subcutaneous tissue, advancement flaps are frequently needed in this area. These flaps bestow the advantages of facial hair confluence and minimize distortion of the vermillion border. Tissue can be mobilized from the lateral lip or from the cheek. Other techniques involve tissue rotation and transposition.

Unilateral advancement flaps can be used on the upper lip if a defect is in one of the lateral subunits and does not involve the medial philtrum. Incisions can be designed to hide within the vermillion border, along the nasal sill, and in the melolabial crease. Maximal mobility must be obtained from the lateral tissue to avoid displacement of the philtrum once the wound is closed. A Burrow's wedge advancement flap is a simple and effective technique to use in this area. Cosmetically, incisions should not disrupt other aesthetic units of the face.

Bilateral advancement flaps can also be employed and are most appropriate for medium-sized defects of the lip. This technique is often used to repair medial upper lip defects, in which lateral symmetry is necessary, or in larger lower lip defects. Incisions can be similarly hidden along the vermillion border, nasal sill, alar crease, and the melolabial fold or hidden in the mental crease for lower lip reconstruction. When lesions occur in the middle of the lateral subunit an O-to-T type flap can be designed with incision lines along the relaxed skin tension lines of the mouth and the vermillion border. Alternately, for partial-thickness defects in the philtrum, closure may be performed by full thickness skin grafts harvested from the periauricular or supraclavicular region and inset into the wound.

To recruit additional tissue and camouflage incisions, an advancement flap can be designed using the contours of the nose, as in the perialar advancement flap (**Figure 7-2**). This technique can be used unilaterally or bilaterally.

Advancement flaps for lateral upper lip reconstruction can also be done using an island pedicle technique. Incisions are made inferior to the defect along the vermillion border and the melolabial fold, and the tissue to be advanced is undermined along its edges. The subcutaneous tissue remains attached centrally to act as a pedicled blood supply that can be advanced into the wound. This technique often risks flap "pincushioning," which may be avoided with minimal undermining leaving a wide subcutaneous pedicle for lymphatic drainage.

Rotational flaps can be used to repair lateral defects in the upper cutaneous lip. The melolabial crease provides a guide for incisions and rotational arc. Standing cones resulting from the use of these flaps can be addressed with excisions along relaxed skin tension lines or by making a back cut along the nasolabial groove. Care must be taken not to distort the vermillion border when these flaps, especially

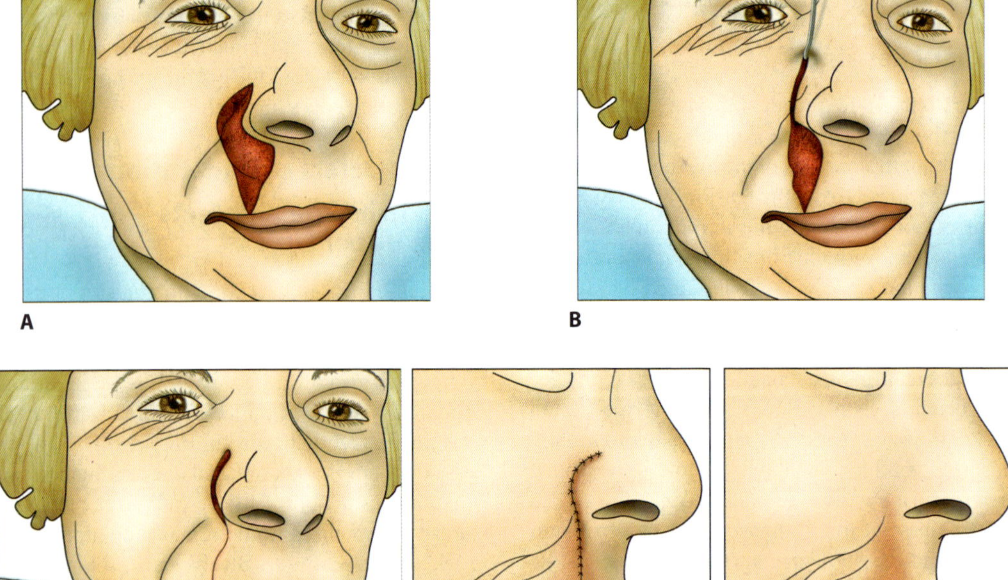


**Figure 7-2.** The final wound defect after excision of the inferior Burow's triangle and superior perialar crescent (A); the first and the key subcutaneous suture to anchor an advance the cheek to the alar crease (B); approximation of the entire would edge with subcutaneous sutures only (C); final wound closure (D); wound appearance at 10 days postoperation (E).

flaps based near the oral commissure. For larger defects in the lateral subunits, the entire subunit should be excised and reconstructed. Potential techniques include an inferiorly based melolabial flap, which may provide coverage of the entire upper lip if there is adequate cheek laxity. The inferior base is preferred to maintain a melolabial crease and to allow lymphatic drainage to minimize flap edema and trap-door deformtiy.

Transpositional flaps for upper lip reconstruction are often based off the melolabial crease and can have a superior or inferior pedicle. This technique transfers stationary tissue into a defect and can alter the tension forces in the anatomic area being reconstructed. Melolabial transposition flaps **(Figure 7-3)** provide an excellent reconstructive option when tension negates a primary closure of a lip defect. This axial flap is based on the facial artery nasolabial branch and is pedicled just superior to the defect. The flap should be elevated above the orbicularis oris muscle and can be inset in a single stage. It is important to inform the patient that this flap has the tendency to swell in the early postoperative period and will initially disrupt the achieved cosmetic results.

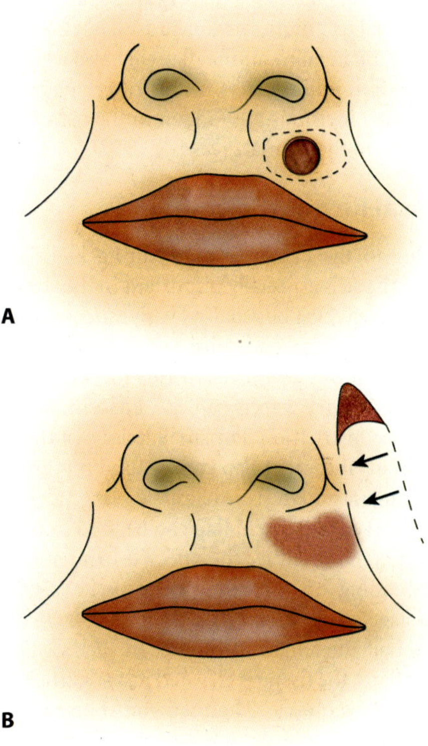


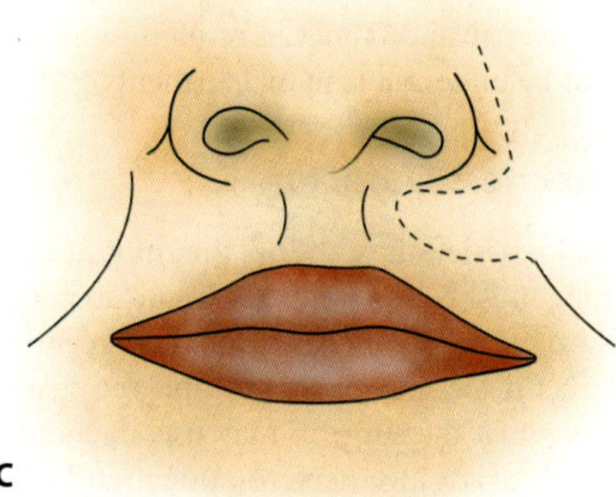


**Figure 7-3.** Melolabial flap for lip reconstruction. Original defect in cutaneous upper lip (A). Defect after resection and planned inferiorly based melolabial flap (B). Final incision and scar lines (C).

## Partial Thickness Defects of the Lower Lip

Superficial defects in the lower lip commonly result from leukoplakia and actinic cheilitis, conditions that can both be associated with squamous cell carcinomas. Given the risk of neoplastic disease associated with these processes, lip shave or excision of the affected vermillion and mucosa are usually done. As in all partial thickness lesions, the primary concern is cosmesis, as function in these defects is usually maintained via intact musculature and sensation.

A partial thickness defect of the lower lip can be closed primarily or with local flaps. Horizontal advancement flaps may be used, similar to the upperlip, with common adjuncts including A–T flaps, in which the base of the A lies along the vermillion. Incisions are created along the vermillion border and once closed the suture line resembles an inverted T. Bilateral advancement flaps can be used for superficial defects. Triangle excisions may be necessary along the labiomental crease in order to achieve tension-free closure.

When lesions involve 50–80% of the lower lip, full thickness excisions including muscle and mucosa often provide the best cosmetic repair. Significant redundancy of the lower lip allows a large amount of lip to be resected without significant cosmetic deformity, microstomia, or functional impairment. Incisions are made in the vermillion border and extend deep through the muscle and mucosa. The laterally based muscle and mucosal flaps are then meticulously repaired to reapproximate both layers.

The remaining cutaneous defects are repaired with conventional techniques as previously mentioned.

O-to-Z bilateral rotational flaps are also a reconstructive option for defects in the lower cutaneous lip, in which incisions are hidden in the vermillion border and in the mental crease.

## Mucosal Restoration

Adhering to the principle of repairing like tissue with like tissue is especially important in the vermillion. This area must be repaired with mucosal tissue to avoid an obvious deformity. Small defects can be repaired with buccal mucosa from the immediate vicinity and larger defects can use adjacent lip mucosa for reconstruction. For small lesions of the lip, a V-to-Y advancement flap can be used mobilizing buccal mucosa into the vermillion. For larger defects, a bipedicled advancement flap can be used from the buccal mucosa of either the affected or unaffected lip, depending on the amount of tissue needed. A two-stage cross lip flap is used for defects encompassing half the length of the lip. In each of these mucosa flaps, the tissue is elevated just superficial to the orbicularis muscle. The tissue must be handled quite carefully to prevent tearing and trauma to the delicate mucosa. Patients must be warned there is a color difference between buccal mucosa and vermillion. Also, overadvancement can result in a fuller lip, which may be undesirable in male patients.

## Full Thickness Defects

In full thickness defects of the lip, the amount of tissue missing must be assessed. Defects involving less than a third of the lip can usually be closed primarily. For larger defects, there are multiple reconstructive options that the surgeon may use, including a combination of advancement, rotational, and transpositional flaps, or, in more severe cases, a composite tissue transfer or free flap.

Familiarizing oneself with different options as well as to the strengths and weaknesses of the flaps is critical to restoring function as well as cosmesis. These flaps are further discussed below, but briefly: the Karpandzic flap manipulates tissues in a way that preserves function, the Abbe flap aims to match tissue components between the unaffected and affected lip, and the Estlander and Gilles fan flaps move tissues, including the modiolus and commissure, from their normal location to the defect. The Karpandzic and Estlander flaps are sliding flaps that are very useful in reconstructing the lower lip.

### *Karpandzic Flap*

The Karpandzic flap was first described in 1974 and is commonly employed to repair large central full thickness defects of the lower lip, with the primary goal of maintaining oral function (**Figure 7-4**). Advantages of the flap include a functional oral sphincter and a sensate lip. The flap involves making bilateral incisions in the nasolabial grooves, and then incising inferiorly in the mental crease. The flap should have uniform width along the entire length of the flap. After the skin is incised, the nerves and blood vessels are bluntly dissected from the surrounding facial musculature to allow greater mobility of the flap without the necessity of transecting these structures. Mucosal cuts are then made separately. Each of the three layers is closed individually.

Disadvantages of the Karapanzic flap include narrowing of the oral aperture, increased scar visibility, and blunting of the oral commissure. Caution should be used in who wear dentures due to the microstomia that can result from large

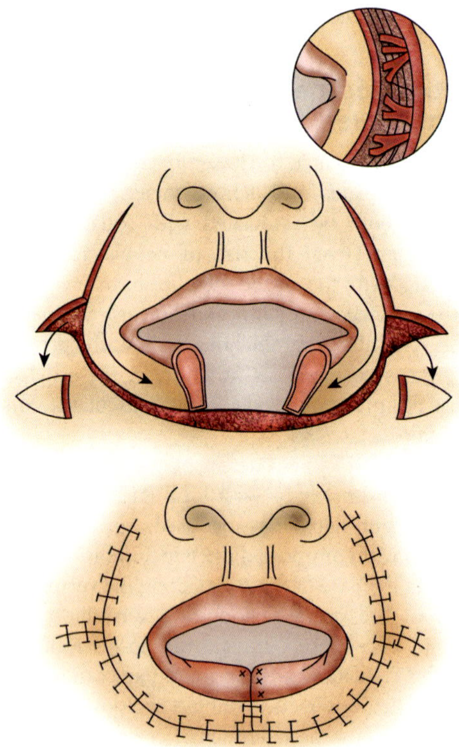

**Figure 7-4.** Bilateral Karapandzic flaps for closure of a large lower-lip defect. The Karapandzic techniques preserves the nerves to the osbicularis muscle.

defects. Lip-stretching devices are available to lessen the restriction and widen the oral aperture.

## *Lip-Switch Flaps (Abbe and Estlander)*

Full thickness defects involving one to two thirds of the lip are often repaired with a pedicled flap from the unaffected upper or lower lip and are referred to as "lip-switch" flaps (**Figure 7-5**). Lip-switch flaps are full thickness tissue transfers that transpose vermillion, muscle, mucosa, and cutaneous lip with the pedicle of the flap containing a blood supply from the labial artery.

The lip-switch flap was first described in 1989 by Dr. Robert Abbe, who desired a reconstructive tool for bilateral cleft lip deformities that would provide a complete philtrum. The original intention of the flap has been liberalized and has been successfully used in both lower and upper lip reconstruction. The Abbe flap is a two-stage procedure, with the first stage involving a pedicled full thickness finger-like flap of tissue being excised from the unaffected lip and then rotated 180 degrees to be set into the defect. The pedicle is then divided after 3 weeks, allowing for inosculation of the transferred tissue. The Abbe flap allows for the replacement of all three tissue layers and also results in shortening of the donor lip that cosmetically improves balance with the recipient lip. An advantage of this flap is that the oral commissure is left intact and is not

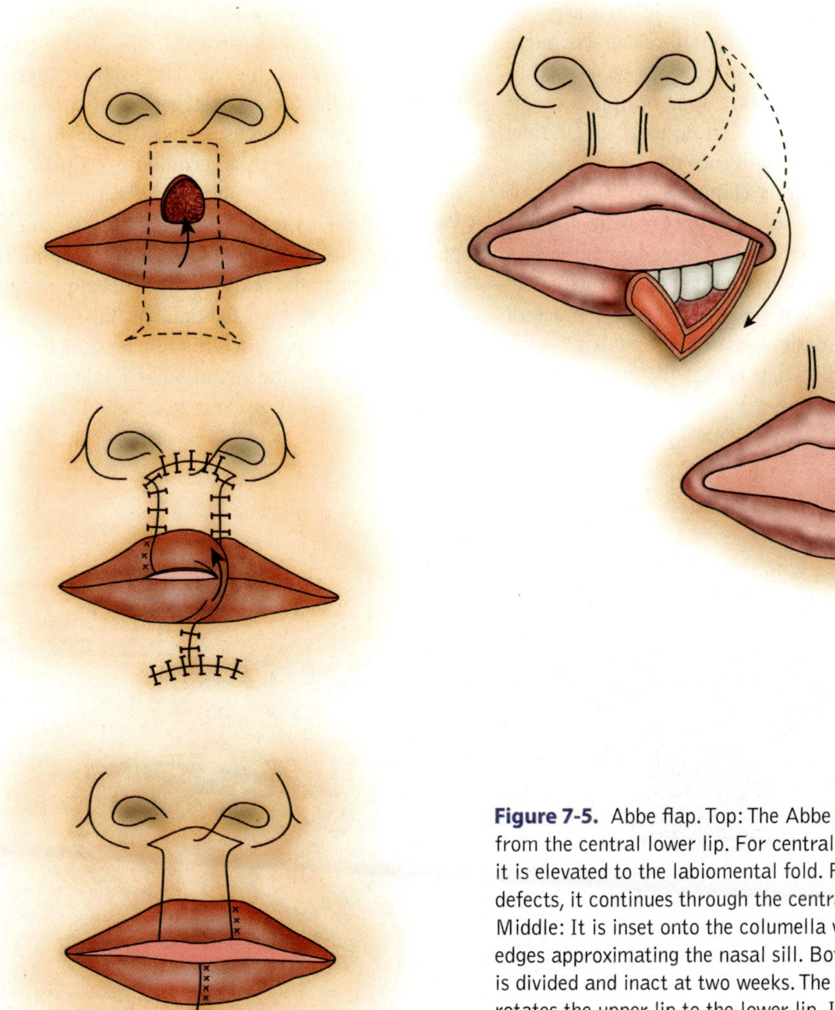

**Figure 7-5.** Abbe flap. Top: The Abbe flap is elevated from the central lower lip. For central upper defects, it is elevated to the labiomental fold. For lateral defects, it continues through the central chin pad. Middle: It is inset onto the columella with lateral edges approximating the nasal sill. Bottom: The flap is divided and inact at two weeks. The Estlander flap rotates the upper lip to the lower lip. It results in a round commissure and loss of the normal taper of the vermilion.

manipulated. However, the transferred lip-switch flap does not retain muscle function, and sensation is decreased.

Unlike the Abbe flap, the Estlander flap is designed as a one-stage technique that is used to reconstruct full thickness lateral lip defects. The resulting rounded neo-oral commissure, however, may require a secondary commissuroplasty. The Estlander flap transfers the lateral upper lip to the lower lip around the oral commissure, resulting in distortion of the vermillion and displacement of the oral commissure.

### *Gilles Fan Flap*

For defects that create a tissue loss of greater than two thirds of the lower lip, local full thickness reconstructive options are limited, and the Karpandzic flap has largely replaced the Gilles flap. For these large defects, adjacent tissue needs to be rotated to obtain a tension-free closure. One option is to use the Gilles fan flap, which can be used unilaterally or bilaterally, and circumvents the reconstructive sequelae of microstomia (**Figure 7-6**). These flaps involve the rotation of full thickness melolabial tissue into the defect and are closed in three layers. The harvest incision is hidden in the melolabial crease. Vermillion can be restored using mucosal advancement flaps or a ventral tongue flap. One disadvantage of this flap is that the rotated tissue does not allow for native oral sphincter competence or sensation.

## Total and Near-Total Lip Reconstruction

Some lip defects are so large that they cannot be reconstructed by manipulating remaining lip tissue. If a defect involves more than 40% of the total lip area, or more than 80% of either lip, any local reconstructive technique will result in undesirable microstomia, and a new lip structure must be created. Reconstructive options include the Webster modification of the Bernard–Burrow flap (Webster–Bernard flap), the McGregor flap, or the Nakajima flap. Free flap tissue transfer can be done as well with tissue from the radial forearm. Reconstruction should aim to recreate the lip subunits using nonlip tissue (cheek or forearm). Optimal functional recovery is rarely achieved. The Webster–Bernard flap has use in the reconstruction of a complete lower lip defect, and uses cheek tissue to reconstruct the defect, with a vermillion reconstruction done with bipedicled mucosal sliding flaps. In the Webster–Bernard technique, bilateral incisions are placed in the melolabial folds, with the incision angled lateral to the oral commissure before angling medially at the level of the oral commissure. A second arc-shaped incision is made extending from the mental crease to the mandibular angle bilaterally

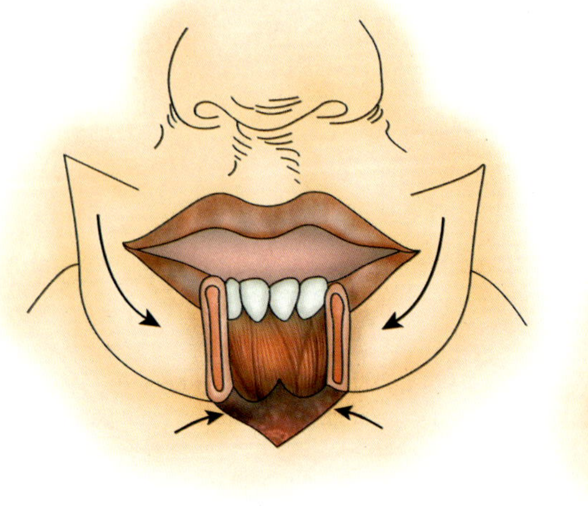

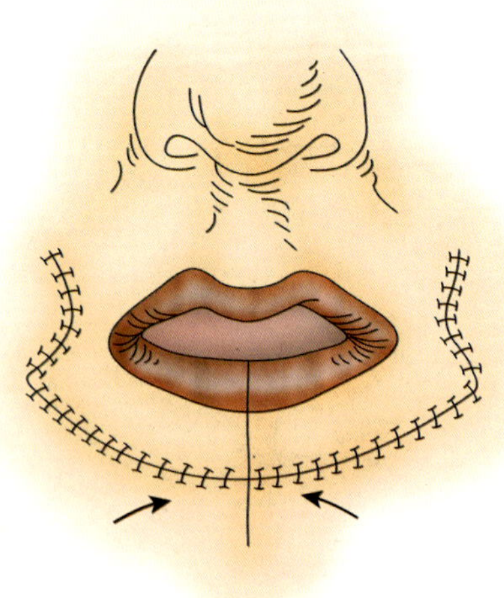

**Figure 7-6.** Gilles fan flap.

and chin and cheek tissues are advanced medially to create a lower lip contour.

## Postoperative Care

Patients should be advised to minimize movement or manipulations of the operative area. Although this is difficult, this means no talking, minimal facial expression, and avoidance of excessive mouth movement.

Oral intake following lip reconstruction is especially challenging, and patients should be instructed to take in only liquids and soft foods for 2–4 days after surgery without using straws.

## Complications

Lip defects from a neoplastic process should not be closed or manipulated until margins are assessed and no active histologic disease is present. Undermining or flap rotations may translocate neoplastic cells if this precaution is not taken. If previous operations have occurred on the lip, the integrity of the labial arteries should be assessed prior to any use of pedicled flaps. Microstomia may result from lip reconstruction and may require surgical revision or lip stretching. Surgical sites are prone to hematoma formation as a result of the rich vascularity in the region and the dynamic nature of the lip tissues. For this reason, surgeons must be vigilant about intraoperative hemostasis.

Antibiotic administration after lip surgery minimizes infection risk from proximity to the oral cavity.

Scar depression can be minimized with proper wound eversion. Hypertrophic scar formation may occur. Distributing tension along the entire wound and not just the distal aspect of the flap will help to minimize scar widening. Patients are also at risk for "pincushioning" particuarly in superior-based flaps with narrow pedicles. Both of these phenomena can be treated with intralesional steroids or surgical revision.

## References


1. Abbe R. A new plastic operation for the relief of deformity due to double hairlip. *Med Record* 1898; 53: 447.
2. Baker SR, Krause CJ. Pedicle flaps in reconstrucion of the lip. *Facial Plast Surg N Am* 1984 Fall, 1(1), 61–68.
3. Boutros, S. Reconstruction of the lips. In Thorne CH, Bartlett SP, Beasley RW, Aston SJ, Gurtner GS, Spear SL, eds. *Grabb and Smith's Plastic Surgery*, 6th ed., Lippincott, Williams and Wilkins, Philadelphia, 2006.
4. Burow CA. Berscheisung einer neuen transplantations methode zum wedersatz. Verlorengeaganener Teile des Gesichts Berlin: Nauck, 1855.
5. Calhoun KH. Reconstruction of small- and medium-sized defects of the lower lip. *Am J Otolaryngol* 1992 Jan-Feb, 13(1), 16–22.
6. Ducic Y, Athre R, Cochran CS. The split orbicularis myomucosal flap for lower lip reconstruction. *Arch Facial Plast Surg* 2005 Sep-Oct, 7(5), 347–352.
7. Estlander JA: Eine methode aus er einen ippe substanzverluste der anderen zu ersetzein. *Arch Klin Chir* 1872, 14, 622.
8. Gillies HD, Millard DR: *The Principles and Art of Plastic Surgery*. Boston: Little, Brown, 1957.
9. Karapandzic M. Reconstruction of lip defects by local arterial flaps. *Br J Plast Surg* 1974, Jan. 27(1), 93–97.
10. Larrabee WF, Sherris DA. *Principles of Facial Reconstruction*. Lippincott-Raven, Philadelphia, 1995.
11. Panje WR. Lip reconstruction. *Otolaryngol Clin N Am* 1982 Feb, 15(1), 169–178.
12. Webster JP. Crescentic peri-alar cheek excision for upper lip flap advancement with a short history of upper lip repair. *Plast Reconstr Surg* 1955 Dec; 16(6): 434–64.
13. Zide B. Deformities of the lips and cheeks. In McCarthy JG, ed. *Plastic Surgery*. Vol 3.WB Saunders, Philadelphia, 1990.
14. Zitelli JA, Brodland DG. A regional approach to reconstruction of the upper lip. *J Dermatol Surg Oncol* 1991 Feb, 17(2), 143–148.

# 8

# Forehead and Brow Reconstruction

Gregory H. Branham, MD, FACS

## Introduction

In this chapter, we discuss the anatomy of the forehead and available reconstructive options. We focus on the most common and best approaches for reconstruction of this region, which encompasses the glabella, forehead, brow and temporal region lateral to the orbital rim. Reconstruction of the forehead presents challenges that are very different than that of a midline three-dimensional structure such as the nose. The broad expanse of tissue of the forehead can be a challenge for hiding incisions, particularly in the younger patient who has not yet developed forehead rhytids. Similarly, a unilateral defect poses challenges for maintaining symmetry of the brows and forehead. Any difference in the height of the brows is readily apparent and must be considered when planning reconstruction in this region.

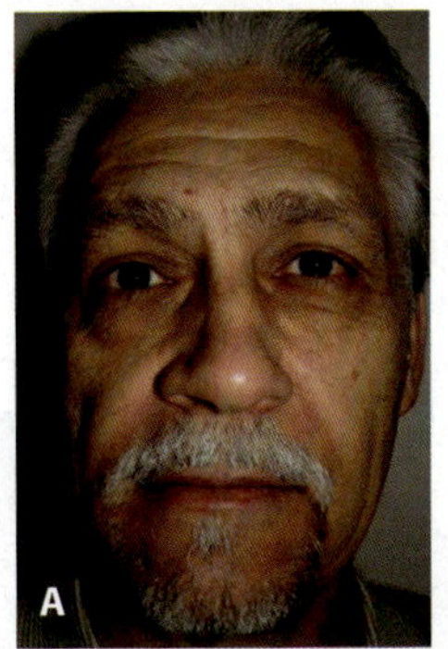


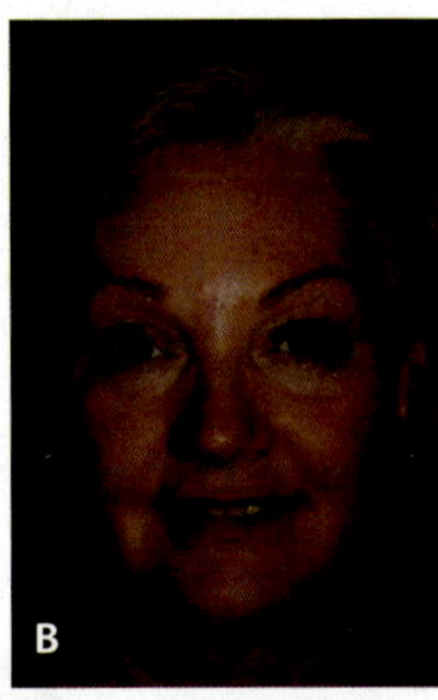


**Figure 8-1.** Topographic anatomy of the forehead and brows in males and females. (A) The male brow is typically more horizontal and fuller. It lies at the bony orbital rim. (B) The female brow is arched at the latter one third of the brow. It is less full and normally lies above the orbital rim.

## Anatomy

The topographic anatomy of the brow and forehead differs in males and females. In males, the brows tend to be thicker, fuller, and rest at the level of the bony orbital rim in what is essentially a horizontal plane. In the female, the brow is thinner and rests above the bony orbital rim with a significant arch that peaks at the level of the lateral limbus or lateral third of the brow. These differences must be considered when planning reconstruction (**Figure 8-1A,B**).

The relaxed skin tension lines (RSTLs) in the forehead run in a horizontal plane, perpendicular to the frontalis muscle, a large sheet of muscle that spans the majority of the forehead (**Figure 8-2**). The relaxed skin tension lines of the temporal region are oriented radially and emanate from the lateral canthus toward the temporal tuft of hair. In the glabellar region above the rhinion, the relaxed skin tension lines are vertically oriented and are created by the action of the paired corrugator supercillii muscles that run nearly horizontally underneath the brow hair. The procerus muscle creates horizontally oriented relaxed skin tension lines at the junction of the glabella and nasion (**Figure 8-3**).

The hairline offers another opportunity to hide incisions and should be kept in mind when planning flaps in this region. It should also be noted

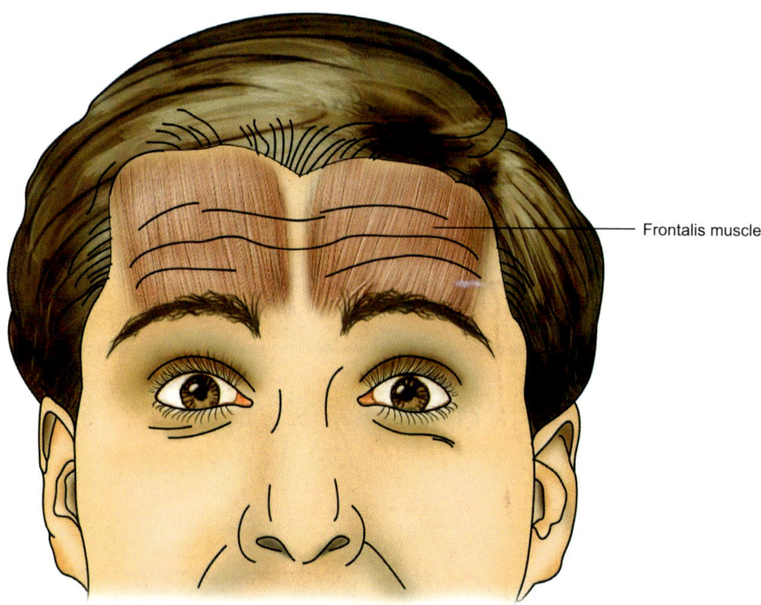


**Figure 8-2.** Frontalis muscle. The frontalis muscle lies within the galea aponeurotic and is a sheetlike muscle that spans from the hairline at the superior forehead to the brows inferiorly. It is divided in the midline to a variable degree and extends laterally to the level of the lateral palpebral fissure; however, this can also be quite variable. It is responsible for horizontally oriented forehead furrows.

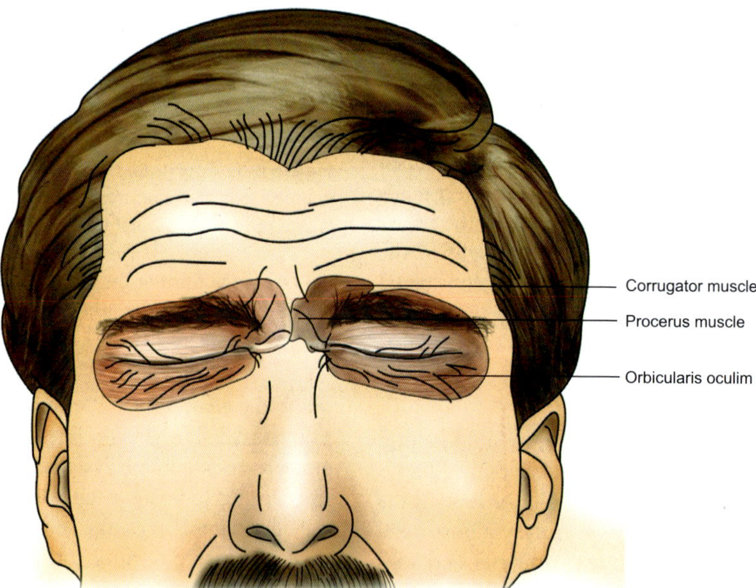


**Figure 8-3.** Corrugator, Procerus, and Orbicularis muscles. The Corrugator muscles are paired muscles that are obliquely oriented and arise from the glabellar area and insert into the medial end of the brow in the dermis. They are responsible for the vertical lines in the glabellar region. The Procerus muscle runs vertically in the glabellar region and is responsible for the horizontal lines found in the nasion. The Orbicularis Oculi muscles surround the eye like a sphincter, and the lines formed by their contraction are radially oriented lines commonly known as "Crow's feet."

that there is significant variability in the position of the hairline between individuals with some having relatively short or narrow foreheads with low hairlines and others with a relatively high hairline. In all males, the hairline changes over time, and this varies from mild temporal recession to complete baldness of the vertex of the scalp. In males, whenever possible, incisions should be placed as high above the hairline as possible to accommodate for future hair loss.

In the forehead and temporal region, the soft tissues are comprised of skin, subcutaneous tissue, fat, gala aponeurotica, loose connective tissue, and periosteum adjacent to the bone. It is the loose connective tissue layer that allows the skin to slide over the skull as the muscles contract. The pericranium adheres tightly to the underlying skull.

The frontalis muscle is contained within the gala aponeurotica. It originates in the galea and inserts into the skin of the forehead, often interdigitating with the corrugator muscles inferiorly. The frontalis muscle is often divided in the midline and can extend as far laterally as the lateral brow or the anterior temporal line.

The temporalis muscle originates in a fanlike fashion over the squamous portion of the temporal bone. The temporalis fascia at its origin is fused with the periosteum creating the conjoined fascia. The location of the conjoined fascia can be determined by having the patient clinch the jaws together to contract the temporalis muscle. It is this anterior temporal line that delineates the temporal region from the forehead.

When elevating forehead and brow tissues for cosmetic or reconstructive purposes, the surgeon must divide the conjoined fascia to adequately mobilize the lateral tissues of the forehead. Similarly, it is critical to release the periosteal attachments of the brow at the superior orbital rim (arcus marginalis) in order to lift the brow adequately (**Figure 8-4**).

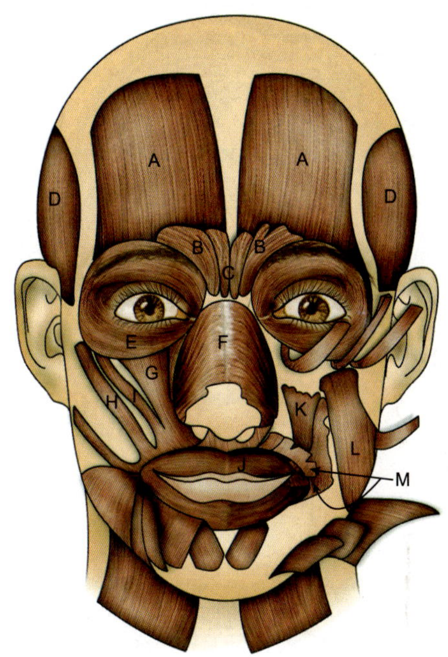


**Figure 8-4.** The facial musculature.

## Vascular Supply

The forehead is supplied by the supraorbital and supratrochlear vessels, which are both terminal branches of the ophthalmic artery, a branch of the internal carotid artery. The supratrochlear artery is located at the medial end of the brow and traverses vertically up the central forehead supplying this region. The supraorbital artery typically arises from the supraorbital notch approximately 1 cm lateral to the supratrochlear artery. In approximately 25% of the time, the notch is a complete foramen, making it harder to locate by palpation. This artery is typically larger than the supratrochlear and supplies the forehead skin lateral to its origin. Branches of the superficial temporal artery supply the temporal region and the most lateral regions of the forehead. The superficial temporal artery is a terminal branch of the external carotid artery (**Figure 8-4**).

## Neural Anatomy

Traveling with the supraorbital and supratrochlear vessels are the nerves of the same name. These nerves carry the sensory fibers that supply the forehead and scalp to the level of the vertex. They are branches of the first division of the trigeminal (V), or fifth cranial nerve. The supratrochlear nerve

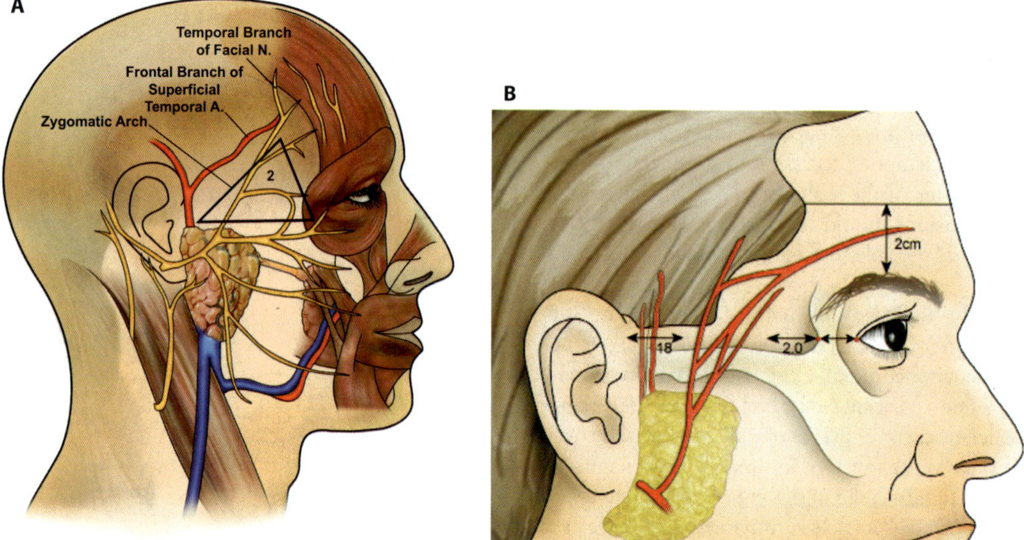


**Figure 8-5.** A facial nerve anatomy of the forehead and temporal region. The frontal branch travels superomedially from the temporal region entering the forehead region approximately 1.5 cm lateral to the orbital rim and innervating the frontalis muscle from its deep surface. As the temporal branch traverses the zygomatic arch, it is quite superficial lying in the subcutaneous plane superficial to both layers of the deep temporal fascia.

supplies the central forehead and scalp and the supraorbital nerve supplies the lateral forehead and anterior and parietal scalp.

The muscles of the forehead are innervated by the frontal branch of the upper division of the facial (VII), or seventh cranial nerve **(Figure 8-5)**. The location of the frontal and zygomatic branches of the facial nerve is essential knowledge for any surgeon operating in this region. Care must be taken to preserve function of these nerves in order to avoid significant functional and cosmetic impairment. The frontal branch travels superomedially from the temporal region entering the forehead region approximately 1.5 cm lateral to the orbital rim and innervating the frontalis muscle from its deep surface. Similarly, the procerus and corrugator muscles are innervated on their deep surface by the frontal branch of the facial nerve. The orbicularis oculi is innervated by the zygomatic branch of the facial nerve.

A detailed discussion of the anatomy of the entire facial nerve is beyond the scope of this chapter; however, it is important to understand the anatomy of the facial nerve as it traverses the temporal region. The temporal region is complicated by the presence of the zygomatic arch and the temporalis muscle, which are responsible for differences in the fascial planes as they split and rejoin to accommodate these structures. There are similarities, however, that make the anatomy of this region easier to understand. As we discussed earlier, muscles of the forehead lie in the plane of the galea aponeurotica. This same plane is evident in the temporal region and is termed the superficial temporal fascia, or the temporoparietal fascia. This fascia is also continuous with the superficial musculoaponeurotic system (SMAS) of the face. Just beneath this fascia in a loose connective tissue layer lays the superficial temporal artery, the frontal branch of the facial nerve and the auriculotemporal nerve. Unlike the forehead musculature, which lies in the galea, the temporalis muscle is encased by a split layer of the periosteum that then fuses at the temporal line to become the conjoined fascia.

The layer of "periosteum" overlying the temporalis muscle is termed the deep temporal fascia, as it cannot be accurately described as periosteum at that point. This layer is thick and dense and has also been called the true temporal fascia. Just superficial to the deep temporal fascia is the superficial temporal fascia or temporoparietal fascia. Approximately 2 cm superior to the zygomatic arch, the deep temporal fascia splits into a superficial layer and a deep layer to invest the superficial temporal fat pad that lies just above the zygomatic arch. The deep layer of the deep temporal fascia at this point dives deep to the fat pad to separate the fat pad from the temporalis muscle and then continues beneath the zygomatic arch with the temporalis muscle. It remains strong and dense. The superficial layer of the deep temporal fascia lies superficial to the fat pad and is thin. It is critical not to confuse the superficial temporal fascia with the superficial layer of the deep temporal fascia.

In order to preserve the facial nerve branches, dissection should be carried out in the temporal region in the plane just superficial to the deep temporal fascia leaving the superficial layer of the deep and superficial temporal fat pads intact. As mentioned earlier, the branches of the facial nerve lie in the plane between the superficial layer of the deep temporal fascia and the superficial temporal fascia and thus, superficial to the superficial temporal fat pad (**Figure 8-6**).

## Defect Analysis

In the forehead and temporal region, special consideration must be given not only to the size, location, and depth of the defect but also to the structures involved and whether there is impairment of function by way of muscle resection or nerve injury. The current position of the hairline is important and how this would change with various reconstructive options must be considered. In general, we want to change existing features as little as possible, but in some cases changing the hairline might be a desirable outcome for the patient. Symmetry is critical not only in the outcome but also in the initial assessment of the patient. More often than not, patients have some innate asymmetry to the brows and this must be considered and pointed out to the patient preoperatively. Sometimes these differences offer opportunities to expand the reconstructive options available to us. Where there is loss of frontal branch function, amelioration of its effects should be a key part of the reconstructive plan. This may include reanimation of the facial nerve depending on the location of the injury/resection or lifting/stabilizing the brow position on the affected side. In the temporal region, the hairline, particularly the temporal tuft, is important considerations. Restoration of the hairline and temporal tuft is an important goal in achieving optimal results.

## Defect Preparation

Defect preparation should ensure that the wound has clean, fresh edges and that there is adequate tissue available for the technique chosen. For example, a vascularized wound bed is essential for successful skin grafting to occur. If there is exposed

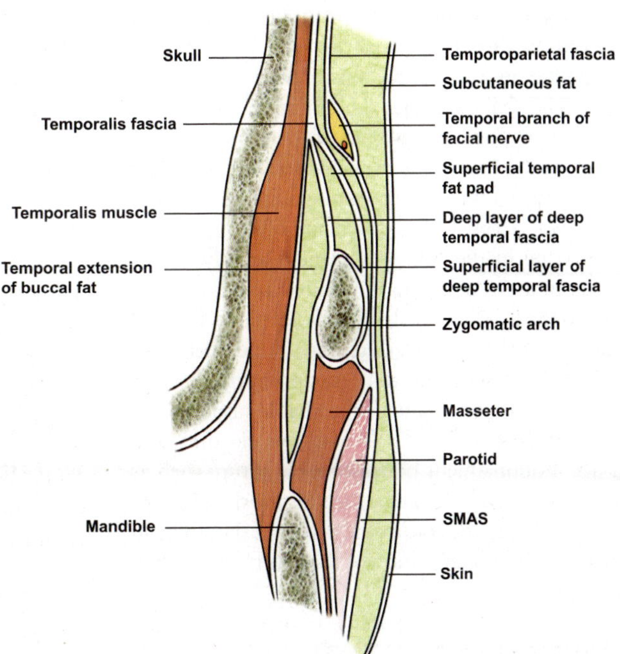


**Figure 8-6.** Cross-sectional anatomy of the facial nerve.

bone in the frontal region, this must be covered prior to grafting or a flap of viable tissue must be used instead. In some cases, defect preparation may involve a period of healing by secondary intention prior to skin grafting to allow the wound bed to fill in and provide a better cosmetic result than immediate grafting.

## Choice of Reconstructive Technique

When considering which technique to use for reconstruction, one must consider the needs and desires of the patient along with their overall health and systemic factors previously discussed in Chapter 4. In this region, unlike many others, a flap may not be the best option for reconstruction if it will create significant scarring or asymmetry. Flaps should also not be used if excess tension will result in compromise of flap viability or if the tissues offer little elasticity such as that seen with extensive actinic exposure. One of the alternatives such as healing by secondary intention or delayed skin grafting may represent a better option for reconstruction.

## Alternatives to Local Flaps

Primary closure represents the best option if it can be performed with little tension and along relaxed skin tension lines. In the forehead and scalp, the skin is not very elastic and primary closure is not an option except for small defects. Undermining is the key to a successful tension-free closure. For small and shallow defects, undermining can be performed in the subcutaneous plane. Undermining greater than 2 cm in the subcutaneous plane offers little if any additional benefit to wound-closing tension. For larger defects, the plane of undermining should be in the subgaleal plane. Care should be taken to avoid injury to the neurovascular bundles and to the frontal branch of the facial nerve. Closure should consist of a layered closure of the galea, subcutaneous tissues, and skin. An appropriately sized (4-0 or 5-0) monofilament absorbable suture works best for the galeal and subcutaneous closures, and a 6-0 monofilament nonabsorbable suture such as nylon or Prolene should be used for the skin. In general, the larger the suture, the deeper it should be in order to prevent extrusion of the suture rather than absorption.

In this region, there are two other options that must be considered and offered to the patient in addition to a flap. In many instances these offer better esthetic results than those that can be obtained by a flap. These include healing by secondary intention and delayed skin grafting. Both of these techniques rely on the presence of a vascularized bed of tissue ensuring that there is no exposed bone.

We know from both the early experience with Mohs surgeries and, more recently, with paramedian forehead flap donor sites that the forehead heals quite well when allowed to heal by secondary intention. Downsides to this are that healing is delayed and patients may be reluctant to socialize or return to work until healing has occurred. It is, easy to care for and has little pain associated with it, however.

A second option to be considered that allows for faster healing with a reasonable cosmetic result is the delayed skin graft. If there is a layer of vascularized tissue present, then granulation tissue will form over the wound over time along with contracture at the wound edges. Once the granulation tissue has filled the depth of the wound, it can then be skin grafted with a split thickness graft to expedite the healing process and lessen wound contracture. This offers a distinct cosmetic advantage over immediate skin grafting, which creates a permanent defect that is not at the same level as the native surrounding tissue and offers no hope of improvement without resection and definitive repair.

Full thickness skin grafting is an option for shallow and small defects. Patients with larger defects who desire immediate reconstruction or who need surveillance of the wound for recurrence may benefit from split thickness skin grafting. In the latter instance, the definitive reconstruction is delayed until the risk of local recurrence is minimized.

## Glabella

The relaxed skin tension lines in the glabellar region are vertically oriented and primary closure in this region should be vertical in orientation. The vertically oriented procerus muscle creates horizontally oriented lines at the rhinion. When considering primary closure, one should consider its effects on the medialization of the brows. This medialization can be avoided by using a V-to-Y technique (**Figure 8-7**) that interposes adjacent tissue between the edges of the defect to allow continued separation of the brows. Transposition flaps in this region should be conceived in such a manner as to not distort the medial head of the brow, rotating it down-

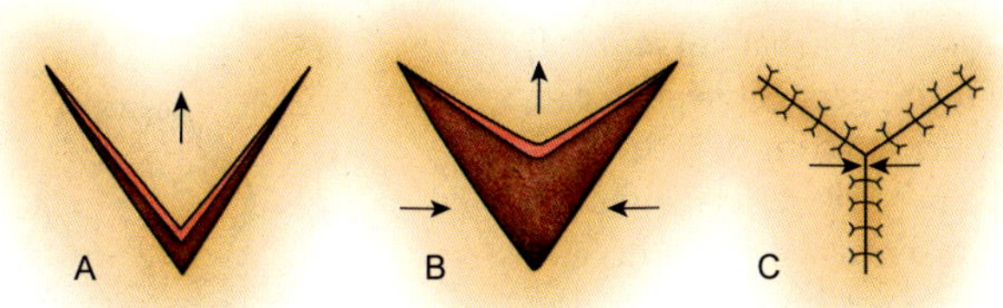


**Figure 8-7.** V-to-Y closure. In the V-to-Y closure, a triangular flap is elevated and pushed away from its apex creating the final Y configuration.

ward. Full thickness skin grafting can be used in this area with reasonably good results.

## Forehead

Although it can be tempting to try many different kinds of flaps in the forehead, there are very few that will yield a truly acceptable cosmetic result. Because the forehead is a broad, rectangular, and relatively flat plane with few wrinkles until later in life, it should be considered as a single esthetic unit and the temptation to subdivide it avoided. Scars on the forehead are quite noticeable unless they are oriented horizontally along the RSTLs. The next best orientation for scars in this region is a vertically oriented scar. This rules out many of rotation and transposition flaps as they often create curvilinear or oblique scars. The tissues of the forehead are thick and relatively immobile. The best option in this area is primary closure if at all possible.

Symmetry of the brows is important when considering primary closure. Most individuals do not have symmetric brows and several millimeters of brow asymmetry is within normal limits. If the arcus marginalis is not released, then the brow is anchored to some extent and can resist upward pull. Relaxation of the brow occurs over several months so that a primary closure that creates some brow asymmetry may relax to an acceptable level. If brow asymmetry is going to create more than 3–5 mm of brow asymmetry once healed, then a different reconstructive option should be considered.

One such option is to close the wound as much as possible and allow the remainder to heal by secondary intention. This routinely occurs at the donor site for the paramedian forehead flap. If primary closure is not possible, unilateral or bilateral horizontal advancement flaps represent the best flap option in this region. As discussed earlier, healing by secondary intention, with or without delayed skin grafting, also yields acceptable results.

Central forehead defects should be closed primarily whenever possible. They can be closed horizontally if small, but if large, they are generally closed vertically, as the entire forehead can be undermined in the subgaleal plane to recruit tissue.

Large lateral forehead defects can be closed by rotating cheek tissue superiorly, using an incision that extends along the hairline or just into the hairline and down along the preauricular crease similar to a facelift incision. This can be extended inferiorly into the neck as a cervicofacial rotation flap that is advanced superiorly instead of medially as in the case of a cheek defect. Care must be taken to leave the temporal branch of the VIIth nerve intact.

## Brow

Defects that involve the eyebrow offer unique challenges. As we discussed in the section on forehead reconstruction, the brow must be within 3–5 mm of the height of the opposite brow. There is also the hair-bearing skin to consider. The brow hairline should be treated much like any other hairline in that care must be taken to align the brow. Misalignment of this important physical landmark is akin to misalignment of the vermillion of the lip. Almost any scar through the eyebrow will result in some hair loss. If the non-hair-bearing scar is wide, then reexcision is in order, making sure that the patient knows that there will continue to be a small area of non-hair-bearing scar present. If a significant portion of the eyebrow is missing, then the primary reconstruction should focus on soft tissue reconstruction with reestablishment of the hair follicles once healing has occurred.

The absence of a portion of the eyebrow hair is quite noticeable and is most disconcerting to females in particular. It is important to be able to offer alternatives for them to help camouflage the defect or restore the hair. If the non-hair-bearing area is small and within the brow, then tattooing of small follicular units into the scar is helpful for camouflage. This is quick and easy for the patient and will make a big difference in their overall appearance. If the defect is larger, then micrografting of individual follicular units should be performed to reestablish the brow. Care must be taken when orienting the follicles so that they are almost horizontal to the skin surface and match the adjacent follicular orientation. Follicular grafts can be placed in scar tissue and usually do very well. The occipital scalp is the best place for obtaining grafts for this purpose. Patients should be advised that they will have to trim the new hair as it is scalp hair and will continue to grow.

## Temporal Region

The temporal esthetic unit is bounded by the temporal line superiorly and the zygomatic arch inferiorly. Anteriorly, it is bounded by the orbital rim and posteriorly by the pinna. There is a curvilinear hairline that runs throughout the extent of the region from the frontal hairline to the sideburn or temporal tuft. This hairline and the pinna offer excellent hiding places for scars but also offer reconstructive challenges when involved in the defect.

In the temporal region, there are many options available for reconstruction, and this area tends to be very forgiving as long as the facial nerve remains intact. The major consideration for the temporal region is the hair-bearing scalp and the sideburn or temporal tuft. This is a region that heals well by secondary intention and, because it is not as noticeable in the frontal view, it is well tolerated esthetically. Secondary intention healing obviously does not restore the hair, and so this must be a primary concern in reconstructing this area. Vertical advancement and or rotation flaps of facial skin are ideal for reconstructing the inferior portions of this region but have limitations superiorly. Parietal scalp and superior temporal hair-bearing defects are best closed by rotating scalp flaps into the defect from above. If the sideburn is involved with the defect, this should be reconstructed with a transposition flap from the adjacent scalp. For anterior temporal (non-hair-bearing) defects, the rhomboid flap is particularly useful. This is one of the few areas that the geometry of the rhomboid flap is ideal, as this subunit is roughly rhomboid in shape and the angles of the flap fit nicely **(Figure 8-8)**.

Large temporal defects that involve significant hair-bearing area can be treated successfully with the use of tissue expanders in the adjacent parietal scalp. This is particularly useful when reestablishment of the hairline and scalp are critical. The obvious disadvantage to this technique is the amount of time required to inflate the expander (usually 8–10 weeks) and the multiple operations required to complete the reconstruction. In well-motivated patients, it is worth the inconvenience to them for the outcome is far superior when the hair is restored in this area.

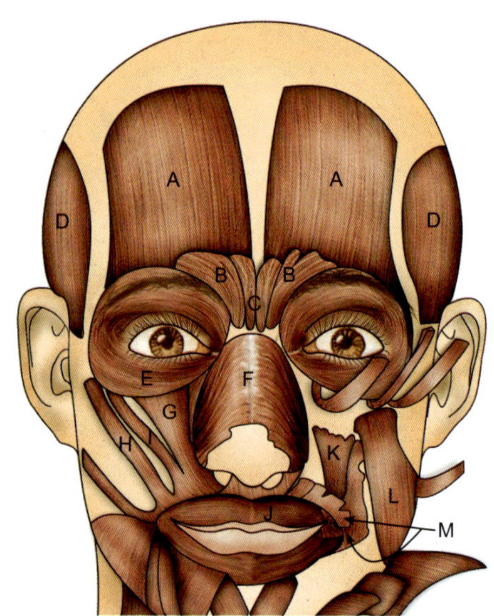


**Figure 8-8.** Rhomboid flap. The Rhomboid flap can have four different variations depending on where the donor flap is easiest to harvest. Shown below the classic 60-degree Rhomboid flap are two variations that can reduce the angle of rotation of the flap and the tension on the closure.

## References

1. Branham GH, ed. Local skin flaps. *Facial Plast Surg Clin N Am* 4(4), 1996.
2. Larrabee, W. et al., eds. *Surgical Anatomy of the Face*, 2nd ed., Lippincott Williams & Wilkins, Philadelphia, 2004.
3. Papel I et al., eds. *Facial Plastic and Reconstructive Surgery*, 2nd ed., Thieme, New York, 2001.
4. Park, SS, ed. Local cutaneous flaps. *Facial Plast Surg Clin N Am* 13(2), 2005.
5. Tardy, ME, ed. *Surgical Anatomy of the Nose*, Lippincott Williams & Wilkins, Philadelphia, 1990.
6. Weerda H, ed. *Reconstructive Facial Plastic Surgery: A Problem-Solving Manual*. Thieme, New York, 2001.

9

# Cheek Reconstruction

Gregory H. Branham, MD, FACS

## Introduction

Like the forehead, the cheek is a large area that is relatively flat and featureless. This absence of features can create a challenge for hiding scars. Unlike the forehead, however, cheek tissues are very mobile. The cheek is bounded by numerous esthetic units that offer excellent hiding places for incisions. The cheek is essentially one esthetic unit that is difficult to divide into subunits based on visual esthetic landmarks; however, it is helpful to consider the cheek as having subunits from the standpoint of reconstruction (**Figure 9-1**). Thus, as a matter of convenience, these subunits can be thought of as reconstructive subunits and not true esthetic subunits.

In males, the majority of the cheek is covered with bearded skin, making the skin thicker and coarser in its features and easier to hide scars within. In females, only a fine vellous hair covers the skin, which is thinner and smoother, making scars more visible. The relaxed skin tension lines in the cheek tend to run in an oblique fashion flowing over the orbital rim in a line parallel to the melolabial fold. Adjacent to the pinna, tension lines tend to be more vertically oriented, following the contour of the preauricular crease.

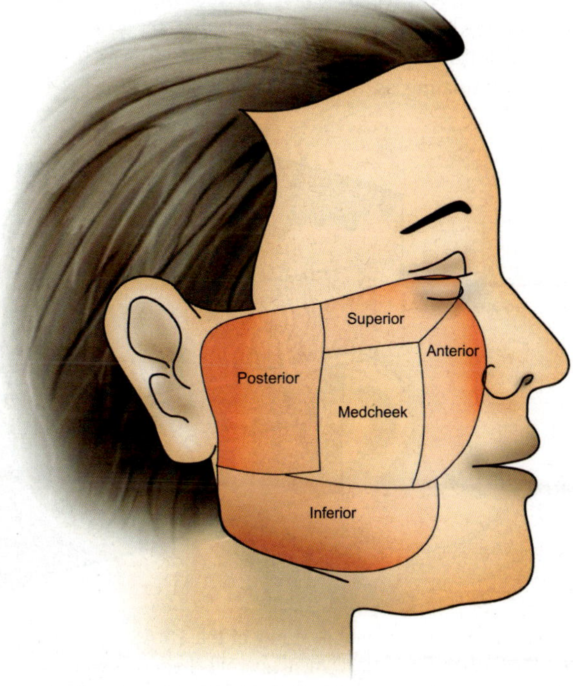


**Figure 9-1.** Cheek esthetic subunits. The cheek can be divided into several subunits, the boundaries of which are not as clear cut, as the cheek has fewer landmarks to divide it naturally. Cheek subunits are more useful in reconstructive planning than actual esthetic subunits.

The cheek is delineated by the melolabial fold and marionette lines medially, the mandible inferiorly, the preauricular crease and angle of the mandible laterally, and the temporal region superiorly in a line extending horizontally along the zygomatic arch to the lateral canthus.

## Anatomy

The skin of the cheek is composed of epidermis, dermis, and subcutaneous tissues that overlie the superficial musculoaponeurotic system (SMAS) (**Figure 9-2**). The SMAS is continuous with the gala aponeurotica in the scalp and the platysma muscle in the neck (**Figure 9-3**). Just deep to the SMAS lie the parotidomasseteric fascia, the parotid gland, masseter muscle, buccal fat pad, and zygomaticus major and minor muscles. The buccinator muscle lies just outside the oral cavity mucosa. It is the zygomaticus major and minor muscles that are responsible for the creation of the melolabial fold and the orientation of the relaxed skin tension lines as they originate from the body of the zygoma and travel anteromedially to insert on the skin at the melolabial fold and modiolus of the lip, respectively.

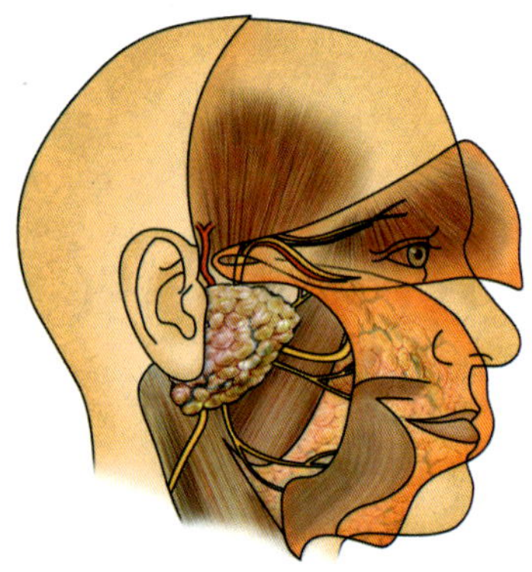

**Figure 9-2.** Superficial Musculoaponeurotic System (SMAS). The SMAS layer is continuous with the galea aponeurotic in the scalp and the platysma in the neck. By plicating the platysma, in older patients in particular, a large amount of skin can be recruited to close cheek defects. This layer is also plicated or resuspended in the most common facelift procedures.

## Vascular Supply

The majority of the cheek is supplied by the facial artery and its branches (**Figure 9-4**). The facial artery is a direct branch from the external carotid artery and gives rise to the superior and inferior labial arteries before terminating as the angular artery running along the nasofacial junction. Cutaneous branches from the infraorbital artery also supply the medial cheek and anastomose with branches of the angular artery. The infraorbital artery is a branch from the third division of the maxillary artery. Branches from the superficial temporal artery assist in the vascular supply to the upper lateral cheek skin.

## Neural Anatomy

Sensory innervation of the cheek is largely from the infraorbital nerve or the second (maxillary)

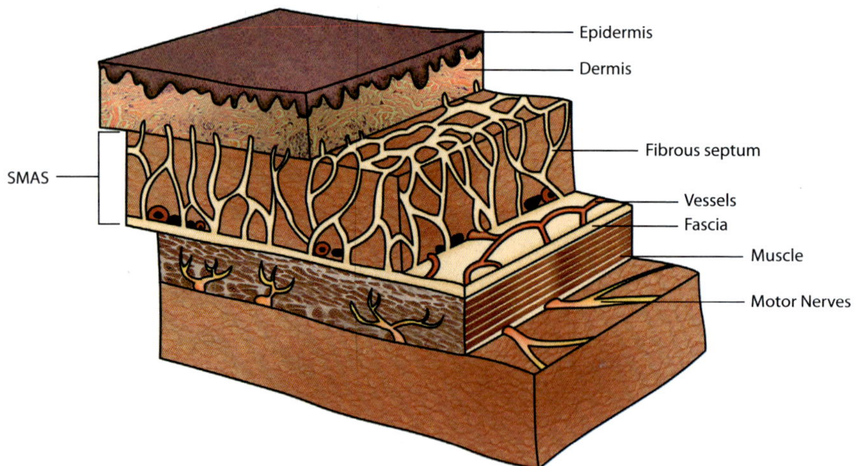


**Figure 9-3.** Cross-sectional anatomy of the SMAS. The SMAS has dermal attachments that connect the skin to the SMAS layer. These attachments permit the recruitment of skin when the SMAS is suspended. The SMAS also provides a layer of cushion to permit the skin to slide as the muscles contract.

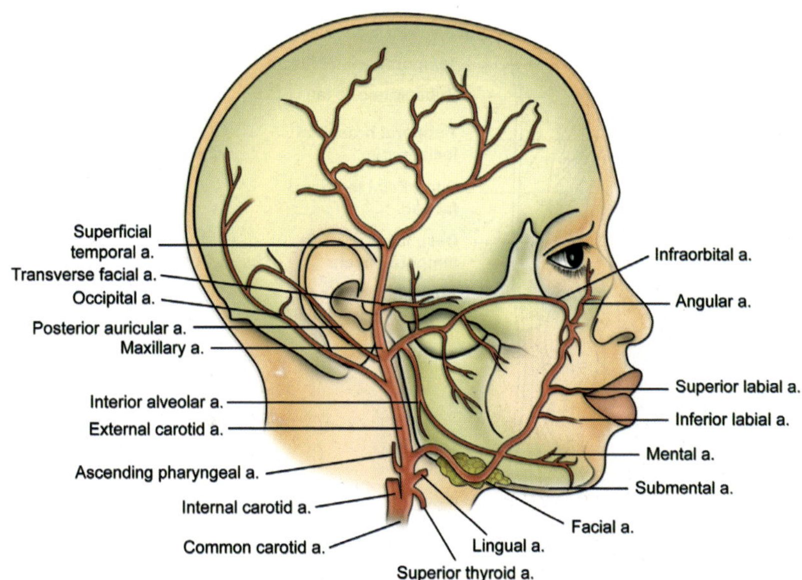


**Figure 9-4.** Vascular anatomy of the face. The cheek is supplied by the facial artery, which is a direct branch from the external carotid artery, and gives rise to the superior and inferior labial arteries before terminating as the angular artery running along the nasofacial junction. Cutaneous branches from the infraorbital artery also supply the medial cheek and anastomose with branches of the angular artery. The infraorbital artery is a branch from the third division of the maxillary artery. Branches from the superficial temporal artery assist in the vascular supply to the upper lateral cheek skin.

division of the trigeminal ($V_2$) nerve. This nerve supplies the skin of the cheek and lateral nasal wall as well as the upper lip to the level of the commissure. The inferior lateral cheek derives its sensory innervation from branches of the cervical plexus. Two small branches of $V_2$, the zygomaticomaxillary and the zygomaticotemporal muscles, contribute sensory innervation to the upper cheek and temporal regions. The auriculotemporal nerve, a branch of the mandibular division ($V_3$) of the trigeminal nerve is responsible for the sensory innervation of the preauricular skin and portions of the pinna. The buccal nerve, a branch of the mandibular division, supplies the skin of the lower cheek along the mandible.

Motor innervation of the cheek musculature is from the VIIth facial nerve. The facial nerve exits the stylomastoid foramen and divides into a superior and inferior division as the pes anserinus. The facial nerve divides the superficial and deep lobes of the parotid and exits just superficial to the masseter muscle and deep to the SMAS. The multiple buccal branches course just anterior to the buccal fat pad and innervate the facial musculature from their deep surfaces. The temporal branch or branches travel progressively more superficially as they ascend to the zygomatic arch. As the temporal branches cross the zygomatic arch, they are just below the subcutaneous fat and thus are quite vulnerable to injury (**Figure 9-5**). A patch of skin overlying the zygomatic arch, known as MacGregor's patch, demarcates the location of the nerves in this area and lies between 2cm posterior to the lateral canthus and 1.5 cm anterior to the edge of the pinna (**Figure 9-6**).

The marginal mandibular nerve divides from the inferior division of the facial nerve and exits the parotid anteriorly. It is generally described as swinging below the level of the mandible as low as 3–4 cm, but this is variable. This nerve travels beneath the platysma muscle and crosses the inferior border of the mandible to innervate the depressor anguli oris from its deep surface. Injury to this nerve creates significant deformity and, due to its lengthy course and lack of cross anastomosis with other branches, rarely regains function once injured.

## Defect Analysis

When analyzing a cheek defect, it is important to evaluate the critical structures that may be involved and create functional problems. The potential

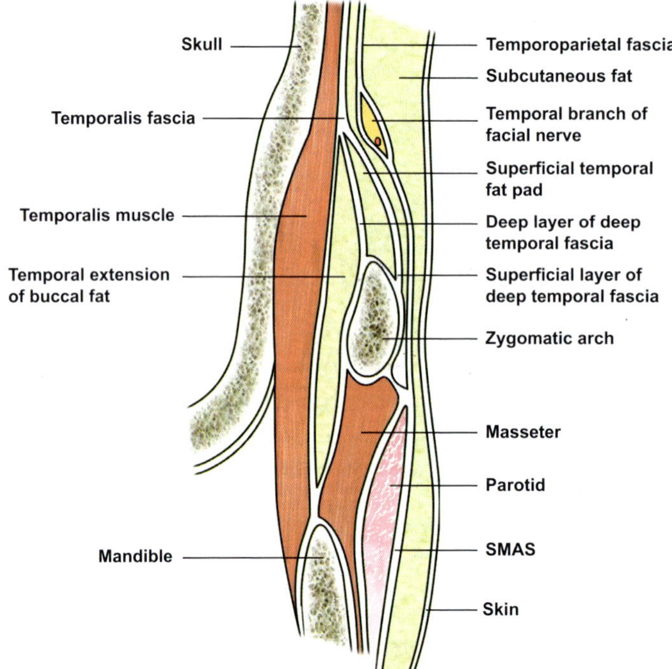


**Figure 9-5.** Cross-sectional anatomy of the facial nerve.

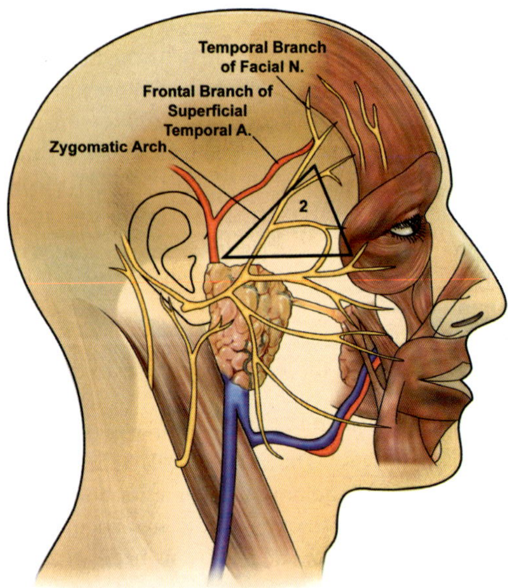


**Figure 9-6.** Anatomy of the facial nerve.

structures involved will depend on the location and depth of the defect. The facial nerve and parotid duct are among some of the most important structures that should be assessed.

The concept of the reconstructive subunit is helpful in determining which technique will be best in reconstructing the defect. Because the cheek abuts several different esthetic units, it is essential to consider how these adjacent esthetic units will be affected by the reconstruction. It is helpful to divide the cheek into central or midcheek, inferior, posterior (preauricular), anterior (melolabial), and superior (infraorbital) subunits.

## Defect Preparation

Fresh cheek defects require little wound preparation. However, if critical structures such as the facial nerve or parotid duct are involved, these should be addressed prior to wound closure. If the reconstruction is a delayed closure of a Mohs defect, for example, then removing fibrinous exudates at the base of the wound and freshening the wound edges is appropriate.

## Choice of Reconstructive Technique

Based on the concept of reconstructive subunits discussed earlier, a reconstructive plan can be generated. Such a plan should consider the age of the patient and relative laxity of the skin as well as the location of the defect. Attention to the adjacent esthetic units and the effect of the reconstruction on them is also critical. Finally, adherence to the orientation of the relaxed skin tension lines is important in achieving the best possible scar, particularly in the primary closure of central cheek defects.

## Alternatives to Local Flaps

In general, primary closure can be accomplished for all small cheek defects with good results. It must be kept in mind that although cheek tissues are mobile and easy to close, they are in constant motion with facial functions such as smiling and chewing and as such are prone to widening. Primary closure is not appropriate if the resulting scar will create too much tension and thereby further widen the scar. Because of this tendency to widen, the incisions should be closed in multiple layers with a meticulous cuticular closure. The use of Steri-Strips is helpful in lessening wound tension once the sutures are removed and should be used for several weeks thereafter.

Full thickness and split thickness skin grafts should be avoided in definitive reconstructions of cheek defects. Because the cheek has no firm surface and is very mobile, these grafts are prone to shearing forces. In addition, because the cheek is flat and featureless, these grafts tend to be quite obvious and have a permanent "stuck-on" appearance. Even the largest of defects can generally be closed with a cervicofacial rotation flap, thus avoiding skin grafts.

## Posterior Cheek

Defects in this location are generally closed by advancing cheek skin posteriorly and placing the scar in the preauricular crease. This is essentially the same concept that is involved in the facelift. In older patients, resuspension of the SMAS layer will also provide more tissue for closure. If the defect is too large or the skin too tight to accommodate an advancement flap, additional tissue must be recruited from adjacent areas to relieve the tension and allow for acceptable closure. This is best accomplished by transposing a flap from the postauricular area to complete the closure. Prior to transposing the flap, however, the defect should be made as small as possible by undermining the wound edges and advancing and securing them. This permits the smallest flap to be used in the transposition. The transposed flap donor site is then closed along relaxed skin tension lines of the neck. In the preauricular area, the relaxed skin tension lines are vertical and the resultant scars should have a vertical orientation with curvilinear lines. The sharp angulation associated with geometric flaps such as the rhombic flap is to be avoided. Similarly, circular lines such as those associated with traditional bilobed flaps are to be avoided. The exception to this would be in the superior aspect of the lateral cheek where it borders the temporal region. This is an excellent place for horizontal scar placement with an advancement or rotation flap. Ideal placement would be along a horizontal line drawn from the lateral canthus and extending posteriorly.

## Anterior Cheek

As previously mentioned, small defects of the anterior cheek can usually be closed primarily. This is done along the melolabial fold or marionette lines or parallel to them. In no instance should tissue be recruited medial to the melolabial fold, as this will result in distortion of the lip and nose. A medium-sized defect may require advancement of lateral cheek tissue known as a cheek advancement flap (**Figure 9-7**).

If the defect is too large to close adequately without distorting the lips or nose, a cervicofacial rotation flap should be used. Depending on the location of the defect, this flap may be a pure rotational flap that has an inferior pivot point or a bilobed flap. For very large cheek defects, the bilobed form of the cervicofacial rotation flap recruits all available cheek tissue to close the defect and postauricular tissue to close the secondary donor site along the preauricular unit. Development of this flap involves extensive undermining in the neck to allow the flap to be advanced superiorly as well as rotated anteriorly. This is generally necessary to permit closure of the secondary donor site.

The incision for this flap extends from the superior aspect of the defect posteriorly across the cheek subunit transversely usually at its most superior aspect. This places the scar along the junction of the cheek and temporal/periorbital esthetic units. The inferior limb of the incision is placed in the preauricular crease and the postauricular flap is designed to the appropriate size to close the remaining secondary defect with the incision usually bordering the hairline in large flaps.

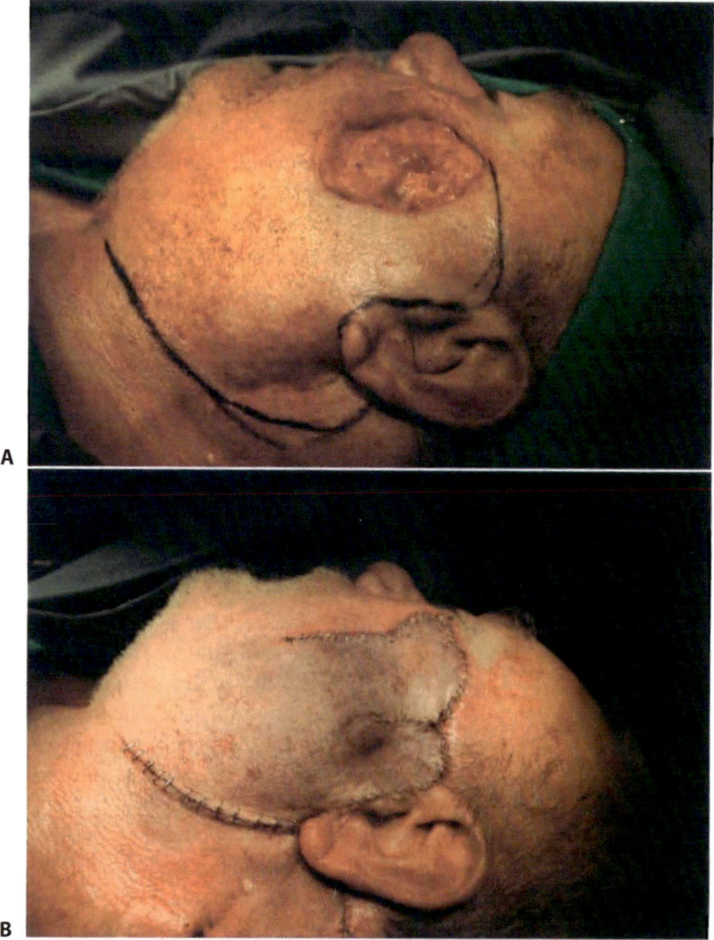

**Figure 9-7.** A large cheek defect from skin cancer resection with bilobed cervicofacial rotation flap outlined as proposed reconstruction. Because the defect is so large, postauricular skin has been recruited as the secondary flap to close the anterior preauricular (secondary) defect. Extensive undermining of the cervical skin is necessary to accomplish adequate rotation. A drain is placed to prevent hematoma formation.

Although extensive undermining is essential for tension-free closure, it is not the only measure that must be used to assure a tension-free result. When closing the wound and insetting the flap, it is necessary to anchor the flap to the deep tissues (often the periosteum). This flap has substantial weight and is constantly being pulled inferiorly. The thin and very elastic periorbital tissues cannot withstand these forces alone, and therefore the flap should be anchored into position. This can be accomplished with a bone anchor that will hold a nonabsorbable suture or with a heavy nonabsorbable suture placed through the periosteum and into the flap. Once the surgeon is assured of appropriate anchoring, the flap can be sewn into position with a typical multilayered closure. Around the periorbital subunit in the thin skin, a 6-0 fast absorbing gut suture is helpful in facilitating closure and avoiding suture removal in this delicate and sensitive area.

The standing cone that results from the rotation of this flap is located at its pivot point in the inferior cheek. This should be excised along relaxed skin tension lines parallel to the marionette lines avoiding backcutting across the pedicle of the flap.

## Central/Inferior Cheek

Although some consider these two areas separately, it is convenient to discuss them together, as the techniques for reconstruction are the same. The inferiormost aspect of the cheek is usually not involved in a defect in isolation and is usually closed by default. In fact, it is the location of the standing cone deformity that is associated with the cervicofacial rotation flap.

When the inferior or midcheek is involved with a small defect, closure along relaxed skin tension lines (RSTLs) is appropriate. When larger defects are involved, advancement of adjacent cheek tissue is appropriate. For larger defects in the midcheek area, the cervicofacial flap as described is useful for closure.

For inferior cheek defects that cannot be closed by simple advancement of cheek tissue, a bilobed flap or posteriorly based transposition flap from cervical tissues is useful. This takes advantage of the relatively loose neck skin and allows the donor site to be closed along the horizontal RSTLs of the neck.

## Superior Cheek

The superior cheek abuts the periorbital subunit, and care must be taken when reconstructing this area so that an ectropion of the lower lid by creating unopposed downward forces on the lower eyelid will not be created. The relaxed skin tension lines in this area are more vertically oriented; however, if the wound can be closed primarily in a horizontal fashion along the junction of the cheek and periorbital units, this should be accomplished. Again, care should be taken not to create ectropion in doing so. If lid retraction occurs, a vertical closure or a combination horizontal/vertical closure such as an O-to-T closure should be used.

Larger defects in this area will require a cheek advancement or a cervicofacial rotation flap as described in the section on anterior cheek defects (**Figure 9-8**). Periorbital reconstruction, including techniques for the lower eyelid, are discussed in Chapter 10.

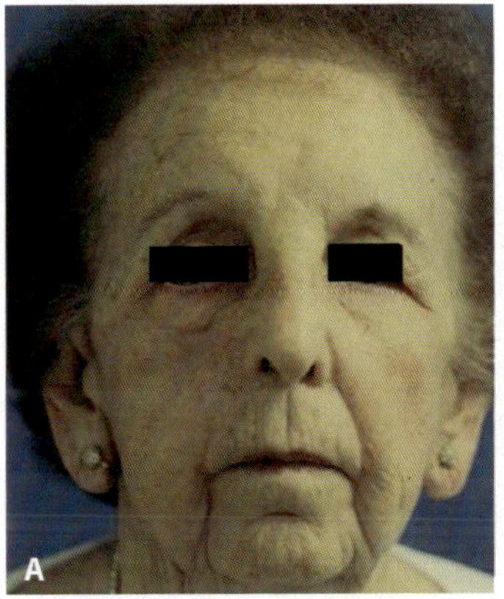


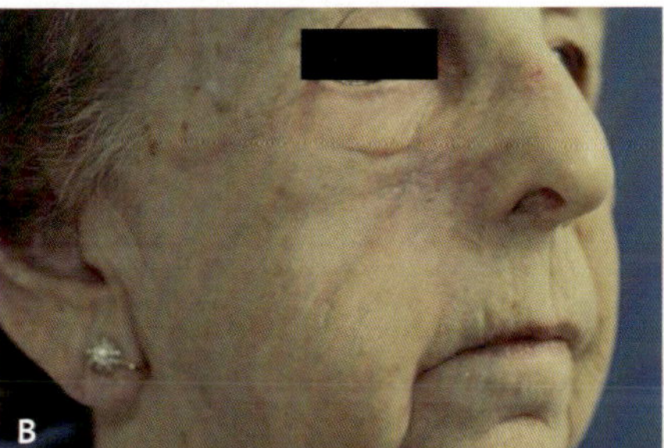


**Figure 9-8.** Cheek advancement flap for anterior/superior cheek defect. (A) Frontal view of a well-healed cheek advancement flap. There is good facial symmetry, but there is also mild lid malposition related to scar contracture and weight of the flap on the lid skin. The advancement flap does not create the significant standing cone deformity of the cervicofacial rotation flap (B) Oblique closeup view. Cheek tissue has been advanced medially to close this anterior and superior cheek defect from a Mohs excision of a squamous cell carcinoma. The lid malposition can be corrected with a tarsal strip canthopexy.

10

# Eyelid and Periocular Reconstruction

Jasmine Mohadjer, MD and John B. Holds, MD, FACS

## Introduction

This chapter focuses on describing surgically relevant eyelid anatomy and highlighting structures and techniques for appropriate reconstruction to maintain function and cosmesis. Most commonly, reconstruction of the periocular area is necessitated in the setting of cutaneous malignancy, but appropriate reconstruction is essential for traumatic and congenital defects as well. Specific surgical principles must be followed in developing a reconstructive plan in this unique area.

## Regional Anatomic Considerations

The following anatomic summary is not intended to be exhaustive, but rather to focus on important issues specific to periocular reconstruction.

### Eyelids

Eyelids protect and lubricate the ocular surface. The anterior lamella, comprising of skin and muscle, provides important support and aid in eye blinking. The posterior lamella conjunctiva is a mucous membrane that contributes to the tear film and wets the globe and the cornea. Both layers are necessary to maintain ocular function and health. In reconstruction of the eyelids, the anterior and posterior lamella must be accounted for separately to preserve ocular function.

The skin in the eyelid is the thinnest skin in the body and continues to thin with age. It is unique in that there is an absence of subcuticular fat between the dermis and the orbicularis muscle. Full thickness skin grafts, advancement, or transposition flaps are necessary for the reconstruction of anterior lamellar defects. Thin, relatively hairless skin is harvested for skin grafts to achieve an appropriate tissue match and avoid symptoms of trichiasis. Common donor sites include redundant upper eyelid skin, pre- or postauricular skin, supraclavicular skin, or inner arm skin.

The orbicularis muscle is a sphincter muscle innervated by the facial nerve surrounding the upper and lower eyelids. It also contributes to the cheek, forehead, and temple area. The orbicularis muscle is divided into pretarsal, preseptal, and orbital portions. The involuntary blink is performed via contraction of the pretarsal and preseptal portions, with the orbital portion allowing forceful eyelid closure along with the corrugator supercilii and procerus muscles (**Figure 10-1**). Significant loss of orbicularis muscle function is uncommon, even with extensive periocular defects and reconstructions.

Each eyelid contains a tarsal plate consisting of dense connective tissue extending up to the eyelid margin that forms the backbone of the eyelid. The upper eyelid tarsus measures approximately 10–12 mm vertically in the central eyelid, whereas the lower eyelid tarsus vertically measures approximately 4 mm in the central eyelid (**Figure 10-2**). Each tarsal plate tapers medially and laterally. There is no tarsus at the medial canthal angle, which contributes to ease of avulsion injuries at this site. The meibomian glands, important holocrine sebaceous glands contributing to the stability of the tear film,

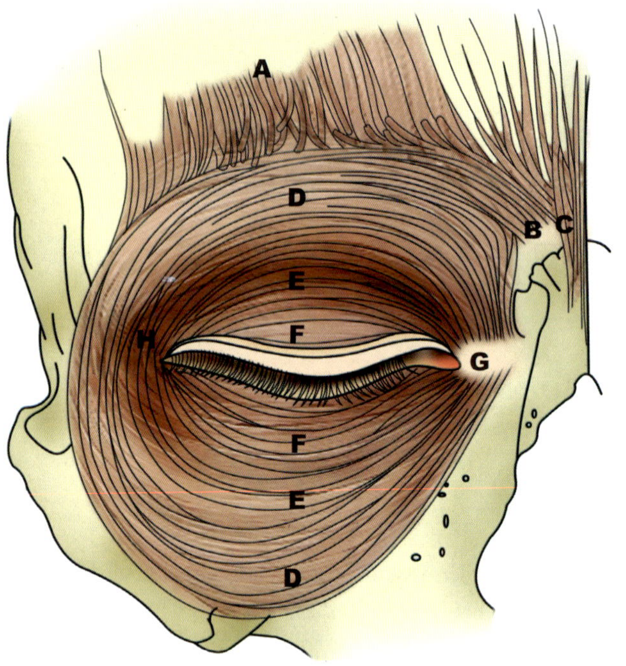


**Figure 10-1.** The Orbicularis muscle and adjacent facial muscles. (A) Frontalis muscle, (B) corrugator muscle, (C) procerus muscle, (D) orbital orbicularis muscle, (E) preseptal orbicularis muscle, (F) pretarsal orbicularis muscle, (G) medial canthal tendon, (H) lateral canthal tendon.

traverse vertically through the center of each tarsal plate. Tarsus may be replaced in the lower lid by hard palate mucosa, although this keratinized tissue is inappropriate for the upper eyelid. Multiple allo- and xenograft materials are available for tarsal replacement. The same or an opposite upper eyelid may be everted and the superior 4–6 mm or tarsus harvested for eyelid reconstruction, leaving a minimum of 2.5–3 mm of tarsus undisturbed at the lid margin.

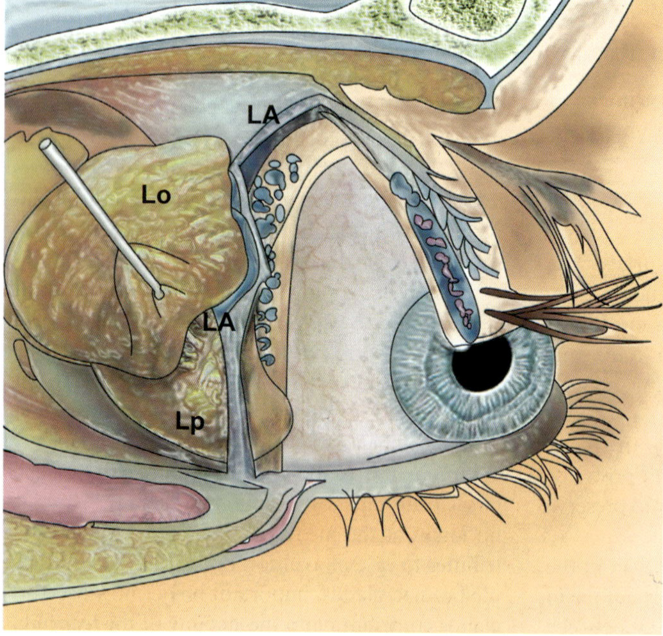


**Figure 10-2.** Cross-sectional upper eyelid anatomy and lateral orbital anatomy showing LO, orbital lobe of lacrimal gland; LP, palpebral lobe of lacrimal gland; LA, levator aponeurosis in a sagittal plane.

The posterior aspect of the eyelid, adherent to the tarsus is a nonkeratinizing mucosa called the conjunctiva. This layer is vital to lubricate and protect the corneal epithelium. Loss of a mucous membrane in a periocular defect must be specifically addressed. Conjunctiva is replaced by other nonkeratinizing mucosa from the opposite eye, buccal or hard palate mucosa of the mouth, nasal turbinate or septum, or historically even anal or vaginal mucosa. Donor amniotic membrane is also commonly used, especially on the ocular surface.

## Canthi

The medial and lateral canthi are unique structures that require specific attention in reconstruction of the periocular area. The medial and lateral canthi are tendinous structures that suspend the tarsus and other eyelid soft tissues allowing proper eyelid position, apposition to the globe and shape of the palpebral aperture. The lateral canthal tendon inserts on Whitnall's tubercle, a bony prominence in the inner aspect of the lateral orbital rim. More anterior suspension during reconstruction will cause vaulting of the eyelid from the globe, an unnatural appearance, and possible tearing or exposure symptoms.

The medial canthal tendon is a highly complex structure encasing the lacrimal system. A well-defined anterior crus of the medial canthal tendon arises from the anterior lacrimal crest, and a more obscure posterior crus arises from the posterior lacrimal crest behind the lacrimal sac **(Figure 10-3)**. Surgical reconstruction must take into consideration the location of the vital canalicular system while maintaining the posteriorly directed vector of the medial canthal tendon for proper apposition of the eyelid to the globe and for appropriate positioning of the punctum to allow tear drainage.

## Lacrimal Drainage System

The lacrimal drainage system consists of a punctum and a canaliculus at each medial upper and lower eyelid, a lacrimal sac within the lacrimal fossa surrounded by the medial canthal tendon, and the nasolacrimal duct within the medial maxilla **(Figure 10-4)**. Proper positioning of the eyelid is crucial for proper lacrimal function. An adequate anterior lamella is necessary to allow blinking and lacrimal pump function to draw the tears into the lacrimal system. Appropriate eyelid and punctal positioning is necessary for tear drainage. A slight outward rotation of the punctum may be enough to cause symptomatic tearing. Appropriate reconstruction of remaining portions of the lacrimal drainage system after tumor excision or trauma will often prevent persistent tearing. This reconstruction is best attempted at the initial repair, or a Jones tube may be necessary to resolve tearing.

## Skin Types and Aesthetic Units

The thin, unique skin of the eyelid aesthetic unit is abutted by thicker skin of the nasal, glabellar, brow, temple, and cheek aesthetic units. Reconstructive results are optimized by creating incisions that follow relaxed skin tension lines. Periocular anterior lamellar defects should be reconstructed with

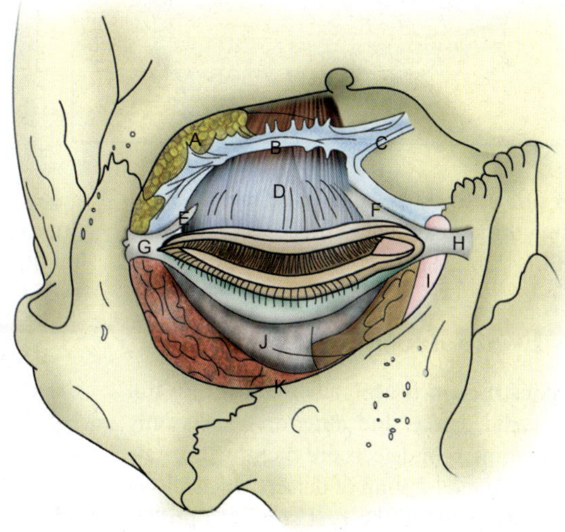


**Figure 10-3.** Anatomic diagram of canthal tendons showing attachments of eyelids to anterior orbital connective tissue structures. (A) Orbital lobe of the lacrimal gland, (B) Whitnall's transverse ligament, (C) superior oblique tendon, (D) levator aponeurosis, (E) lateral horn of levator aponeurosis, (F) medial horn of levator aponeurosis, (G) lateral canthal tendon, (H) medial canthal tendon, (I) lacrimal sac, (J) capsulopalpebral fascia, (K) lockwood's suspensory ligament.

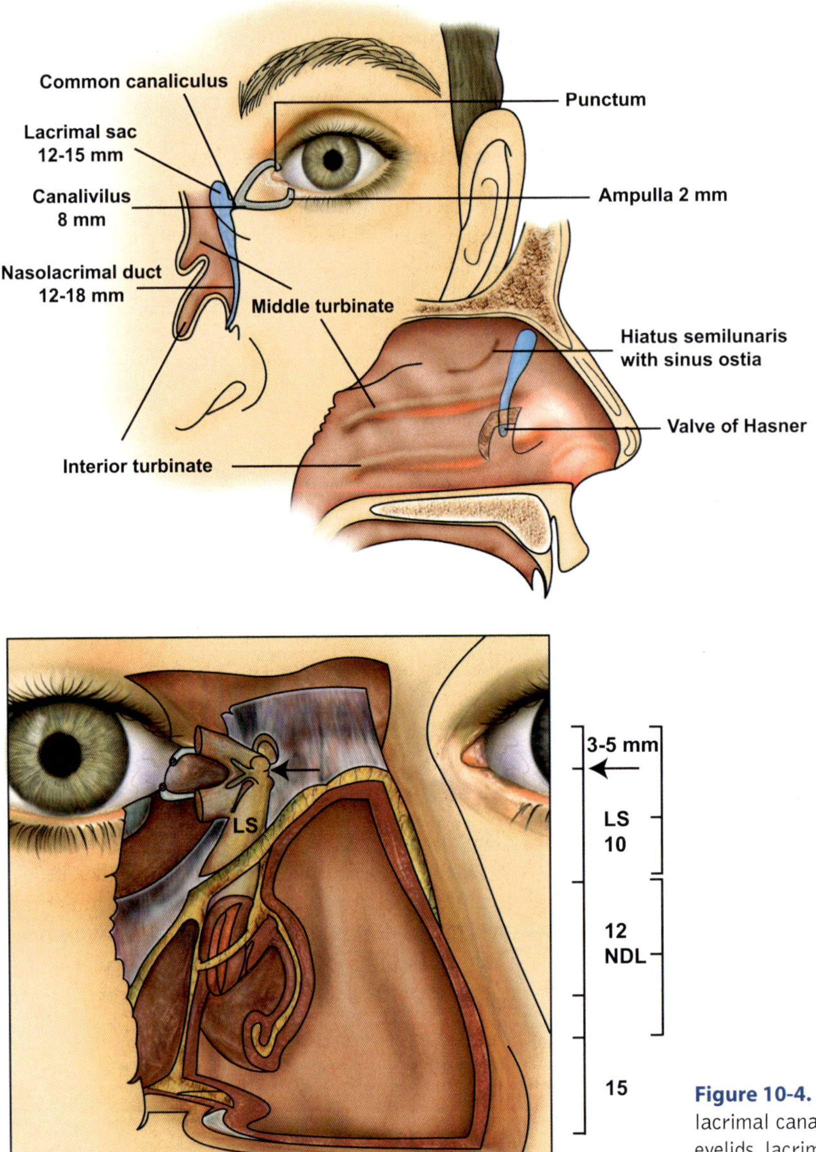


**Figure 10-4.** Anatomy of the lacrimal canaliculi relative to the eyelids, lacrimal Sac (LS), and bony nasolacrimal duct (NLD).

tissues of similar thickness. It is important to avoid transposing thicker adjacent tissue (cheek, glabella) into the thin-skinned periocular area if possible.

## Eyelid Reconstruction

Eyelid reconstruction is generally divided into full thickness eyelid defects and anterior lamella-only defects. Eyelid margin defects are then further categorized by size and location of defect, which allows the surgeon to examine the best surgical options. A key concept in eyelid reconstruction is to allow appropriate horizontal tension in closure while minimizing vertical tension. Vertical tension causes eyelid retraction or ectropion and may result in an aesthetically and functionally poor result.

Reconstructive options are more numerous for defects not affecting the eyelid margin. Depending on location, size, and depth of the defect, reconstruction may use rotational, advancement, or transposition flaps depending on the availability of adjacent tissue. A full thickness skin graft is often appropriate for anterior lamella defects without an ideal adjacent flap site. Ideal donor sites involve non-hair-bearing sites such as the same or adjacent upper eyelid if the patient has sufficient dermatochalasis. The second preferred donor site is healthy retroauricular tissue. If that is unavailable, other hair-free donor sites may be considered including preauricular, supraclavicular, or inner arm skin.

## Lower Eyelid Marginal Defects

Full thickness defects involving one fourth or less of the horizontal length of eyelid margin are oftentimes repaired by direct closure. This provides a continuous eyelash line and the best cosmetic result. If there is a significant amount of tension or distraction of the lateral canthus, a superiorly directed canthotomy and cantholysis at the inferior limb of the lateral canthal tendon allows 2–4 mm more advancement. Care must be taken to ensure the tarsal edges are cut perpendicular to the margin of the eyelid for proper alignment. Squaring of the tarsus and lid margin from the original defect may be necessary. The tarsus is approximated with a 6-0 polyglactin (Vicryl) suture in robust bites from just beneath the skin to the deep tarsus. Care must be taken to ensure proper alignment of the eyelid margin. A 6-0 or 7-0 silk suture is used to realign the lashes and skin, incorporating long tails into each subsequent inferior knot to ensure that the knots do not abrade the cornea. Alternatively, especially in children in whom future suture removal is difficult, 7-0 or 8-0 plain or chromic gut suture is used for anterior lamellar closure with compact knots and suture ends cut on the knot (**Figure 10-5**). Rearrangement of residual excess skin (dog ears) is performed as necessary along relaxed skin tension

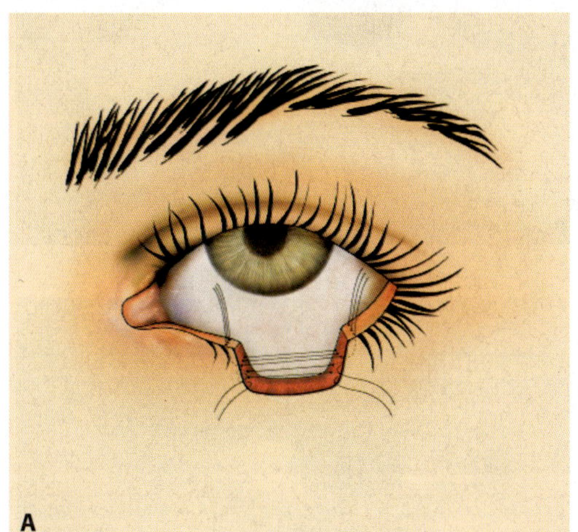


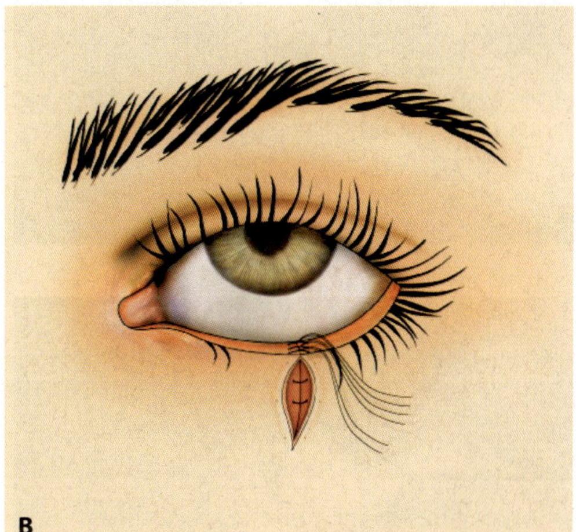


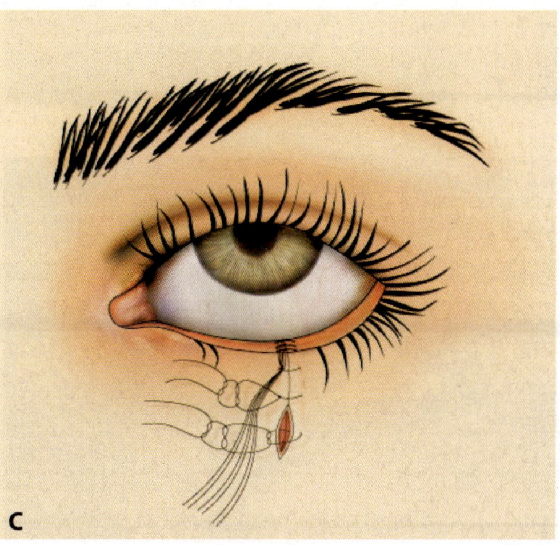


**Figure 10-5.** Full-thickness lid margin repair showing appropriate wound construction and closure.

lines. Marginal sutures are removed 10–12 days postoperatively as needed.

Full thickness defects involving one quarter to one half of the lower or upper eyelid margin usually require advancement of lateral tissues via a Tenzel-type semicircular advancement flap from the lateral canthus. As before, the tarsal edges of the defect are squared as necessary to allow proper alignment. For lower eyelid reconstruction, an initially nearly vertical incision is made upward through the lateral canthus, curving toward the lateral brow. It is generally not necessary to curve the flap around in a full semicircle, and the total length of the canthotomy incision is usually only 10–12 mm. When sharply dissecting beneath the orbicularis muscle and leaving the muscle undisturbed except for the canthotomy incision, the inferior limb of the canthal tendon is lysed in an *en glove* fashion. The flap is elevated in a submuscular plane. Cautery is limited on the flap to ensure proper vascular supply. The flap is undermined inferiorly and laterally until the cut edges of tarsus are reapproximated without excess tension (**Figure 10-6**). The eyelid margin defect is repaired as noted previously. The canthal angle is reformed with a Vicryl suture passing through the upper limb of the canthal tendon near the canthal angle, through the periosteum, then through the orbicularis muscle in the advancement flap lateral to

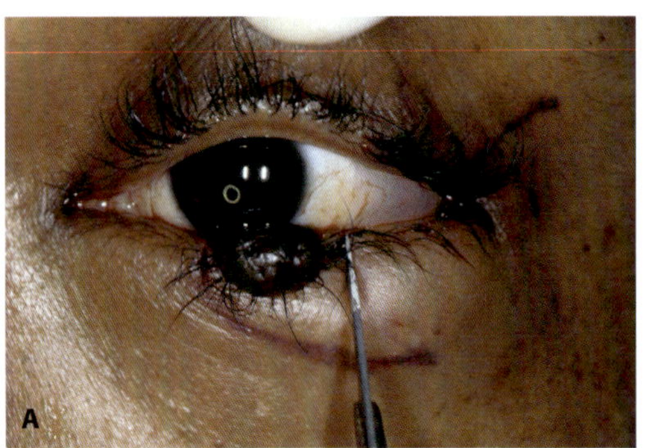


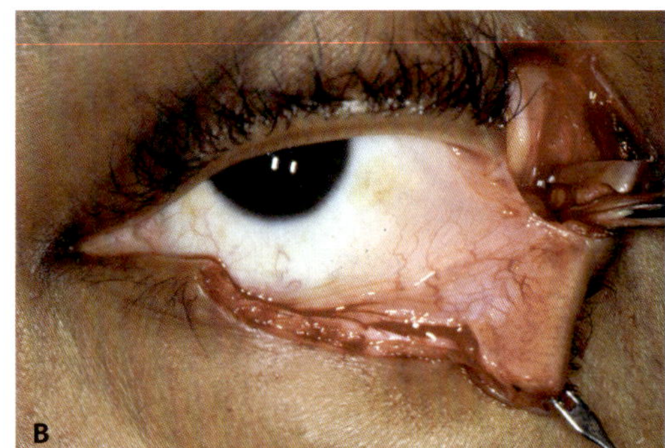


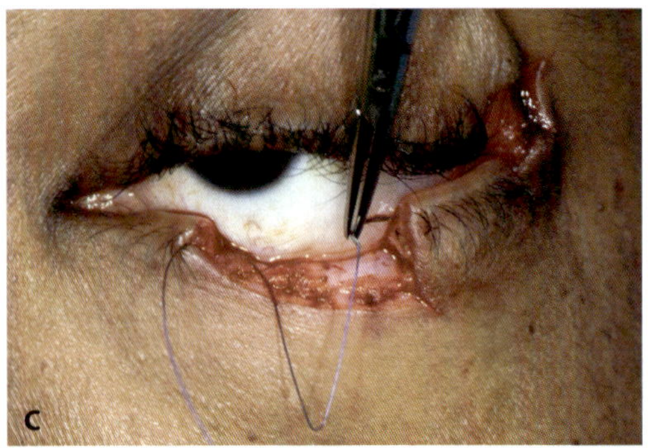


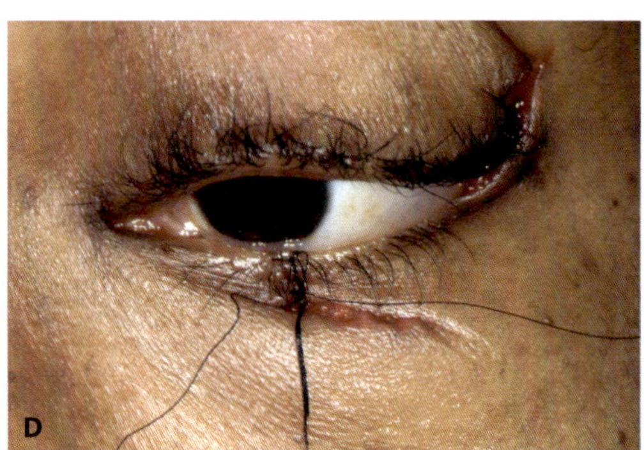


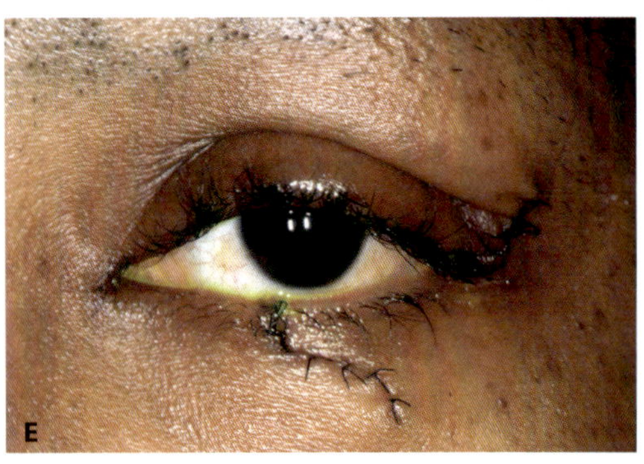


**Figure 10-6.** Modified lateral advancement flap for lower eyelid reconstruction. The lateral canthal incision is rearranged into the upper eyelid crease as necessary to rearrange redundant skin.

the original canthal angle. Redundant tissue is rearranged with Burrow's triangles laterally.

Defects in the lower eyelid involving more than 50% of the eyelid margin are more challenging with fewer options. With a preexisting lax eyelid, an advancement flap may be used for defects up to three fourths of the eyelid margin. The traditional approach to repairing these large full thickness lower eyelid defects is to perform an eyelid sharing procedure such as the Hughes tarsoconjunctival flap. This procedure involves transversely incising the tarsus of the upper eyelid, leaving the inferior 2.5–3 mm for upper eyelid stability. The upper eyelid tarsus is released as a conjunctival-based flap that is advanced into the defect of the lower eyelid and sutured to the residual medial and lateral tarsus of the lower lid and inferiorly to the conjunctival border. Proper flap construction with recession of the Müller's muscle is essential to prevent postoperative eyelid malposition or retraction. A full thickness skin graft or an advancement skin flap is placed covering the anterior lamella defect (clinical photos or a diagram is available—contact the author). The eye is occluded by the flap, and the flap is opened 3–6 weeks later. Another option to consider, especially for monocular or poorly sighted patients, is to harvest a free tarsal graft from the opposite eyelid and advance an adjacent vascularized skin flap. A transposition flap from the upper or lower eyelid is also an option in this case.

## Upper Eyelid

Full thickness marginal defects of the upper eyelid are similar to lower eyelid defects with some specific caveats. Defects up to one quarter of the eyelid are repaired with direct closure as previously described for the lower eyelid. The tarsal plate is much higher vertically, so care should be taken to extend the vertical incision the full height of the tarsus, squaring the edges. Furthermore, the tarsal sutures must not extend through the conjunctiva to avoid corneal abrasion during healing. Residual dog ears are rear ranged in the upper eyelid along the eyelid crease to conceal the incision.

Larger defects of the upper lid (33–50%) are repaired by performing a lateral canthotomy and cantholysis of the upper limb of the canthal tendon or extending this with an upper lid version of a semicircular flap for more advancement. Defects larger than 50% of the eyelid margin, although rare, are challenging. Reconstructive options include creating a Hughes tarsoconjunctival flap transposed medially or laterally in the same lid if there is enough remaining tarsus, or use of a free tarsal graft from the opposite upper eyelid with a vascularized flap to the anterior lamella. A Cutler–Beard-bridged pedicle flap may be advanced from the lower eyelid, but this is usually reserved as a last option, as functional and aesthetic outcome is often suboptimal.

## Lateral Canthus

Small lateral canthal defects are often repaired by advancing the remaining stump of lower or upper eyelid to fixate at the periosteum near Whitnall's tubercle. If the marginal defect is too large to advance, or there is no remaining nearby tarsus, a strip of periosteum is elevated from the lateral orbital rim and zygoma to attach to the remaining tarsus medially. Larger defects require the reconstruction of one lamella with a flap and typically the other with a graft, as described for large marginal eyelid defects.

## Medial Canthus

The medial canthus is structurally the most complicated area of eyelid, which makes it a challenging area to reconstruct. Small anterior lamella defects may be allowed to granulate, but this may lead to webbing or hypertrophic scarring that is aesthetically unacceptable. Smaller defects of one or both eyelids extending into the medial canthus are repaired by advancing adjacent eyelid with canthal tendon fixation. In deeper defects lacking a periosteum, a drill hole may be necessary through the bone of the anterior lacrimal crest for suture fixation of the medial eyelid and canthus. Attempts should be made to direct the repair posteriorly to recreate the natural position of the posterior limb of the canthal tendon. Alternatively, a microplate can be run vertically from the maxilla and frontal bone or anterior-posteriorly from the nasal bone to appropriately position suture attachment of the reconstructed canthus.

Large deep defects may require a glabellar flap or median forehead flap for reconstruction. These flaps are reserved for situations when other options are not available, as thicker skin is transferred into the eyelid area. Although these flaps may be cosmetically undesirable, they are necessary to provide a good functional outcome in certain cases.

## Lacrimal Drainage System

Canalicular lacerations and defects occur with trauma or as a result of excision of skin cancers in the medial canthal area. A canalicular laceration should be suspected with avulsion-type injuries. Any laceration or incision of the eyelid margin medial to the punctum should raise suspicion for a canalicular laceration. To identify the location of laceration, a Bowman probe is passed through the canaliculus. Lacerations found deeper and more medial are often associated with medial canthal ligament trauma requiring a challenging repair. Reconstruction of the canalicular system is performed in a timely manner (preferably within 24 hours) to increase the likelihood of success. Lacrimal drainage function is adequate in most cases of trauma or with small surgical defects with appropriate repair.

Canalicular reconstruction is performed by most surgeons under general anesthesia. Afrin spray is instilled in the nose preoperatively and the inferior turbinate is packed with cottonoids soaked in Afrin or 4% cocaine solution. A silicone lacrimal stent (Crawford, FCI Ophthalmics) is first passed through the punctum and retrieved through the cut end of the canaliculus. The medial cut end of the canaliculus is located and the stent is passed through the cut end, into the lacrimal sac, and then down the nasolacrimal duct. The stent is retrieved in the nose beneath the inferior turbinate, preferably using a specialized Crawford hook. A pig-tailed probe or fluorescein irrigation through the opposite canaliculus may help to locate the cut end in difficult situations. The other half of the stent is passed through the opposite canaliculus and also retrieved in the nose. A square knot tie is placed in the stent and the position checked. The stent is secured intranasally with a polyglactin (Vicryl) or gut suture to the lateral nasal sidewall to prevent prolapse, if needed. Alternatively a monocanalicular stent (Monoka, FCI Ophthalmics) may be passed through just the lacerated canaliculus. The stents are removed after 3–6 months.

The only option for complete canalicular loss is a conjunctivodacryocystorhinostomy with insertion of a Jones tube to allow for tear drainage. This is often delayed until the patient has healed from other reconstruction and/or trauma. In cases of malignancy, it is best to ensure that there is no concern about residual or recurrent tumor before proceeding in creating a tract between the orbit and the nose. If there is any significant risk of recurrence, surgery is delayed.

## Periocular Reconstruction

The options for the repair of nonmarginal periorbital defects are generally more intuitive to the non-ophthalmic surgeon. Factors to consider include defect location, size, and availability of adjacent tissue. Direct closure is an excellent option for small defects when similar skin types are opposed, assuming that there is minimal vertical tension. Full thickness skin grafts in the lower eyelid usually heal well and have an excellent tissue match when harvested from retroauricualar areas, upper eyelid, and supraclavicular or medial arm skin.

Flaps are very commonly used in periorbital reconstruction. Final cosmesis is optimal when similar tissue is approximated and incisions are placed appropriately along relaxed skin tension lines. Common flaps in the periocular area include advancement flaps where tissue is undermined and brought together to close a linear defect **(Figure 10-7A)**, rotational flaps in which tissue is advanced to fill a defect , and transposition flaps that involve transfer over normal tissue to fill a defect **(Figure 10-7B)**.

Flap types with particular utility in periocular anterior lamella reconstruction include the rhombic flap **(Figure 10-8)**, glabellar, median forehead, Mustarde, and bilobed flaps. Opposing island pedicle flaps are useful in reconstructing small- to medium-sized defects that span the junction of the eyelid–cheek aesthetic units.

## Postoperative Care

Postoperatively, patients are instructed to ice their incisions for up to 48 hours. After that time, a warm, wet washcloth soak helps to keep the incisions clean and is soothing. Patients are instructed to use an ophthalmic antibiotic ointment three to four times a day for up to 2 weeks on the incision and in the eye as necessary, especially if there is any ocular irritation or lagophthalmos.

Patients continue normal ocular medications (glaucoma drops) and lubricant eye drops (artificial tears) as needed. Anticoagulants are generally resumed directly after surgery unless there is persistent postoperative bleeding. Patients are also prescribed a light narcotic if necessary, although pain is generally minimal in the periorbital area and most patients obtain excellent relief with acetaminophen alone.

## Ocular Issues

### *Dry Eye/Exposure Keratitis*

It is important to inquire about dry eye symptoms prior to surgery. A Schirmer's test may provide

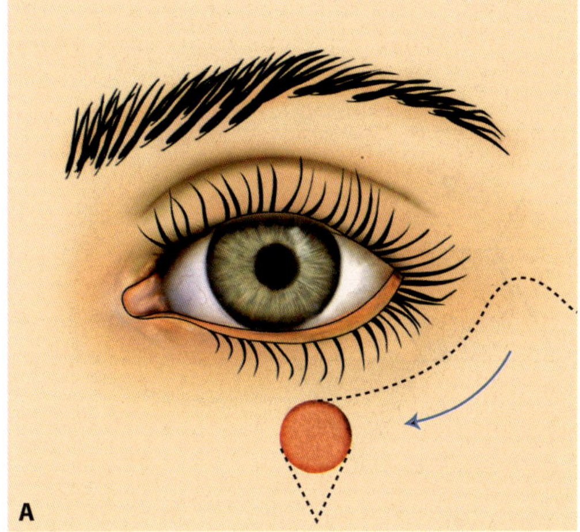


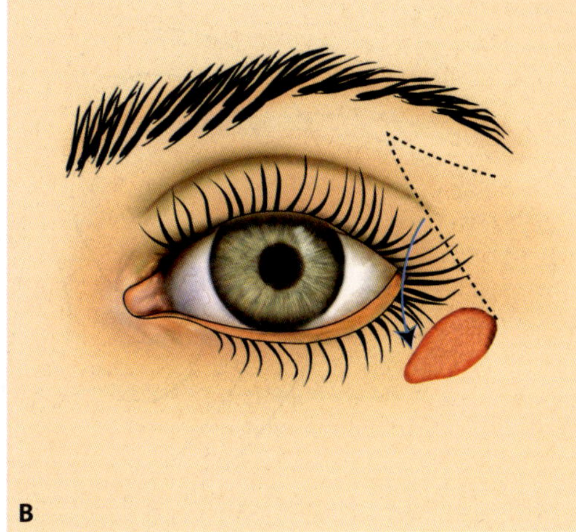


**Figure 10-7.** (A) Advancement along the relaxed skin tissue lines allows closure of a lower eyelid defect without vertical tension. (B) Laterally situated defects are amenable to a transposition flap from the upper eyelid.

objective data on tear production. Reconstructive surgery may worsen dry eye signs and symptoms temporarily or permanently. Exposure keratopathy may occur if there is lagophthalmos. The routine use of an ophthalmic ointment in the eye for the first 24 hours postoperatively and at night along with artificial teardrops during the day lessens the severity of signs and symptoms in patients prone to these complaints. Rarely do patients need to continue ocular lubrication indefinitely.

### *Restrictive Strabismus*

Reconstructive surgery may rarely be a source of temporary or permanent diplopia. If the conjunctiva is not adequately reconstructed, symblepharon or scar tissue may cause a restrictive strabismus limiting ocular versions. Adequate conjunctival lining of the eyelids and eye socket are necessary to allow for normal ocular versions. Restrictive strabismus may respond to symblepharon lysis and mucous membrane grafting as previously described. Sutures in Tenon's fascia or a rectus muscle may limit motility resulting in postoperative diplopia.

## Revision Surgery

In most cases, definitive therapy is performed during the initial reconstruction. With very large defects or in areas of recurrence where adjacent tissue is limited, final reconstruction may be delayed or staged. Flaps such as the Hughes tarsoconjunctival flap or median forehead flap require an expected second stage to divide and inset the flap.

# Eyelid Malpositions

## Ectropion

Ectropion after periocular reconstruction may be secondary to involutional, cicatricial, paralytic, or mechanical forces. Older patients generally have laxity of the eyelid prior to surgery. A canthoplasty suture placed at the time of surgery may prevent future ectropion. A tarsal strip procedure usually improves the lid position if an involutional ectropion develops. After larger reconstructions, it is common to have an orbicularis paresis that improves without intervention. Permanent facial nerve damage is uncommon in reconstruction of the periorbital area and significant permanent orbicularis weakness is rare. Cicatricial ectropion is common after eyelid reconstruction due to residual vertical tension. This may respond to a Z-plasty or secondary flap placement but usually will require a full thickness skin graft to the eyelid.

### *Lid Retraction*

Eyelid retraction after periorbital reconstruction is often secondary to scarring at the level of the orbital septum. The orbital septum is never repaired or sutured to prevent eyelid retraction. Repair requires release of this scar tissue and usually a posterior or anterior spacer graft to prevent recurrence.

### *Canthal Malposition*

Canthal malpositions usually are due to inferior displacement of the canthus. The lateral canthal angle

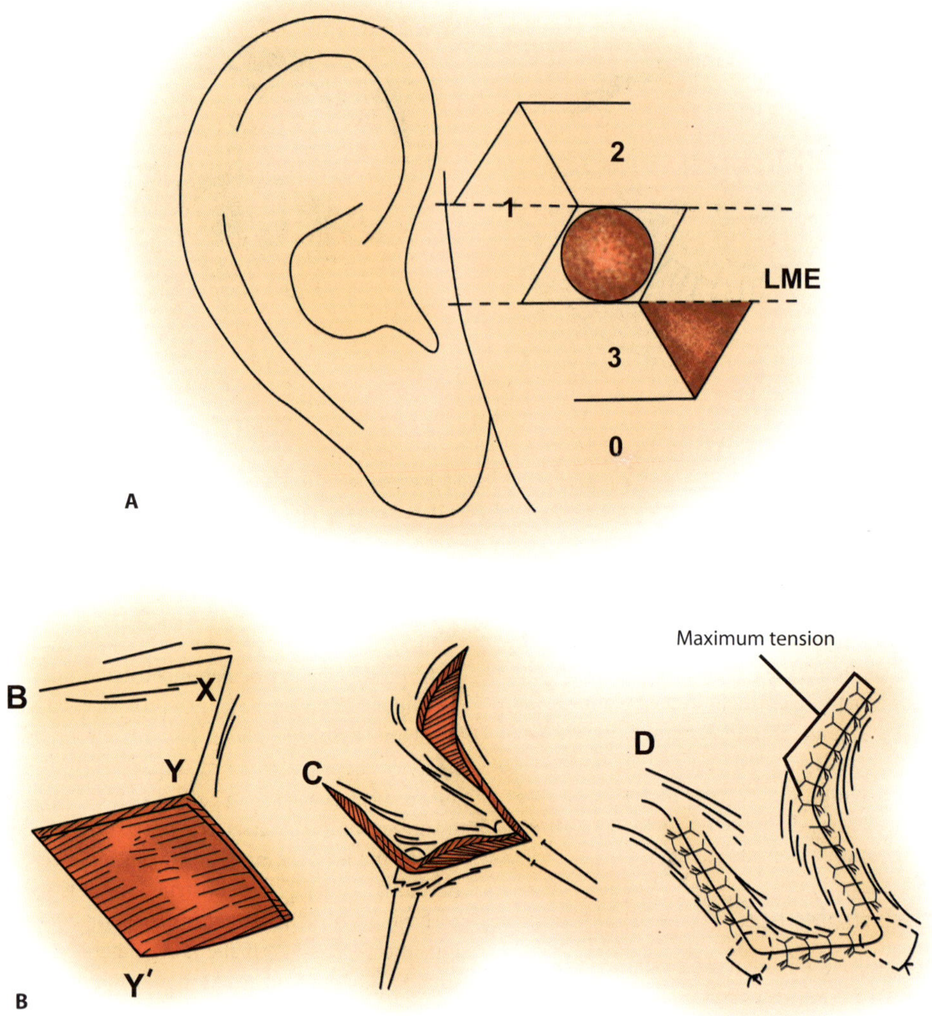


**Figure 10-8.** The Limberg Rhomboid flap has tremendous utility in the periocular area. (A) Ovoid skin defect allows multiple orientations of the flap. (B) Flap is elevated with closure of the donor site and carefully inset.

is naturally 1–2 mm superior to the medial canthus, and this is accounted for with lateral canthal reconstruction. The medial canthus is very challenging to repair and when the medial canthal tendon is deficient, care must be taken to reform and reattach superiorly and *posteriorly.* Revision will usually require a more complex reconstruction with periosteal or bony fixation.

## *Prominent Scar*

Incisions in the periorbital area usually heal very well due to the highly vascular tissues. Healing is enhanced by good wound design and closure, as well as timely removal of nonresorbable sutures. Skin sutures are removed between days 6–8, with the exception of eyelid margin sutures, which remain in place for 10–12 days. However, wound contracture may occur and full thickness skin grafts often hypertrophy and contract to some extent as they heal. Reassurance, massage, and time improve scarring. Occasionally, a steroid injection is necessary to relax scar tissue beginning 4–6 weeks postoperatively. Small amounts (0.05–0.2 ml) of triamcinolone 5 mg/ml are injected intradermally. Rarely is scar revision necessary, and techniques including direct excision and closure, Z-plasty, V–Y-plasty, or M-plasty may be useful.

## Conclusion

Optimal reconstruction in the periorbital area is enhanced by proper understanding of the anatomy and functional demands of this region. Proper reconstructive planning and execution enhance the function and cosmesis of the repair. Optimal outcomes are desirable, as vision and comfort are dependent on eyelids and adjacent structures.

## References


1. Nerad JA. Eyelid reconstruction. In *Oculoplastic Surgery, The Requisites*, Mosby, St. Louis, 2001, pp. 282–311.
2. Stephenson CM, Brown BZ. The use of tarsus as a free autogenous graft in eyelid surgery. *Ophthal Plast Reconstr Surg* 1985, 1, 43–50.
3. Cohen MS, Shorr N. Eyelid reconstruction with hard palate mucosa grafts. *Ophthal Plast Reconstr Surg* 1992, 8(3), 183–195.
4. Wenkel H, Rummelt V, Naumann GO. Long term results after autologous nasal mucosal transplantation in severe mucus deficiency syndromes. *Br J Ophthalmol* 2000, 84, 279–284.
5. Tseng SC, Di Pascuale MA, Liu DT, Gao YY, Baradaran-Rafii A. Intraoperative mitomycin C and amniotic membrane transplantation for fornix reconstruction in severe cicatricial ocular surface diseases. *Ophthalmology* 2005, 112, 896–903.
6. Howard GR, Nerad JA, Kersten RC. Medial canthoplasty with microplate fixation. *Arch Ophthalmol.* 1992 ;110: 1793–7.
7. Custer PL, Vick V. Repair of marginal eyelid defects with 7–0 chromic sutures. *Ophthal Plast Reconstr Surg* 2006, 22, 256–258.
8. Jordan DR, Anderson RL, Holds JB. Modifications to the semicircular flap technique in eyelid reconstruction. *Can J Ophthalmol* 1992, 27, 130–136.
9. Patrinely JR, O'Neal KD, Kersten RC, Soparkar CN. Total upper eyelid reconstruction with mucosalized tarsal graft and overlying bipedicle flap. *Arch Ophthalmol* 1999, 117, 1655–1661.
10. Leone CR Jr. Periosteal flap for lower eyelid reconstruction. *Am J Ophthalmol* 1992, 114, 513–514.
11. Della Rocca DA, Ahmad SM, Della Rocca RC. Direct repair of canalicular lacerations. *Facial Plast Surg* 2007, 23, 149–155.
12. Patrinely JR, Marines HM, Anderson RL. Skin flaps in periorbital reconstruction. *Surv Ophthalmol* 1987, 31, 249–261.
13. Jordan DR, Anderson RL. The lateral tarsal strip revisited. The enhanced tarsal strip. *Arch Ophthalmol* 1989, 107, 604–606.

# 11

# Scalp Reconstruction

Michael J. Brenner, MD, FACS

## Introduction

The need for scalp reconstruction most commonly arises from malignancy, trauma, infection, or burns. The limited elasticity of the scalp, coupled with the potential for sizable defects, makes repair particularly challenging. Due to the fibrous character of the galea, scalp flaps tend to be relatively indistensible and usually require a large surface area of dissection relative to the size of defect. The anatomy of the scalp is also distinctive in that it possesses a convex surface, has hair-bearing regions, and serves as the sole coverage for the cranium. Given these considerations, each rung of the reconstructive ladder has a role in successful reconstruction of scalp defects. With careful surgical planning and execution, even large and complex defects may be managed successfully. This chapter presents the surgical anatomy of the scalp, analysis of the various types of scalp defects, and the range of techniques that may be used for repair.

## Facial Analysis

### Surgical Anatomy

#### *Overview*

The scalp extends in the anteroposterior dimension from the supraorbital margin to the superior nuchal line and extends transversely on either side through the frontal process of the zygoma, along the zygomatic arch, and to the mastoid process. The anatomic layers of the scalp are shown in (**Figure 11-1**) and are easily remembered by the mnemonic "SCALP," corresponding to **s**kin, sub**c**utaneous tissue, galea **a**poneurotica and muscle, **l**oose areolar tissue, and **p**ericranium. The outermost layer of the scalp consists of skin and subcutaneous tissue. There is no natural plane of cleavage between these layers, which contain hair follicles, sebaceous and sweat glands, and other integumentary structures. Fibrous attachments exist between this layer and the underlying galea aponeurotica, or musculoaponeurotic layer. The galea consists of fibrous tissue extending from the frontalis muscle anteriorly to the occipitalis muscle posteriorly and laterally becomes the temporoparietal fascia. Deep to the galea is subgaleal fascia, consisting of loose areolar tissue. The deepest layer of the scalp is the pericranium, the periosteal layer of the calvarium. The neurovascular and muscular anatomy of the scalp is shown in (**Figures 11-2, 11-3, and 11-4**).

#### *Vascular Anatomy*

Although the scalp has a rich vascular supply, the surgeon should consider the course of the principal arterial supply to maximize flap viability. The external carotid artery is the dominant blood supply to the scalp, via the superficial temporal, posterior auricular, and occipital arteries. The contribution of the internal carotid system includes the supraorbital and supratrochlear arteries. This vascular network has abundant anastomotic connections, although connections are more limited across the midline. As a result, flaps extending well across the midline may benefit from delay. A Doppler probe may prove helpful in identifying the vascular supply. Because many arterial branches run within the galea and temporoparietal fascia, the subgaleal plane of dissection is often used. Under the galea is a loose layer of areolar tissue known as the subgaleal fascia, which can be elevated as a separate, fine layer of vascularized tissue. Deep to the subgaleal fascia, the periosteum is tightly adherent to the cranium and possesses its

*(Text Continued on page 114)*

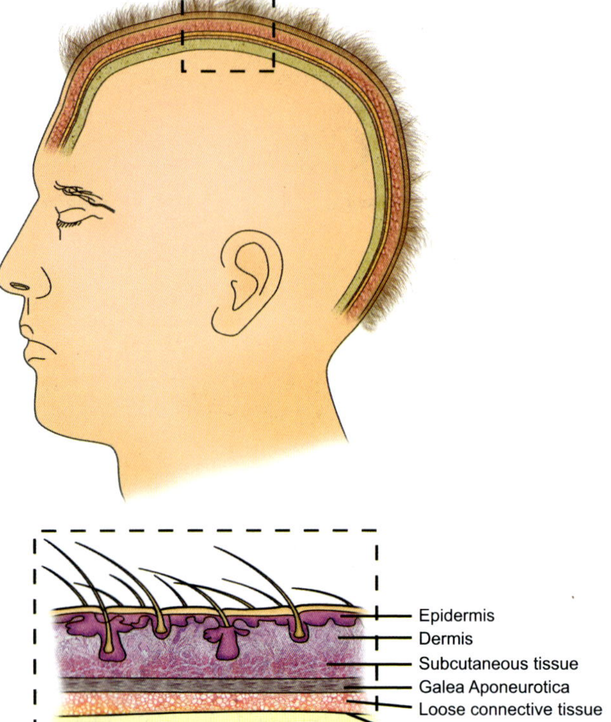


**Figure 11-1.** Scalp layers. The anatomic layers of the scalp may be easily remembered by the mnemonic "SCALP," corresponding to skin, subcutaneous tissue, galea aponeurotica and muscle, loose areolar tissue, and pericranium.

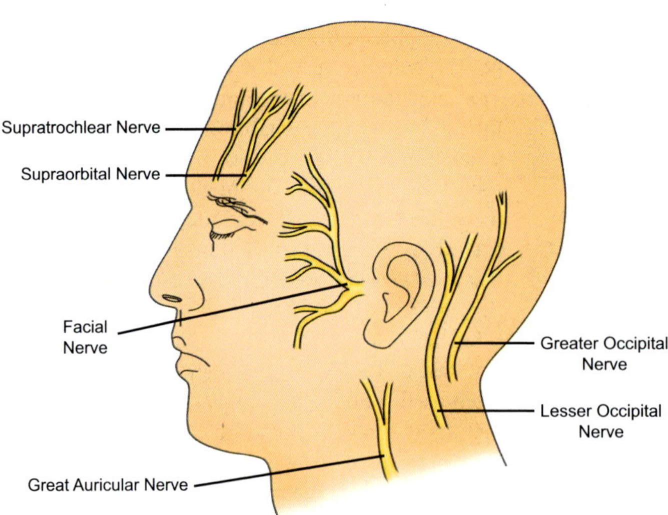


**Figure 11-2.** Neural anatomy of the scalp.

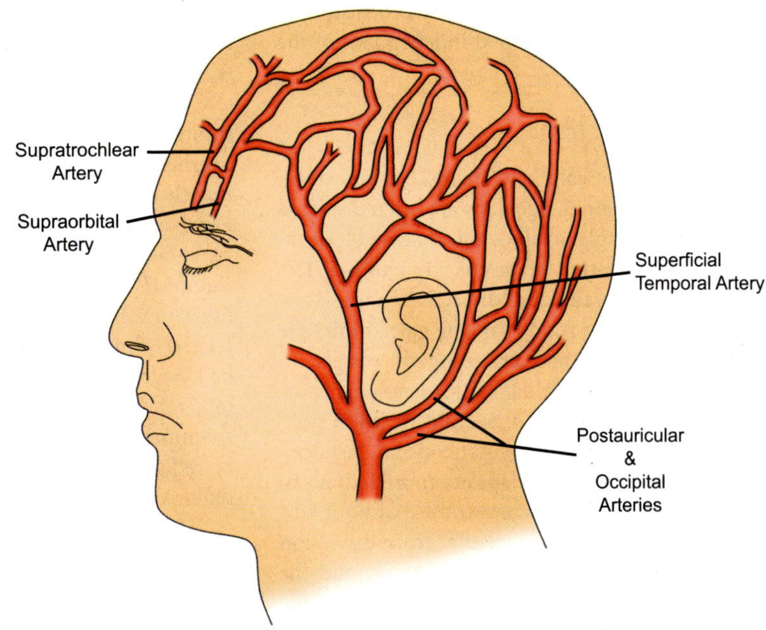


**Figure 11-3.** Vascular anatomy of the scalp.

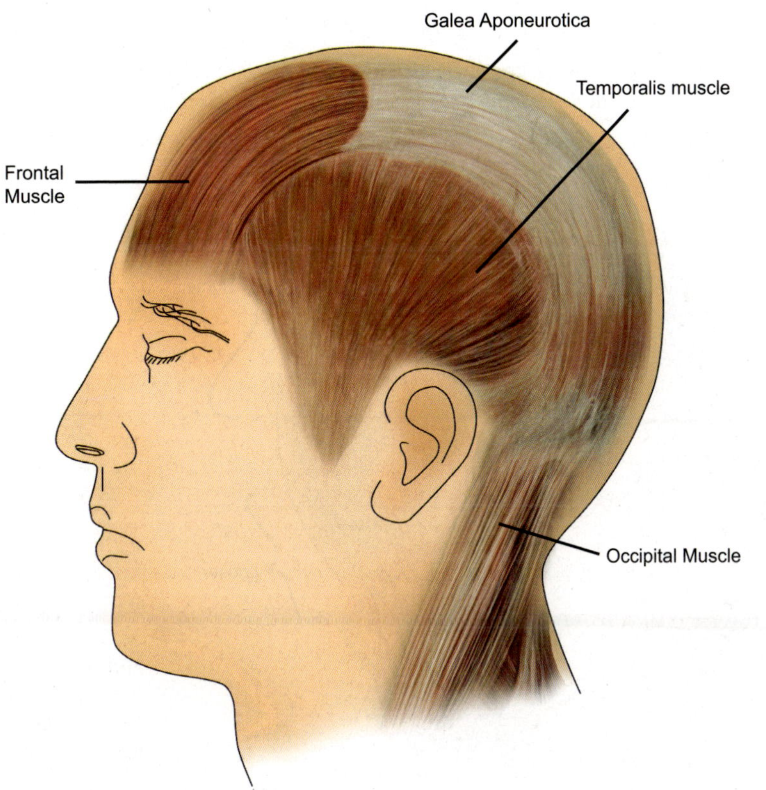


**Figure 11-4.** Muscular anatomy of the scalp.

own vascular supply. As a result, flaps consisting of periosteum may be developed independent of the overlying scalp tissues.

## Planes of Dissection

The layers of the scalp lend themselves to certain planes of dissection. Large flaps are often dissected in the subgaleal plane, allowing for ease of elevation and preservation of vascularity and hair follicles. Another advantage of dissection in this plane is that the intrinsic rigidity of the galea limits the stretching, torsion, and crimping of vessels. In contrast, subcutaneous flaps afford no such protection, requiring sharp dissection in a less anatomic plane within the subcutaneous fat, just deep to the hair follicles. Such flaps are more tedious to elevate and may involve compromise of both hair follicles and flap vascularity either from dissection or from efforts to maintain hemostasis amid the numerous small vessels encountered. Laterally, the temporoparietal fascia may be raised as a pedicled flap or used as a free flap based on the superficial temporal artery, taking care to remain posterior to the frontal branch of the facial nerve.

## Regional Scalp Mobility

Although the scalp is thick and inelastic compared to other areas in the head and neck, its mobility is variable across different regions of the scalp, as shown in (**Figure 11-5**). The tight region of the scalp has a dense galeal layer, no underlying muscle, and poor distensibility. The galea becomes thinner in those portions of the scalp where it overlies muscle, both laterally over the temporalis muscle as well as posteriorly below the nuchal line. For example, flaps incorporating the temporoparietal fascia of the lateral scalp are associated with significantly greater mobility than those that span the vertex. Because flaps are more distensible in the relatively loose regions of the scalp, flaps can often be designed over the underlying musculature to repair smaller defects. In contrast, large flaps, often spanning several different regions of the scalp, may be required to repair defects that involve the tight regions of the scalp.

## Motor Nerve Anatomy

To avoid injury to the frontal branch of the facial nerve during scalp reconstruction, the surgeon must have a solid understanding of the anatomy of temporal-parietal region, which is illustrated in coronal section in (**Figure 11-6**). The temporal branch of the facial nerve and the superficial temporal artery both run within the temporoparietal fascia. The temporoparietal fascia is the lateral extension of the galea. The temporalis fascia is deep

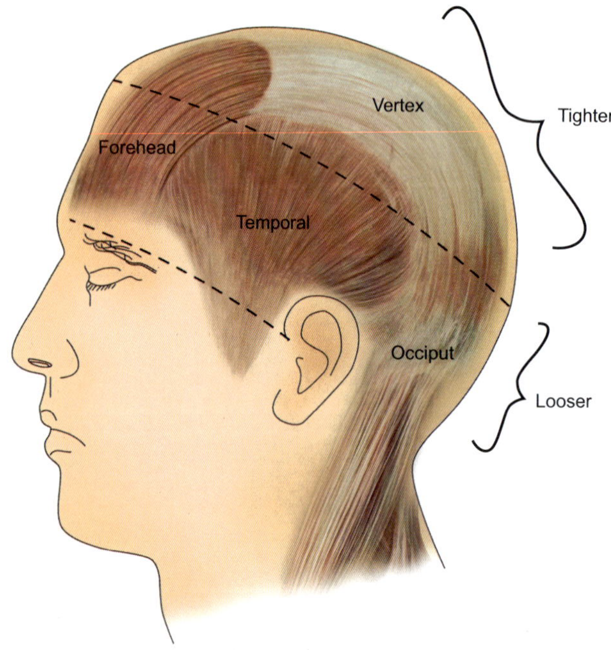


**Figure 11-5.** Tight and loose regions of the scalp. Although the scalp is thick and inelastic compared to other areas in the head and neck, there is more mobility across areas of the scalp with underlying muscle.

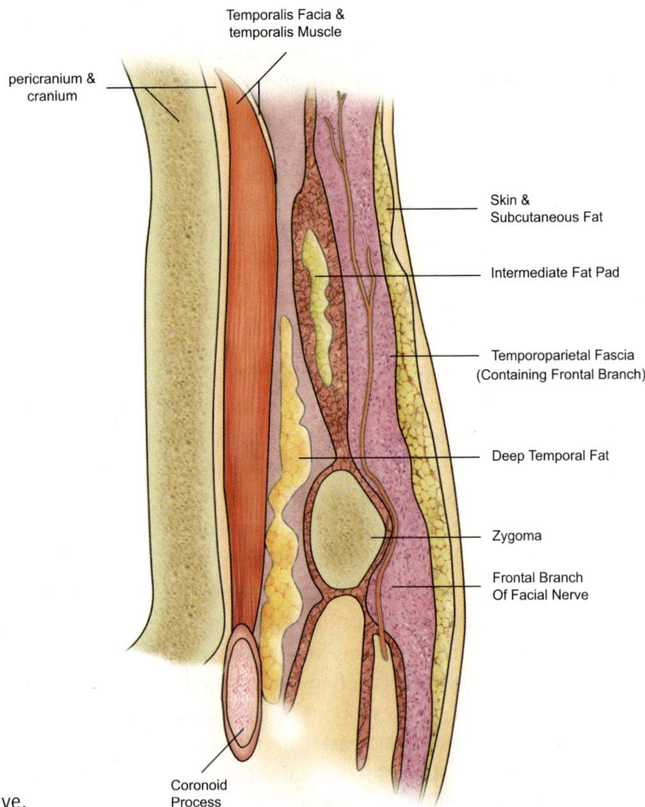


**Figure 11-6.** Anatomy of the temporal region and frontal branch of the facial nerve.

to this layer. A few centimeters above the zygomatic arch, this fascial layer splits to encase the temporal fat pad. Incision of the fascia and dissection within this fat pad predisposes to temporal atrophy but does allow for protection of the frontal branch. For this reason, this plane of dissection is common when raising bicoronal flaps to avoid injury to the frontal branch. At the level of the zygomatic arch, there is fusion of the temporoparietal fascia, superficial layer of the temporalis fascia, and periosteum into a single dense layer. The frontal branch is most vulnerable to injury at this site where the branch passes over the arch on its way to the frontalis and corrugators forehead muscles.

### *Sensory Nerve Anatomy*

Branches of the trigeminal nerve provide sensory innervation to the scalp. Injury to these nerves by transection, traction, or cautery may be associated with numbness, itching, or paresthesias. Although some degree of denervation is often inevitable with scalp flap reconstruction, consideration of this anatomy minimizes morbidity. The supraorbital nerve traverses the supraorbital region through either a supraorbital notch or foramen, extending superiorly up the forehead and anterior scalp. The supratrochlear nerve passes through the corrugators muscle to provide sensation to the central forehead. The temporal, auricular, and occipital sensory nerves provide sensory innervation to the lateral and posterior scalp.

## Evaluation of the Defect

### *Achieving Functional Closure*

The primary objective of scalp reconstruction is to provide stable coverage of the cranium. The size, depth, and location of the defect are all of critical importance. Small defects may be amenable to primary closure or secondary healing, whereas intermediate to large defects are more likely to require local tissue rearrangement or more extensive reconstruction. If the periosteum has been lost and there is substantial bone exposure, flap reconstructions are often preferable to skin grafting due to lack of a vascular bed. Due to the inelasticity of the scalp, scalp flaps are usually large relative to the size of the defect. These flaps tend to tolerate more wound closure tension than flaps elsewhere on the face. If a bony defect is present, consideration should be given to cranioplasty. The location of the defect over a tighter or looser area of the scalp will also affect the size of the flaps required to achieve an acceptably low tension closure.

### *Achieving Aesthetic Reconstruction*

The secondary objectives of scalp reconstruction involve restoring scalp contour, maintaining the hairline, and restoring aesthetic boundaries. Replacing like tissue with like is desirable whenever possible,. For example, when performing reconstruction for a resected region of the hair-bearing scalp, the surgeon should consider whether adjacent hair-bearing tissue may be transposed into the defect. Particular attention is given to the position of the anterior hairline, which can often be preserved with appropriate flap design, as depicted in (**Figure 11-7**). Respecting the aesthetic subunits of the forehead decreases the risk of an unsightly patchwork appearance. One should also consider the effect of reconstruction on nearby mobile structures, such as the hairline and the brow. Tissue expansion can prove helpful as an adjunct procedure if there is a stable wound; this requirement is less likely to be met in the case of a fresh wound resulting from surgical resection or trauma. Preferences of the patient are an important factor. Some patients may have little concern for the cosmetic aspects of the procedure, as long as a functional reconstruction is achieved. In such cases, there may be greater flexibility in the reconstructive approach.

## Preoperative Considerations

### Patient Characteristics

Individual patient characteristics inform the reconstructive approach. For example, the patient who is unwilling or unable to tolerate a prolonged duration with scalp expanders is not a suitable candidate for controlled tissue expansion. Prior external-beam radiation therapy or scarring from prior scalp incisions will also limit reconstructive options, particularly if important vascular pedicles have been transected during previous surgery. Similarly, diabetes, smoking, hypothyroidism, and cachexia all profoundly affect wound-healing capacity. To the extent that the adverse effects of these predictors of poor wound healing can be mitigated, the likelihood for successful reconstruction improves. When impaired healing is anticipated, extra care should be taken to widely undermine flaps to minimize tension across the closures. There is poor tolerance of tissues for ischemia at the distal tips of flaps. One approach to decreasing tension is to skin graft the donor site scalp defects that are secondarily created by flap rotation.

## Techniques

### Healing by Secondary Intention

When scalp defects are allowed to heal by secondary intention, wound healing proceeds more slowly than in other areas of the head and neck.

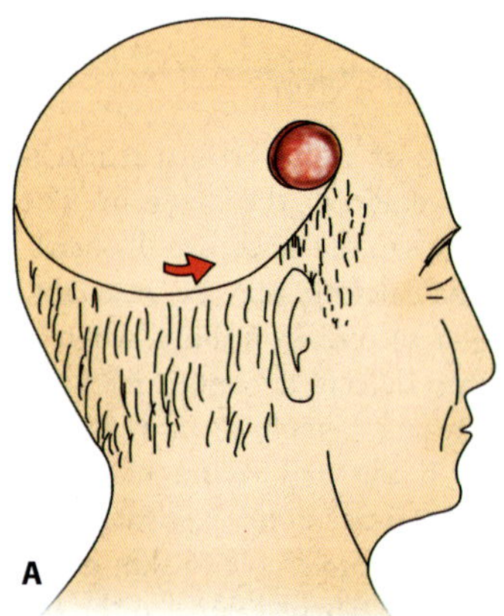


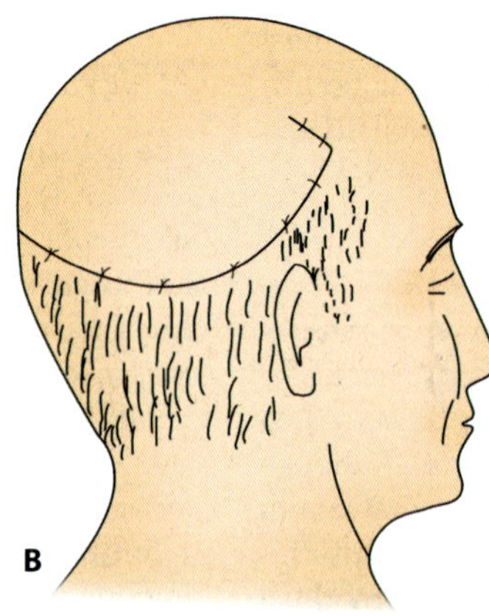


**Figure 11-7.** Preservation of the anterior hairline. The anterior hairline is an important aesthetic landmark that can often be preserved with appropriate attention to flap design. (A) Scalp defect and flap design. (B) Reconstructed scalp.

This delay occurs because of the inelastic nature of the scalp's galeal layer, which resists wound contracture. Before opting to proceed with healing by secondary intention, the surgeon should consider whether the final result is likely to be satisfactory. The healed area will not be hair bearing, and the epithelialized surface will usually be very thin with a far greater susceptibility to injury and breakdown than the surrounding scalp. Healing by secondary intention is most likely to be successful when the pericranium is preserved, but it may still require several weeks of attentive wound care. In some nonirradiated patients, granulation tissue will gradually extend over areas of bare bone given sufficient time; however, granulation over bare bone from the periphery of the defect is time consuming and tedious for patients with uncertain prospects for success. If the decision is made to attempt healing by secondary intention over bone, burring down the outer table of the cranium to expose the diploic space will promote formation of granulation tissue. In selected patients, this approach yields acceptable results.

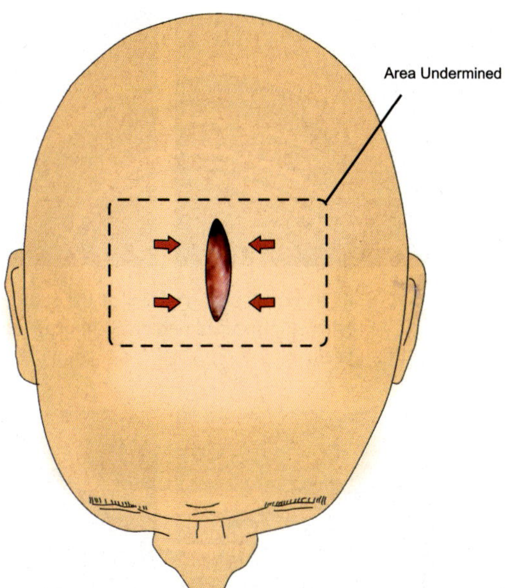


**Figure 11-8.** Primary closure of a midline scalp wound. Generous undermining in the subgaleal plane facilitates closure. The galea aponeurotica, rather than the skin of the scalp, should bear most of the tension on the closure to minimize the risks of wound dehiscence, scarring, and alopecia.

## Primary Wound Closure

Although scalp elasticity varies with age and between individuals, the general dictum is that primary wound closure is best reserved for defects of the scalp that are 3 cm wide or less. In order to accomplish primary closure, generous undermining in the subgaleal plane is performed, as depicted in (**Figure 11-8**). After adequate undermining, the defect is closed with the galea bearing most of the tension on closure. This approach substantially decreases the tension across the skin closure, conferring benefits of decreased risk of dehiscence, less scarring, and reduced risk of alopecia.

## Skin Grafting

### *Skin Grafting Alone*

Split thickness skin grafting is an important tool in treatment of scalp defects, but it generally provides less satisfactory aesthetic and functional results than flap repair when used alone. Skin grafts provide a far less robust buffer to injury and everyday wear and tear than does the normal scalp. For example, skin grafts are quite susceptible to trauma, may be painful, and are often too fragile for use of a hairpiece. Skin graft reconstruction of the scalp is particularly fraught with problems when it is attempted over bare bone or when postoperative radiation therapy is necessary. In addition to these significant functional considerations, the grafts are not hair bearing, are associated with contour deformity, and are often unsightly. Nonetheless, skin grafts do have a reliable take when the pericranium is present, and they are appropriate as a sole reconstruction in selected patients. Such an approach is best suited for patients who are poor candidates for a local flap reconstruction and who are accepting of a less than optimal aesthetic outcome. One of the preferred locations for use of a skin graft is in the repair of a scalp defect involving the vertex in a balding patient. Clinical examples of skin grafting of scalp defects are shown in (**Figures 11-9** and **11-10**).

### *Skin Grafting as an Adjunctive Technique*

Despite its limitations as a "stand-alone" technique, split thickness skin grafting is quite versatile as part of a larger reconstructive approach. For example, skin grafts serve a valuable role as temporary scalp coverage while preparations are being undertaken for either expansion or free

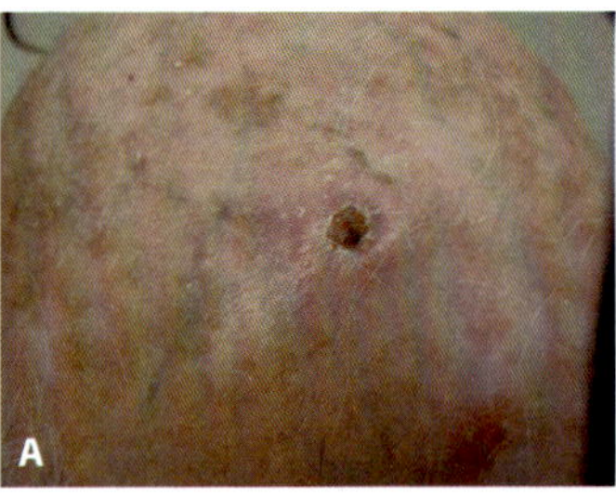
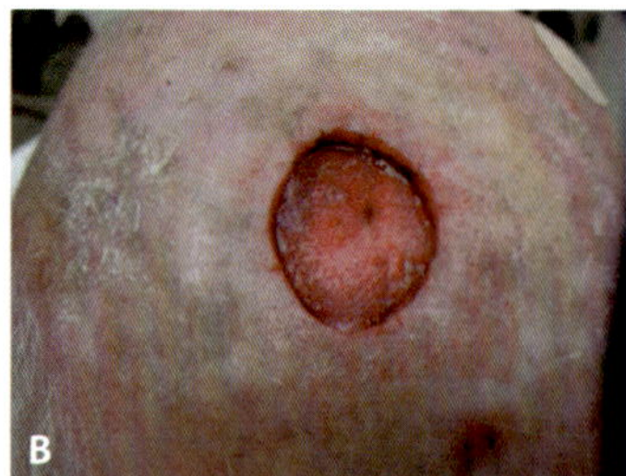
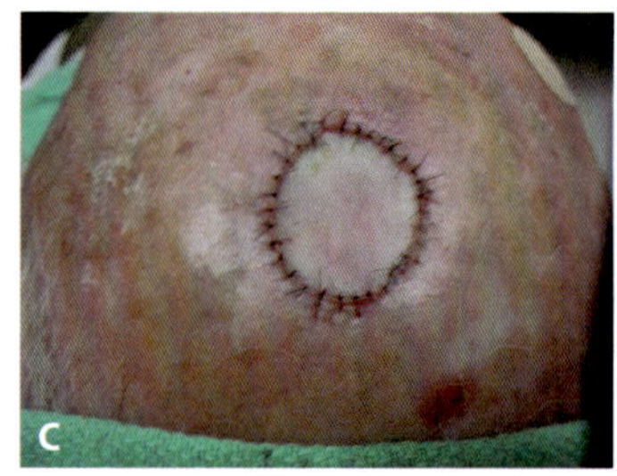

**Figure 11-9.** Split thickness skin grafting of the scalp vertex. (A) Original lesion. (B) Defect after Mohs resection. (C) Freshly skin-grafted defect. Skin grafting is most frequently performed in the vertex region in patients with alopecia.

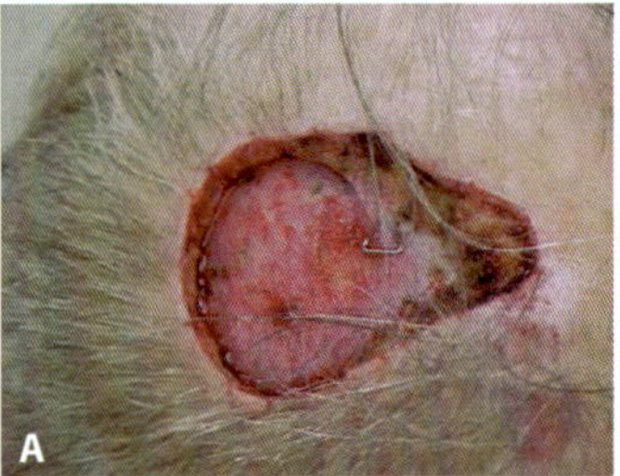
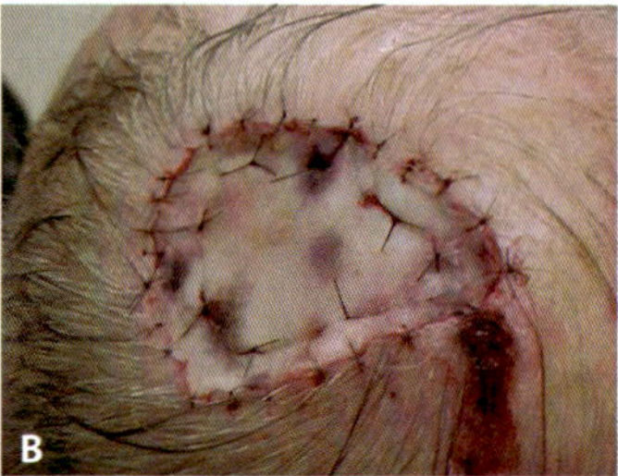
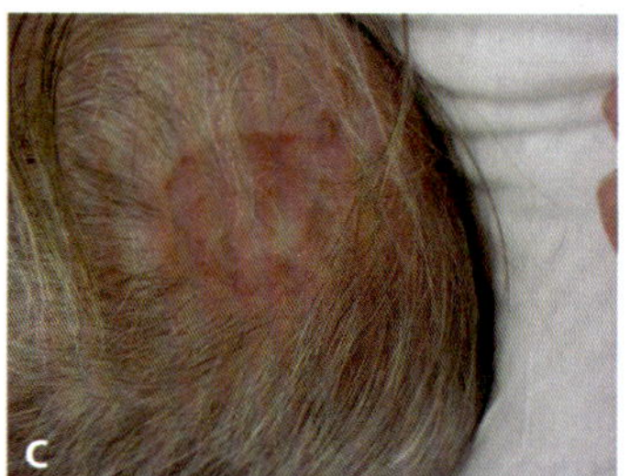

**Figure 11-10.** Split thickness skin grafting of the hair-bearing scalp. (A) Defect after Mohs resection. (B) Freshly skin-grafted defect. (C) Result at follow-up shows successful take of graft, although there is persistent alopecia and the grafted site remains fragile and susceptible to trauma.

flap reconstruction. Skin grafting should also be considered when there is a high risk of local recurrence. Once an adequate waiting period has elapsed, more definitive reconstruction may be undertaken. Skin grafts are effective for resurfacing temporoparietal fascia flaps or latissimus free flap reconstructions for extensive scalp defects. Skin grafts are also useful in closure of secondary defects after flap closure of a defect. These secondary donor site defects can often be camouflaged in relatively inconspicuous sites with careful flap design or, alternatively, are later removed by serial excision. Exposure of the diploic space allows for a bed of granulation to develop and may be helpful in the setting of a denuded cranium.

## Local Flaps

### *Overview*

Hosts of local tissue rearrangements for scalp reconstruction have been described. These approaches have included various permutations of rotational, advancement, and transposition flaps both alone and in combination. Larger flaps with broad bases are generally preferable to smaller flaps given the relative inelasticity of the scalp. Unlike other areas of the face, the scalp does not have relaxed skin tension lines to camouflage incisions. Therefore, the placement of incisions is most influenced by the position of the anterior hairline and the need to maintain vascularity with maximal tissue recruitment. The use of large flaps and generous undermining of the surrounding scalp serves to distribute wound closure tension over a wide area. In some cases, a secondary defect may be created by the local flap. This defect may be covered with a skin graft and, if desired, excised at a subsequent point once the scalp has healed.

If the scalp defect involves the anterior hairline, the flap should be designed to restore the natural hairline. It is helpful to bevel incisions at the hairline to facilitate growth of hair through the incision, thereby camouflaging the scar. Incisions within the hair should be made parallel to the hair follicles and electrocautery used discreetly to minimize alopecia. Atraumatic handling of tissue, particularly at the distal tip of the flap, will minimize the risk for focal flap ischemia, breakdown, and unsightly scars. Flap inset is facilitated by suturing the leading border first. Often a back-cut along the

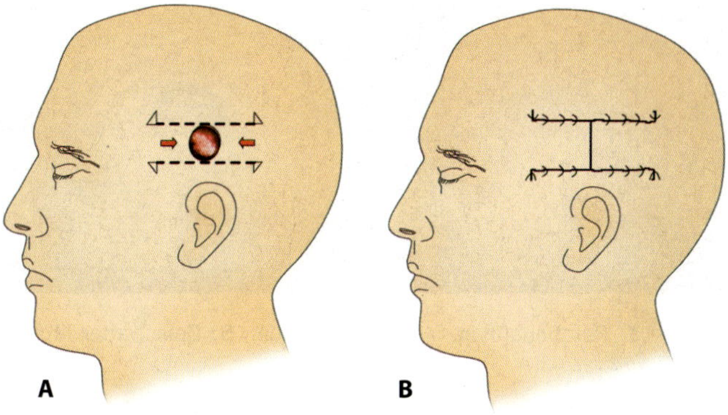

**Figure 11-11.** Bilateral advancement flaps. Advancement flaps are most useful in the lateral scalp, where there is favorable mobility. Flaps may be used as single or bilateral flaps. (A) Scalp defect and flap design. (B) Reconstructed scalp.

base of the flap will serve to reduce tension; however, this maneuver has the adverse effect of narrowing the base of the flap. Such relaxing incisions must be made judiciously, so that flap perfusion is not compromised. As a general rule, it is usually preferable to leave standing cutaneous deformities to maximize vascularity of the flap. Many such deformities resolve spontaneously and, if persistent, are easily removed at a later point.

## Scalp Advancement Flaps

Advancement flaps are most useful in the lateral scalp, where there is greater mobility than over the vertex. Two opposing advancement flaps may be combined to facilitate reconstruction, as shown in (**Figure 11-11**). In addition, wide undermining and advancement of opposing edges of scalp tissue is routinely performed during primary closure of the scalp. Some scalp advancement flaps incorporate varying degrees of rotation, as shown in (**Figure 11-12**). Due to the inelastic nature of most of the scalp, advancement flaps have a relatively limited role in scalp reconstruction when compared to elsewhere in the face. Advancement flaps are most practical for small lateral defects, usually less than 3 cm. Galeal relaxing incisions may be used to facilitate stretch; however, this added stretch inevitably comes at the expense of an increased tendency for ischemia of the distal aspect of the flap edge.

## Single Rotational Flaps

Rotational flaps have proven the most useful and versatile reconstructive option for the majority of scalp defects. A clinical example of a rotational flap closure is shown in (**Figure 11-13**). The natural convexity of the scalp is well suited to the curvilinear incisions used in rotation flaps. Furthermore, contour of the anterior hairline often lends itself to flaps that follow the hairline, thereby camouflaging scars. In most cases, the flap and the surrounding scalp are widely undermined in the subgaleal plane in order to minimize tension along the line of closure. Advantages of these flaps include favorable cosmesis, ability to replace hair-bearing defects

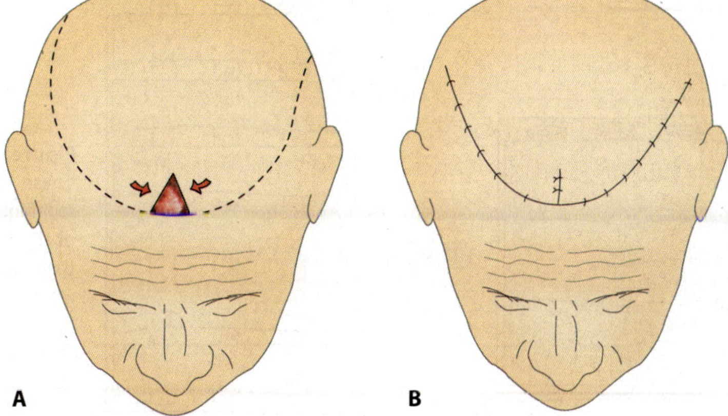


**Figure 11-12.** Combined rotation and advancement flaps. (A) Scalp defect and flap design. (B) Reconstructed scalp.

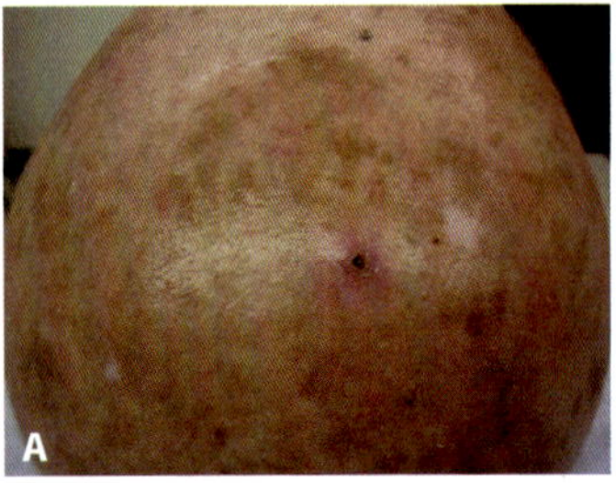


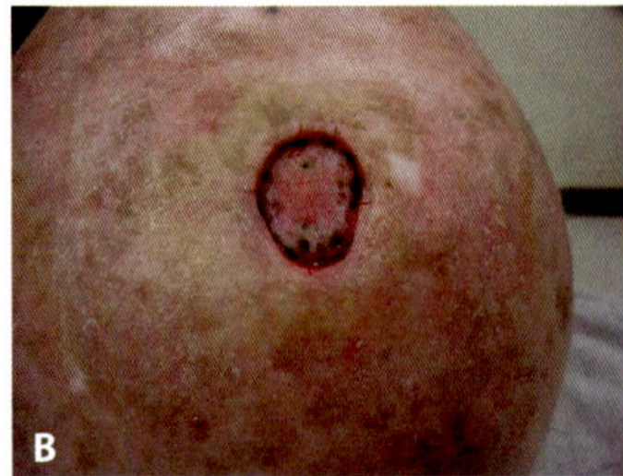


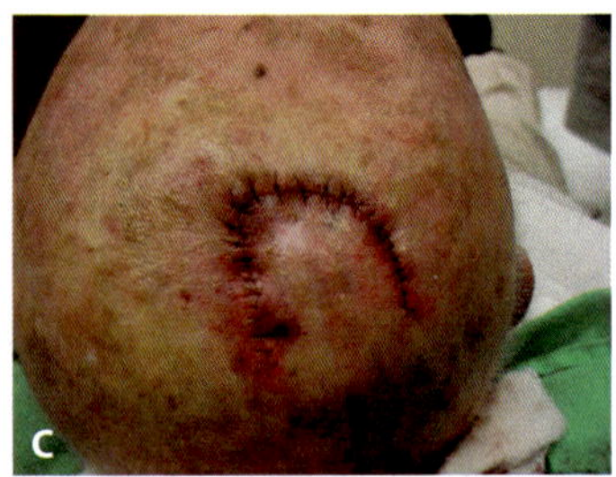


**Figure 11-13.** Rotational flap. (A) Original lesion. (B) Defect after Mohs resection. (C) Local flap reconstruction of scalp.

with hair-bearing scalp, and minimal donor site morbidity. The principal drawback is the potential to displace adjacent mobile structures, such as the eyebrow or hairline. Galeal relaxing incisions allow additional stretch, but they must be used with caution. Galeal-relaxing incisions may decrease vascularity either by direct vessel injury or by impairing the galea's natural protection of vessels against stretch and contortion, as shown in (**Figure 11-14**). The surface area of the flap is routinely far greater than that of the defect and may require a back-cut, as shown in the examples in (**Figure 11-15**).

## *Multiple Rotational Flaps*

Frequently, multiple rotational flaps are used simultaneously. The most commonly used technique involves use of two opposing rotational flaps that allow for an O-to-Z type closure of the defect, as shown in (**Figure 11-16**). These double flaps can be quite effective in the hair-bearing scalp (**Figure 11-17**), but they are especially well suited to the repair of large scalp defects of the inelastic and convex vertex (**Figure 11-18**). These more complex reconstructions distribute wound closure tension over a larger area of the scalp and allow for recruitment of scalp tissue from multiple donor areas, some of which may have greater elasticity (e.g., scalp covering the temporalis muscle and occiput). In addition, such flaps may decrease the need to span a large area of convex scalp. The disadvantage of using multiple flaps is the greater complexity of the flap design, which entails more incision with the potential for alopecia and greater interruption of scalp vascularity if planning is inadequate. A variety of configurations may be used, often involving two or three rotational flaps that are oriented in a pinwheel fashion and closed in a manner analogous to the iris of camera lens. An example of a three-flap pinwheel configuration is shown in (**Figure 11-19**).

## *Flaps Based on the Superficial Temporal Artery*

The temporoparietal fascia flap, based on the superficial temporal artery and vein, is a thin, pliable, and highly vascular flap. It has proven useful in

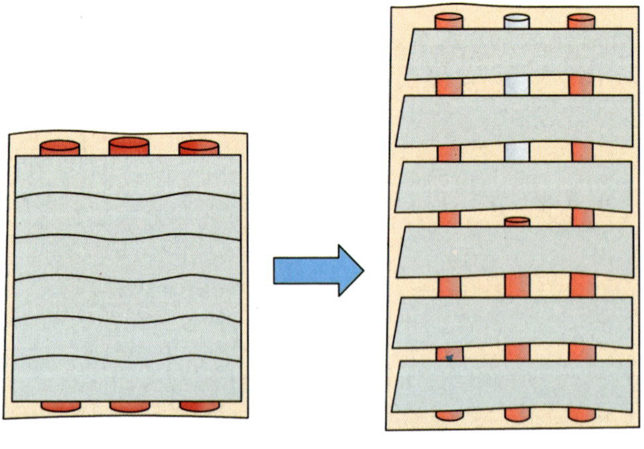

**Figure 11-14.** Galeal relaxing incisions. These incisions are a well-accepted technique for achieving additional stretch of the relatively indistensible scalp, but they must be used with caution. Galeal relaxing incisions have the potential to decrease vascularity both by direct vessel injury and by attenuating the galea's ability to safeguard vessels against excessive stretch and contortion.

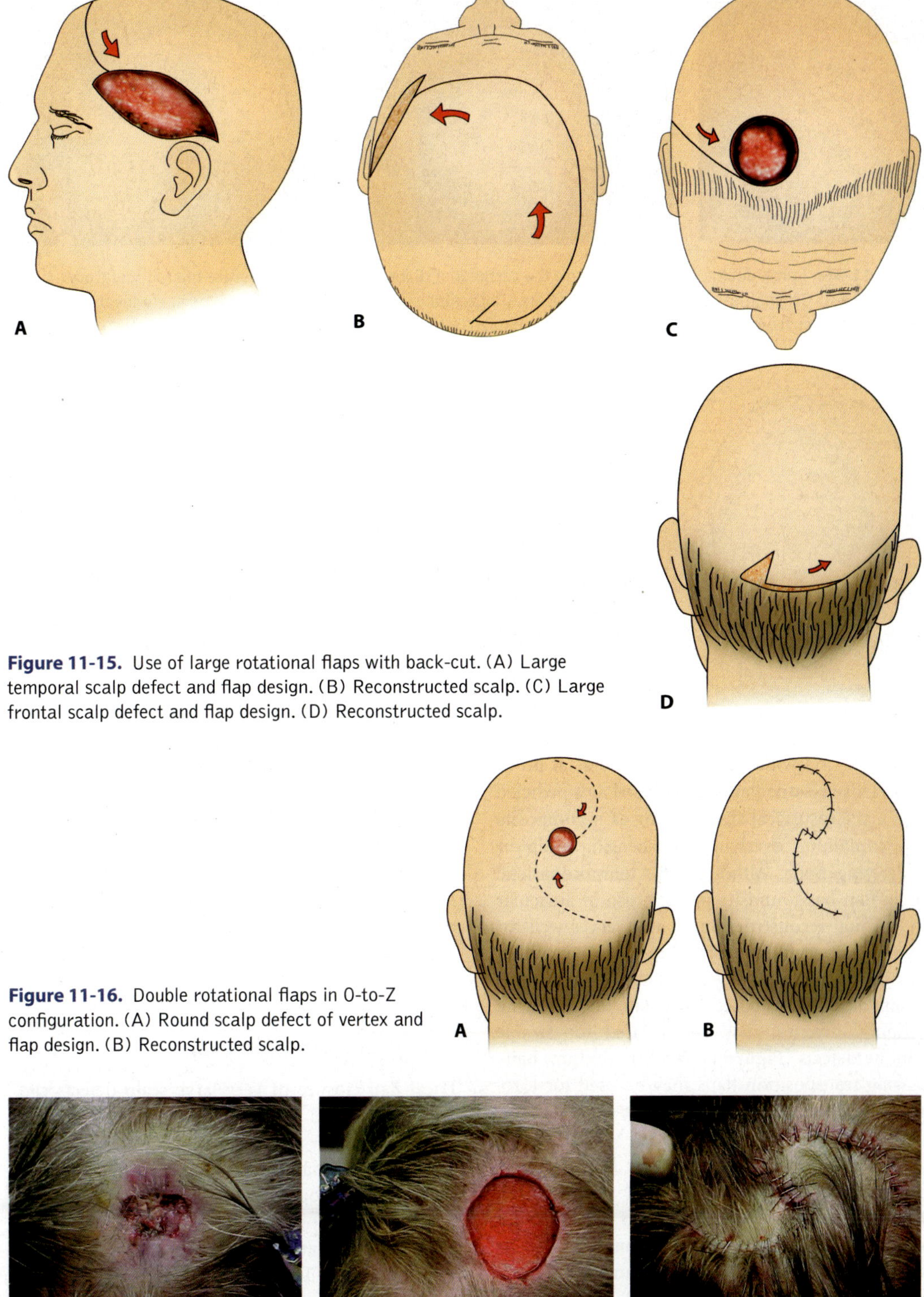

**Figure 11-15.** Use of large rotational flaps with back-cut. (A) Large temporal scalp defect and flap design. (B) Reconstructed scalp. (C) Large frontal scalp defect and flap design. (D) Reconstructed scalp.

**Figure 11-16.** Double rotational flaps in O-to-Z configuration. (A) Round scalp defect of vertex and flap design. (B) Reconstructed scalp.

**Figure 11-17.** Small double rotational flap in the hair-bearing scalp. (A) Original lesion. (B) Defect after Mohs resection. (C) Reconstruction of scalp.

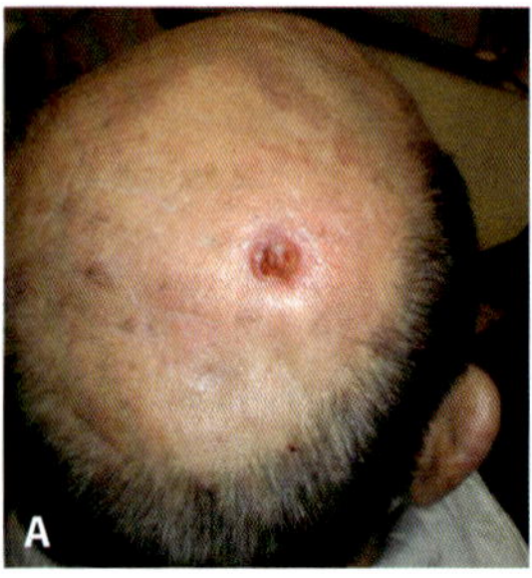

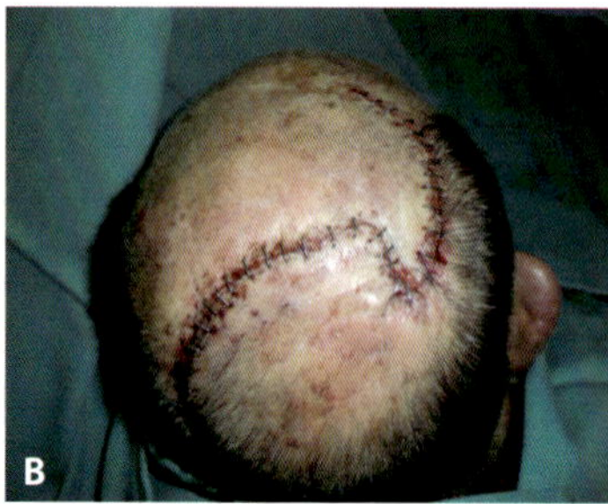

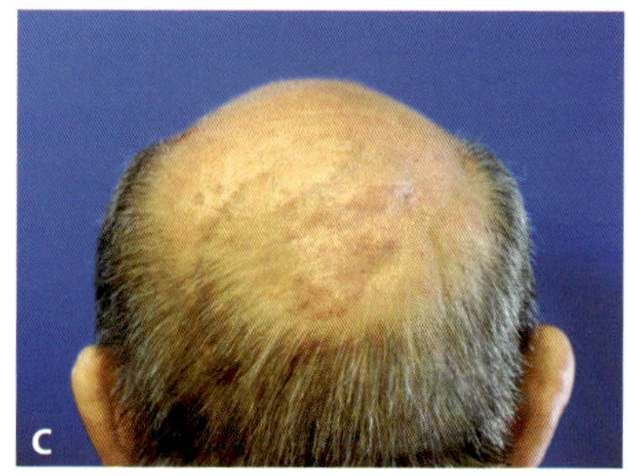


**Figure 11-18.** Large double rotational flap on the vertex in a diabetic patient with severe microcirculatory pathology. (A) Original lesion, which had significant subdermal extension. (B) Reconstructed scalp involved recruiting tissues from a wide region of scalp to minimize ischemia and tension. (C) Result at 6 weeks.

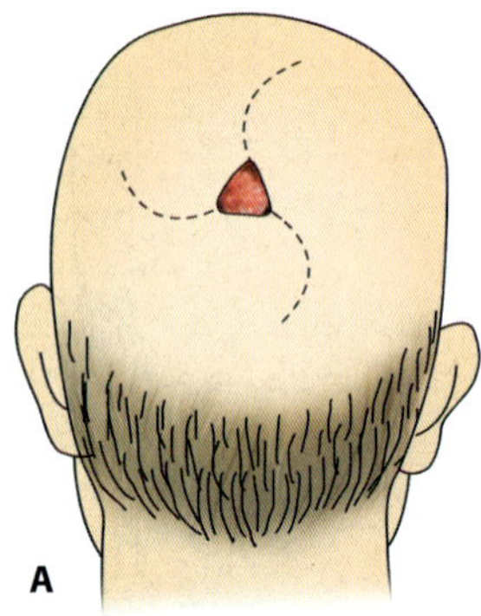

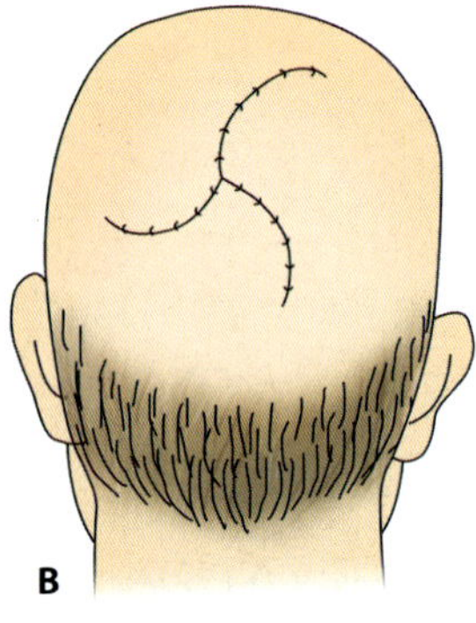


**Figure 11-19.** Pinwheel flap. (A) Triangular scalp defect of vertex and flap design. (B) Reconstructed scalp.

treatment of a wide variety of craniofacial problems. This versatile flap may be used as a pedicled flap, a microsurgical free flap, or as a composite flap containing overlying hair-bearing scalp or underlying bone. Although the temporoparietal fascia flap has found its greatest use in auricular and orbital reconstruction, it also serves well for a variety of scalp reconstructions. It may restore hair-bearing scalp or cover areas of exposed bone. A bipedicled flap, based on bilateral superficial temporal arteries, may be elevated for sizable midline defects (**Figure 11-20**). In addition, hair-bearing transposition flaps may be used for forehead and lip reconstruction (**Figure 11-21**).

A few technical considerations warrant mention. Because the vascular pedicle is tortuous, a Doppler probe is used to map the course of the superficial temporal artery prior to injection of a local anesthetic or creating incisions. The flap is usually based on the posterior branch of the superficial temporal artery to avoid injury to the frontal branch of the facial nerve and to preserve the anterior hairline. Alternatively, the flap may be based on the anterior branch or both branches of the artery, as well. The fascia-only temporoparietal flap provides a reliable means for covering exposed bone with highly vascular tissue that readily supports skin grafting. The flap is elevated in a plane just deep to the hair follicles to avoid alopecia. When planning a hair-bearing flap, the surgeon may wish to consider preoperative controlled tissue expansion of adjacent scalp to facilitate closure of the secondary defect.

## *Multiple transposition flaps*

Local flap closure of very large scalp defects can be accomplished by using a "banana peel" flap in which essentially the entire scalp is mobilized as a series of flaps that are transposed to resurface the scalp. This approach, first described by Orticochea (1971), allows for reconstruction of scalp defects up to approximately 100 $cm^2$ in appropriately selected patients. This approach is most useful for defects involving the anterior scalp and hairline and may be combined with controlled tissue expansion (**Figure 11-22**). The corresponding flaps for large posterior scalp defects have also been

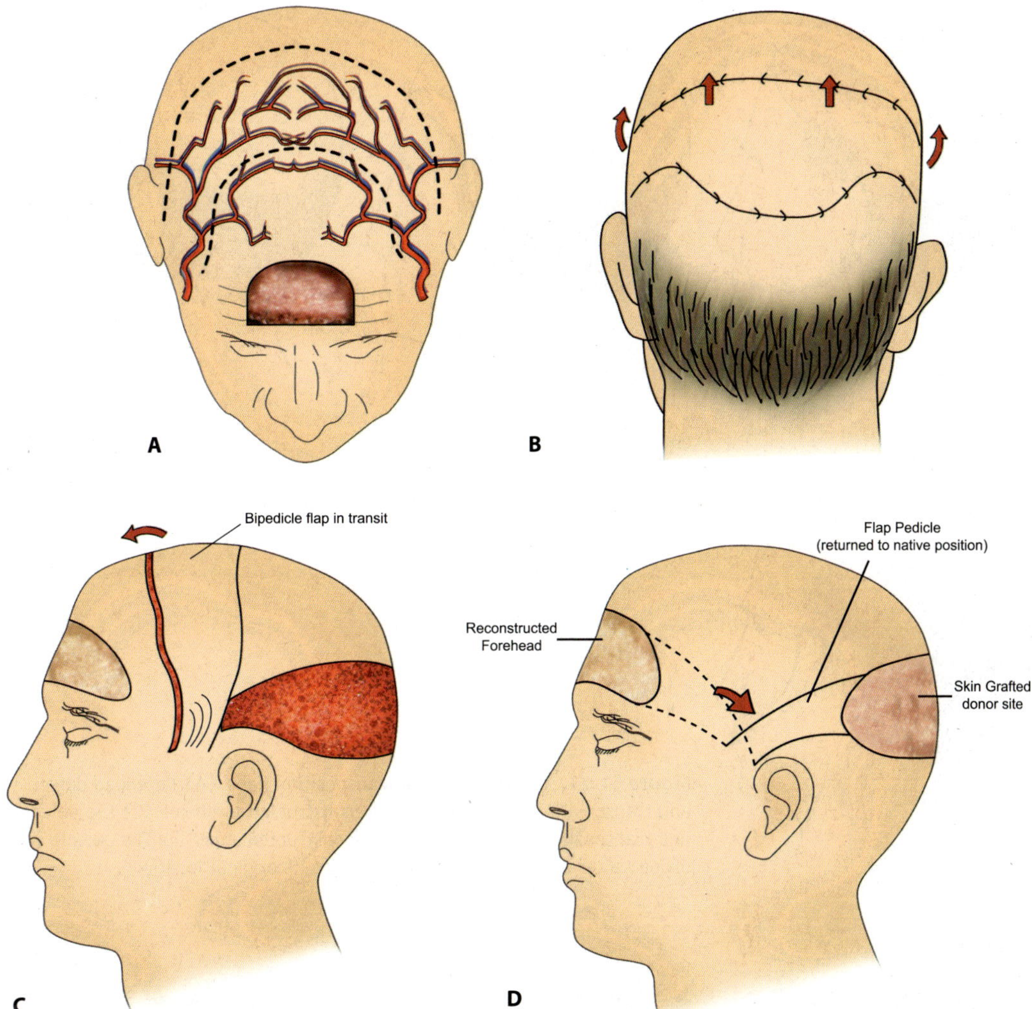


**Figure 11-20.** Bipedicled flap based on superficial temporal arteries for reconstruction of a large forehead defect. (A) Flap shown is based on the posterior branches of bilateral superficial temporal arteries. (B) Performing flap in delayed fashion improves vascularity of midline region. (C) Bipedicled scalp flap in transit, pivoting anteriorly toward forehead and then inset into defect. The posterior scalp defect is skin grafted. (D) After delay, bilateral pedicles are divided and returned to their native positions.

described **(Figure 11-23)**. Although this type of reconstruction has become less common with the advent of microvascular techniques, it continues to have a useful role in patients who either are not candidates for a prolonged anesthetic or who desire hair-bearing flaps and are not willing to undergo tissue expansion procedures (described subsequently). It warrants mention that recurrent disease will be difficult to identify beneath such complex reconstructions, and therefore it is best to delay repair if there is a question as to whether a persistent tumor may be present.

## Regional Flaps

Regional flaps are used relatively infrequently in scalp reconstruction due to the limited reach of their vascular pedicles. Nonetheless, several options may be considered for repair of defects involving the inferior occipital or temporal regions of the scalp. The most commonly used pedicled flaps include the latissimus dorsi, pectoralis major, trapezius, and splenius capitis flaps. The pedicled latissimus flap is passed through the axilla, allowing for correction of temporal and orbital defects.

*(Text Continued on page 132)*

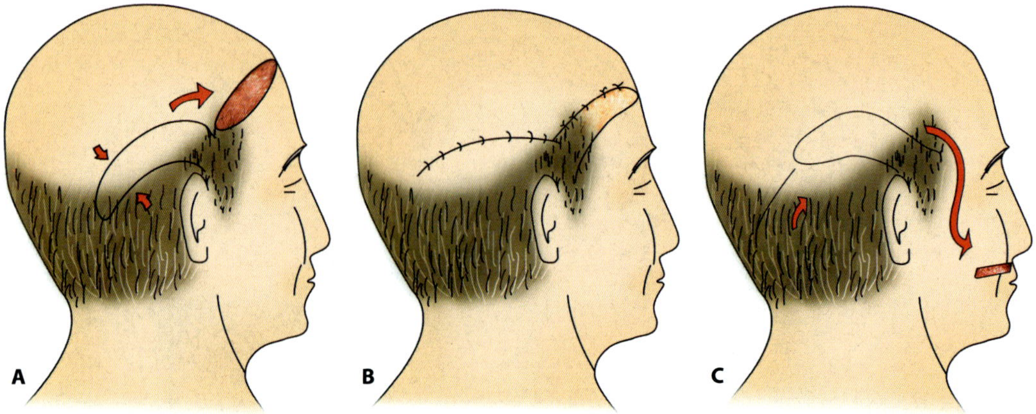

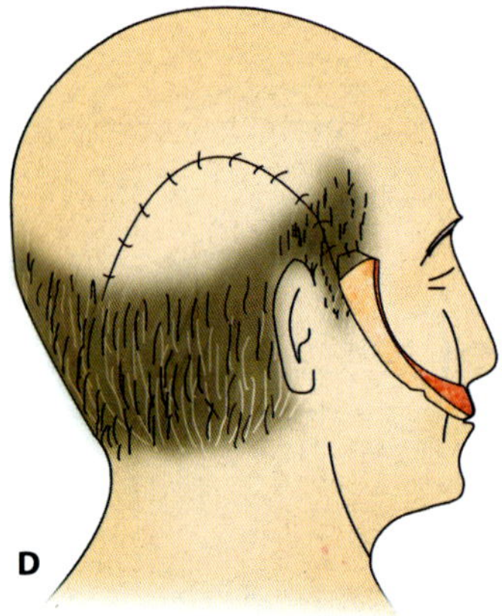

**Figure 11-21.** Temporoparietal transposition flaps. (A) Forehead defect and transposition flap design. (B) Reconstructed forehead. (C) Lip defect and transposition flap design. (D) Reconstructed upper lip. The pedicle is divided after a delay and then returned to its original location.

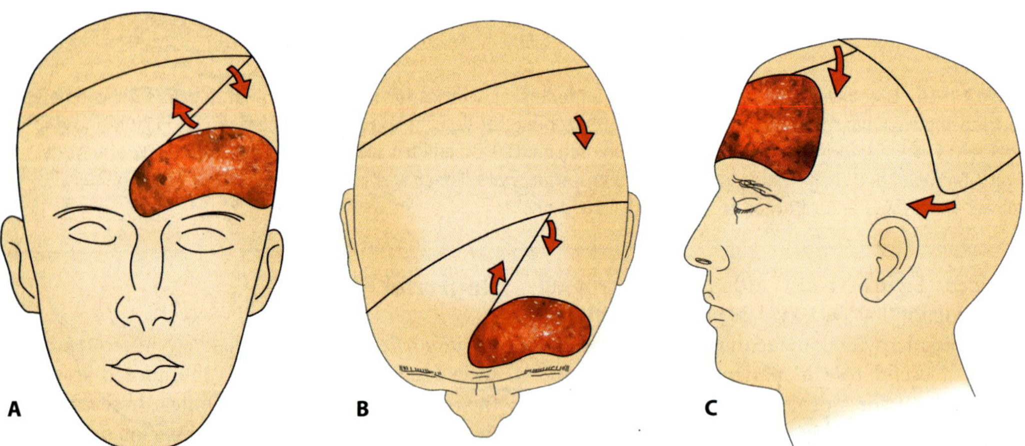


**Figure 11-22.** Anterior defect reconstruction with the three-flap technique. (A) Frontal view of defect and flap design. (B) Superior view. (C) Lateral view *(Continued)*

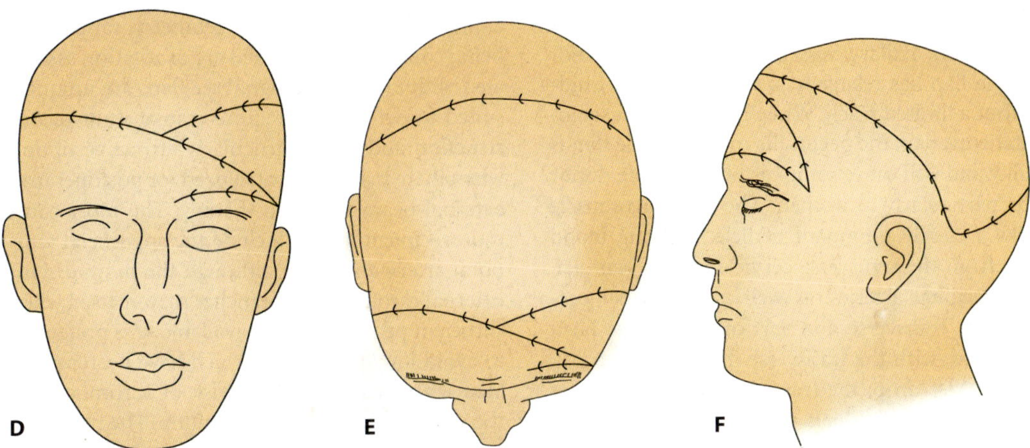


**Figure 11-22.** *(Continued)* (D) Frontal view of reconstructed scalp. (E) Superior view. (F) Lateral view.

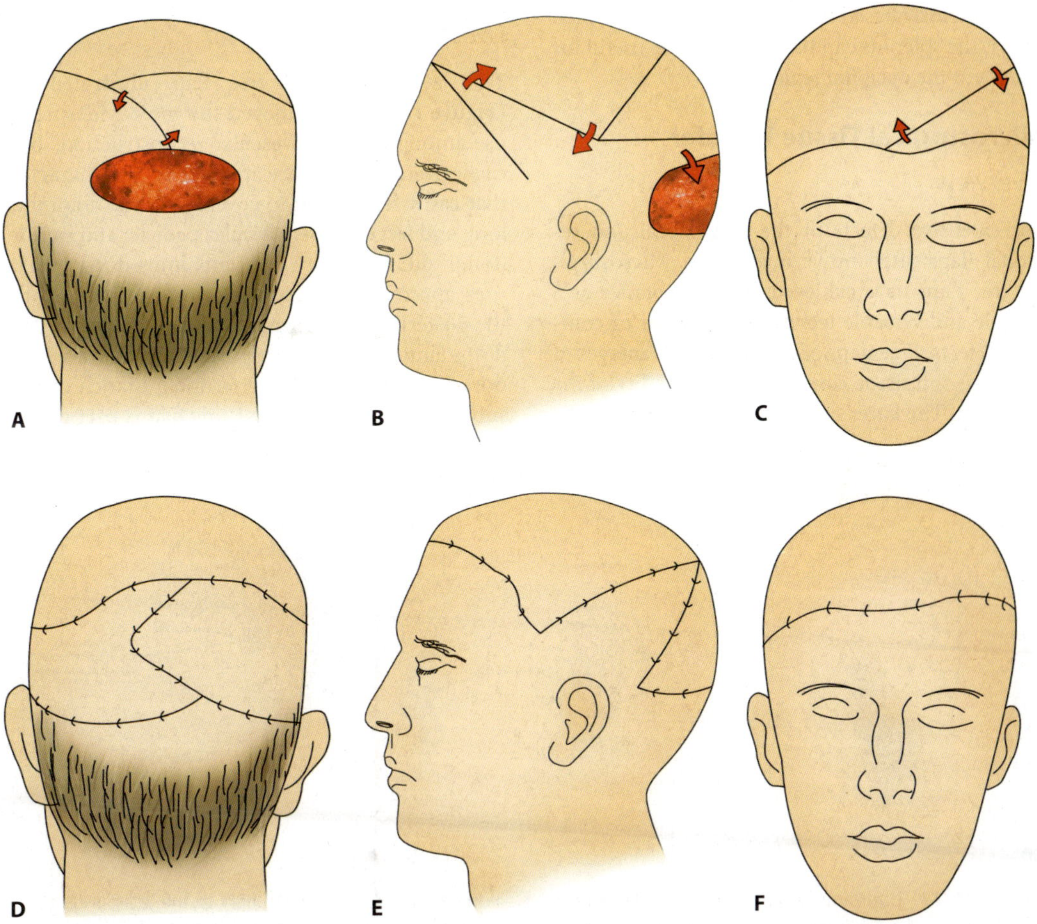

A B C

D E F

**Figure 11-23.** Posterior defect reconstruction with the three -flap technique. (A) Posterior view of defect and flap design. (B) Lateral view. (C) Frontal view. (D) Posterior view of reconstructed scalp. (E) Lateral view. (F) Frontal view.

Care must be taken to avoid injury to the brachial plexus and axillary vessel. The pectoralis major muscle flap has relatively low donor site morbidity, but a limited reach. When raised as a musculocutaneous flap, the pectoralis major muscle flap is bulky and will cause some distortion of the donor site, particularly in women. The trapezius muscle lacks a clearly dominant pedicle, deriving blood flow from the transverse cervical, dorsal scapular, and occipital arteries, as well as paraspinal perforators. Transverse and vertical flaps have been described, with the transverse flap carrying a risk of shoulder drop; the transverse flap is thus best reserved for individuals with a previous sacrifice of the spinal accessory nerve. The splenius capitis muscle also has a complex vascular anatomy, receiving its blood supply from the occipital, transverse cervical, and vertebral arteries. When raised as a superiorly based flap supplied by the occipital artery, the splenius capitis muscle can be useful for defects in the occipital region.

## Microsurgical Tissue Transfer

### *Overview*

For extensive defects of the scalp, local and regional flaps often prove inadequate. Microsurgical free flaps have achieved wide acceptance as a reliable and versatile technique for repair of complex defects. Free flaps offer the dual advantages of generous soft tissue coverage with flexibility of the flap inset. The latter benefit is primarily due to the ability to manipulate vessel geometry, rather than being constrained by a fixed arc of rotation associated with local flap design. Free flaps are uniquely suited to defects that require cranial vault reconstruction and are a particularly attractive option when there is an anticipated need for postoperative external-beam radiation therapy. The most common recipient vessels include the superficial temporal artery and veins, although the more distant external carotid artery branches may be used when sufficient pedicle length is available. It is preferable to avoid long vein grafts, which have been associated with an increased the risk of thrombosis of the vascular pedicle and flap failure. The main disadvantage of microsurgical free flaps in the scalp is the lack of hair replacement, although this consideration may be of lesser concern to patients with the need for such extensive scalp reconstruction.

### *Latissimus Dorsi Free Flap*

The latissimus dorsi free flap, illustrated in (**Figure 11-24**), has enjoyed the most widespread use among the microvascular reconstructions because of its large surface area; broad, flat character that easily lends itself to coverage of the cranium; long and large-caliber vascular pedicle; and minor donor site morbidity. The latissimus dorsi measures approximately 20 × 40 cm, extending from the posterior axilla to the midline of the back. The dominant arterial supply arises from the thoracodorsal artery, which is the terminal branch of the subscapular artery. Because this flap is part of the

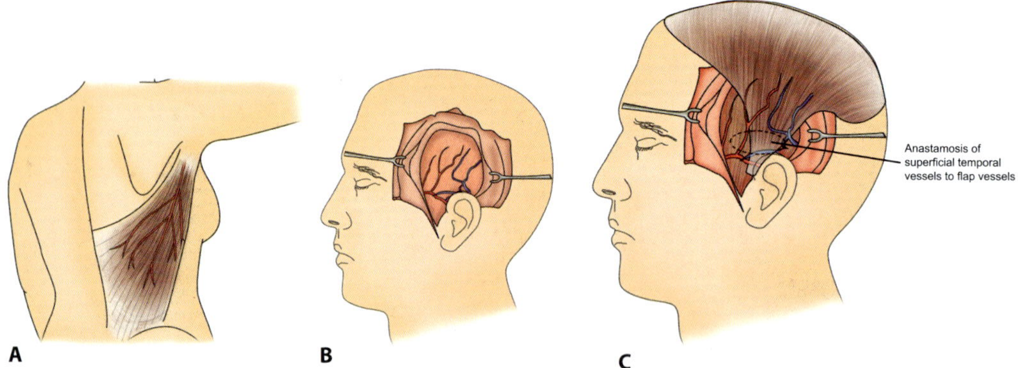


**Figure 11-24.** Latissimus flap reconstruction for massive scalp defect. (A) Arterial supply to the latissimus flap is provided by the thoracodorsal artery, arising from the subscapular artery. Note the large surface area and thin, sheetlike character of the latissimus muscle. (B) Superficial temporal artery and vein recipient vessels are exposed and a large scalp defect is demonstrated. (C) Reconstructed scalp with latissimus inset, which will support skin grafting.

subscapular system, it can be harvested not only as a muscle or myocutaneous flap but also as an osseomyocutaneous flap in combination with the serratus anterior, or even as a scapular/ parascapular (osteo) fasciocutaneous flap. Often, the latissimus muscle is harvested alone and skin grafted. This flap is well suited to massive defects of the skull, and the intramuscular blood supply allows the flap to be split into two musculocutaneous flaps. The most common complication with this flap is seroma formation at the donor site, the risk of which is decreased with use of suction drain and fixating skin flaps with tacking sutures.

### *Other Microvascular Free Flaps*

A variety of other flap types have also been described for reconstruction of extensive scalp defects, each with its own benefits and drawbacks. Among these are the anterolateral thigh, scapula, rectus abdominus, and radial forearm flaps. In addition, a temporo-occipital microvascular free flap that is based on the superficial temporal artery and vein has been used to achieve hair restoration. Typically, controlled tissue expansion is performed on the donor side, allowing for transfer of the hair-bearing scalp to the contralateral side with primary closure of the secondary defect at the donor site. The selection of flap type is based on the size of defect, tissue components absent, and aesthetic and functional objectives of surgery.

## Scalp Replantation

Scalp replantation is the treatment of choice for complete or nearly complete avulsions of the scalp. No other method of scalp reconstruction can match the results of successful replantation, either in terms of restoration of avulsed hair-bearing scalp, eyebrows, and portions of the ear and forehead musculature or in terms of avoidance of a large secondary donor site and the ability to perform a single-stage procedure. The main contraindications include hemodynamic instability or other severe life-threatening injuries that preclude lengthy surgery. Scalp avulsion injuries most commonly result from the entanglement of long hair in moving machinery, resulting in an oblique shearing force. Scalp avulsions follow a predictable pattern beginning at the site of the shearing force and propagating along the natural cleavage plane between the galea and the periosteum. Shearing will often extend until the fascial attachments in the supraorbital, temporal, auricular, and occipital regions are reached. Temporal tears frequently include the superior portion of the ear. High-volume blood loss at time of injury is the rule with such injuries. Primary vein grafting is often necessary due to damage of the large vessels by avulsive forces. Arterial repair is performed first to minimize ischemia time and to facilitate identification of veins. Most commonly, the superficial temporal artery is used, as this artery has good vessel caliber, and a single superficial temporal artery can often support survival of the entire scalp. To minimize flap congestion, two venous repairs are recommended.

## Adjuvant Techniques

### *Controlled Tissue Expansion*

Controlled tissue expansion allows for the creation of large areas of hair-bearing scalp with good tissue match to the surrounding scalp. It thus overcomes one of the cardinal limitations of most microvascular flaps. This technique has been used successfully for decades. Tissue expansion induces increased vascularity in the overlying flap, and the thinning of the expanded scalp makes the flap more elastic than the normal scalp. Although transient alopecia may be observed with prolonged expansion, this problem is usually only transient. Because the cranium provides a smooth and rigid foundation for the expander, tissue expansion is more predictable in the scalp than in other areas of the head and neck. Furthermore, the naturally tough and vascular character of the scalp resists breakdown in the later stages of expansion.

Prolonged tissue expansion does have several important limitations, both from the standpoint of the surgeon and of the patient. First, tissue expansion exerts considerable mechanical stress on the adjacent tissues. Therefore, expansion must either be performed weeks prior to resection or after a stable wound has been established. This consideration limits the applicability of tissue expansion in reconstruction of acute traumatic defects or a malignancy for which resection is best not delayed. Second, patients may be understandably reluctant to undergo several weeks of expansion. Careful patient counseling prior to the procedure is mandatory, and frequent office visits are necessary. During expansion, the number of hair follicles is not increased; therefore, hair density diminishes proportionately as the scalp surface area increases.

Expander exposure is also a frequent complication. Finally, the capsule that forms around the expander tends to induce flap contraction after the expander has been removed. Conservative resection of this capsule may be considered, but care must be taken not to inadvertently compromise flap vascularity.

A few technical considerations should be kept in mind. Two or more expanders are usually used to allow for design of multiple flaps. Often, one expander is placed on each side of the head to allow for maximal defect coverage using bilateral local flaps. Because the majority of scalp flaps are rotational flaps, oval or crescent-shaped expanders correspond well to the curvilinear incisions usually required. The location of the future flap incisions should be taken into consideration when deciding where to make the incision for expander placement. The preferred placement for the expander is in the subgaleal plane, just deep to the galea and superficial to the periosteum. Inflation is best begun approximately 2 weeks after initial placement. The expanders are injected via a remote port under the scalp that is easily accessed, and the expander is inflated twice a week until the desired amount of expansion has occurred.

## *Intraoperative Tissue Expansion*

Intraoperative tissue expansion is mechanistically distinct from controlled tissue expansion, and it may be considered when tissue expansion is desirable but a prolonged duration of expansion is not possible. With this technique, the scalp tissue is rapidly stretched over a period of a few minutes prior to raising the flap. Usually, a couple of iterations of inflation are preformed, with the scalp being expanded until it blanches, maintained on stretch for 3 minutes, and then afforded intervening "rest periods." This approach does not induce the same metabolic and physiologic changes achieved with controlled tissue expansion, and there is greater potential for flap necrosis with this technique. Some surgeons believe that the mechanical changes induced by rapid expansion are beneficial in scalp reconstruction, but it remains unclear whether this technique provides an advantage over well-designed and widely undermined flaps.

## *Wound Vacuum-Assisted Closure*

Wound <u>V</u>acuum-<u>A</u>ssisted <u>C</u>losure (e.g., "Wound V.A.C.") refers to negative pressure wound therapy and was introduced roughly two decades ago. Originally developed for treatment of chronic, nonhealing wound beds, as seen with pressure ulcers in patients with microcirculatory pathology, this technique has an evolving role in scalp reconstruction. The wound is sealed with either gauze or foam dressing and a vacuum is applied continuously or intermittently. Vacuum-assisted closure is thought to promote tissue granulation and to decrease wound volume by debriding devitalized tissue, decreasing bacterial colonization, promoting blood flow, and removing excess serous fluid that might inhibit wound healing. V.A.C therapy is contraindicated in patients with grossly contaminated wounds, malignancy in the wound bed, fistula, necrosis, and osteomyelitis, thus narrowing its role elsewhere in the head and neck.

## *Hair Transplants*

Hair transplants are a useful adjunct to scalp reconstruction. Follicular unit transplantation, which involves restoration of hair by transplanting hair in groups of one to four hairs along with sebaceous glands, has largely supplanted other techniques due to its aesthetic superiority over earlier techniques that often left patients with an unnatural "pluggy" appearance. In order for hair transplantation to be successful, a vascular recipient bed must be available. Wounds that heal by secondary intention will often accept hair transplants as a secondary procedure. Multiple stages of grafting are usually necessary, but good hair density can often be achieved even over large areas of alopecia. Transplantation may be used in conjunction with hair-bearing flaps or delayed scalp reduction to decrease the area requiring coverage.

## *Dermal Regeneration Templates*

Collagen-based scaffolds may also have a role in scalp reconstruction. Bilayer membrane constructs that include a dermal replacement layer (cross-linked bovine collagen and glycosaminoglycan) and a thin epidermal substitute layer (polysiloxane/silicone) have been applied in treating burn patients. Although these frameworks are relatively inert, they do provide a potential substrate for ingrowth of blood vessels and gradual migration of tissue from the periphery of the scalp defect. The silicone surfacing helps to protect the treated area from desiccation and, in doing so, may foster granulation and/or epithelialization over areas with limited bone exposure. The collagen matrix is slowly resorbed as tissue ingrowth proceeds. Experience with this material in scalp reconstruction remains limited, and the utility of this approach for supporting healing in regions lacking a well-vascularized bed continues to be studied.

## Postoperative Care

Requirements for postoperative care following scalp reconstruction vary with the complexity of the repair. Many scalp repairs may be performed on an outpatient basis, whereas more extensive surgery, such as free flap reconstruction, necessitates closer surveillance in the hospital. Because small amounts of serous fluid tend to pool under dependent areas of scalp flaps, use of prophylactic antibiotics with Gram-positive coverage are recommended for the first postoperative week. Closed suction drains are often helpful in larger reconstructions, particularly in the case of a "banana peel" flap type reconstruction that involves mobilizing essentially the entire scalp surface in the course of reconstruction. Drains are also advised for other large local, regional, or free tissue reconstructions. Drains may usually be removed in the first few days once the volume of drainage has decreased. A notable exception is the latissimus dorsi flap donor site, which should be drained for closer to a week to minimize the risk of seroma formation.

Wound care is another important consideration. Tight dressings are to be avoided. Excessive external compression predisposes to flap ischemia. Covering the wound with an opaque dressing will also delay the diagnosis of hematoma. Use of injection (containing 1:100,000 epinephrine) prior to incision followed by discreet use of bipolar electrocautery during surgery maintains good hemostasis and, with closed suction drainage, should obviate the need for compressive wraps. Dried blood and crusts along incision lines are atraumatically removed with half-strength peroxide to promote reepithelialization. Antibiotic ointment is helpful during the first few days in preventing fresh wound edges from desiccating. However, many scalp reconstructions—particularly those involving granulation or healing by secondary intention—require significant time to fully heal. Prolonged use of antibiotic ointments may cause contact dermatitis or predispose to redness and irritation from secondary fungal overgrowth. Nonantibiotic-containing ointments, such as Aquaphor, are preferable for ensuring hydration of the tissues.

## Complications

Although excellent aesthetic and functional results may be achieved in the majority of patients undergoing scalp reconstruction, a variety of problems may be encountered. Most complications reflect the inherent challenges that are imposed by the rigid, inelastic character of the scalp, the natural convexity of the cranium, and the difficulty of restoring hair-bearing tissue. Ischemia of distal flaps, particularly at the convergence of multiple flaps, may result in focal wound breakdown or dehiscence. Wounds that heal by secondary intention or that are skin grafted may develop into chronically troublesome sites that are prone to bleeding. Loss of distant flaps is a rare, but serious, complication that usually requires secondary reconstruction. Infection and hematoma may occur either at primary or secondary donor sites. If a portion of the calvarium has been removed, the potential morbidity of a scalp wound infection is magnified by the potential for meningitis or intracranial extension. Controlled tissue expansion poses a significant risk of scalp breakdown and may require expander removal if significant infection is present. Future progress in tissue engineering may broaden available reconstructive options and decrease the risk of complications.

## References


1. Beasley NJ, Gilbert RW, Gullane PJ et al. Scalp and forehead reconstruction using free revascularized tissue transfer. *Arch Facial Plast Surg* 6, 2004, 16.
2. Cox AJ, Wang TD, Cook TA. Closure of a scalp defect. *Arch Facial Plast Surg* 1, 1999, 212.
3. Hoffmann JF: Management of scalp defects. *Otolaryngol Clin N Am* 34, 2001, 571.
4. Hoffman JF. Reconstruction of the scalp. In Baker SR, *Local Flaps in Facial Reconstruction*, Elsevier Inc., Philadelphia, 2007, 637–663.
5. Jurkiewicz MJ. Scalp reconstruction with multiple flaps. In Brent B, ed., *The Artistry of Reconstructive Surgery*, CV Mosby, St. Louis, 1987.
6. Lesavoy MA, Dubrow TJ, Schwartz RJ, et al. Management of large scalp defects with local pedicle flaps. *Plast Reconstr Surg* 91, 1993, 783.

7. Ling EH, Wang TD: Local flaps in forehead and temporal reconstruction. *Facial Plast Surg Clin N Am* 4, 1996, 469.
8. Lipa JE, Butler CE. Enhancing the outcome of free latissimus dorsi muscle flap reconstruction of scalp defects. *Head Neck* 26, 2004, 46.
9. Marathe US, Sniezek JC. Use of vacuum-assisted closure device in enhancing closure of a massive skull defect. *Laryngoscope* 114, 2004, 961.
10. Mehrara BJ, Disa JJ, Pusic A. Scalp reconstruction. *J Surg Oncol* 94, 2006, 504–508.
11. Newman MI, Hanasono MM, Disa JJ, et al. Scalp reconstruction: A 15 year experience. *Ann Plast Surg* 52, 2004, 501.
12. Orticochea M. Three flap scalp reconstruction technique. *Br J Plast Surg* 24, 1971, 184.
13. Sasaki GH. Tissue expanders and general guidelines for tissue expansion technique. In *Tissue Expansion in Reconstructive and Aesthetic Surgery*, Mosby, St. Louis, 1998.
14. Seline PC, Siegle RJ. Scalp reconstruction. *Dermatol Clin* 23, 2005, 13.
15. Tanaka Y, Miki K, Tajima S, et al. Reconstruction of an extensive scalp defect using the split latissimus dorsi flap in combination with the serratus anterior musculo-cutaneous flap. *Br J Plast Surg* 51, 1998, 250.
16. TerKonda RP, Sykes JM. Concepts in scalp and forehead reconstruction. *Otolaryngol Clin N Am* 30, 1997, 519.
17. Wax MK, Burkey BB, Bascom D, Rosenthal EL. The role of free tissue transfer in the reconstruction of massive neglected skin cancers of the head and Neck. *Arch Facial Plast Surg* 5, 2003, 479.

12

# Postoperative Care, Complications, and Adjunctive Scar Camouflage

Gregory H. Branham, MD, FACS

## Postoperative Dressings

Once reconstruction is completed, the healing process begins and it is critical to enlist the assistance of the patient in properly caring for the wound. In the head and neck, infection is not common, and therefore a dressing is not required during the course of the healing process. However, it is preferable to have the patient wear a dressing in the immediate postoperative period. This will keep the wound edges occluded and will help to maintain the coating of antibiotic ointment that is routinely used to cover the wound. It is also helpful in providing support and pressure if needed and serves as a way to absorb any immediate postoperative oozing of blood from the incision lines. A simple nonadherent gauze pad affixed to the skin with a nonreactive paper tape works nicely in most cases. However, if support of the wound or pressure is desired then an elastic dressing or an elastic tape is useful. Gauze may also be used to provide bulk to the dressing to increase pressure on the wound. Care should be taken not to place too much pressure over flaps as the risk of exceeding the capillary filling pressure will cause flap necrosis.

In the case of skin grafts, a bolster-type dressing that applies constant pressure to the graft to permit it to adhere to the wound bed may be necessary. The most common type of bolster is one that is fashioned from a nonadherent dressing material such as Xeroform (cotton gauze impregnated with iodinated petrolatum) or adaptic gauze, a woven nonadherent gauze that is impregnated with petrolatum. If additional bulk is needed, sterile cotton balls can be placed inside the core of the dressing and then wrapped in several layers of Xeroform. Once the dressing is made, it is sutured to the wound edges with a nylon or other nonabsorbable suture and the sutures are tied over the bolster to apply pressure to the graft. Typically, sutures are placed on opposing sides of the bolster in pairs and tied together over the bolster. Some surgeons prefer to suture the bolster directly to the wound edges as an alternative method. In either case, the bolster is then maintained by keeping it from getting wet and applying a new coat of antibiotic ointment or petrolatum to keep it from desiccating and adhering to the wound edges or the graft itself. The bolster may be covered for esthetic purposes, but this is not necessary. At 1 week, the bolster is removed, as the graft should have had sufficient time to adhere to the recipient bed.

All sutured incisions should be cleaned twice daily, or as often as necessary, with a dilute mixture of hydrogen peroxide and water. The patients are instructed to keep any crusting or dried blood off of the incision so that individual sutures are visible

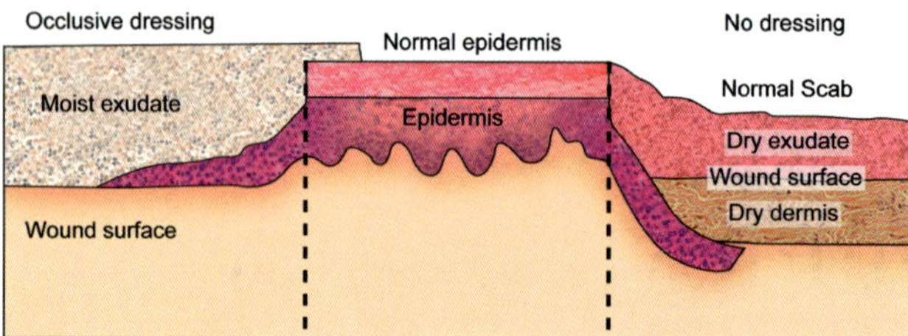


**Figure 12-1.** Effect of occlusive dressing on wound healing. An occlusive dressing allows the wound matrix or incision line to remain moist, which promotes reepithelialization at a more superficial level yielding a more acceptable scar. It essentially raises the water table in the wound to promote better healing.

and separately distinguishable. Patients are instructed to apply a fresh coat of ointment after cleaning the incisions. This regimen should be maintained until 2 days after suture removal in order to allow the suture tracks to seal over. The occlusive dressing, whether ointment or bandage, raises the humidity level at the wound surface and allows the wound/incision to reepithelialize at a level closer to the normal skin surface than an open wound allowed to heal without being occluded **(Figure 12-1)**.

## Tissue Adhesives

2-Octylcyanoacrylate (Dermabond) was approved by the Food and Drug Administration as the first medical-grade topical skin tissue adhesive for wound/incision closure in 1988. Skin tissue adhesives offer a number of advantages over suture approximation. When applied properly, adhesives are less time consuming and offer greater early wound strength when compared to comparable suture techniques. In addition, they seal the wound and act as a barrier against bacterial contamination of the wound and provide an occlusive, moist environment in which the edges may reepithelialize. In addition, adhesives offer an opportunity to avoid suture track marks that can occur if sutures are left too long, are too large, or closed too tightly at the wound edges.

Skin tissue adhesives should only be used in low tension wounds that can be easily approximated with fingers or forceps. This does not exclude the use of deep dermal sutures or subcutaneous sutures as long as the epithelial edges can be easily approximated with low tension once the sutures have been placed. Adhesives have been used successfully on the face and most other areas of the body. They can be used in the cuticular closure of local flaps but have not gained popularity with most surgeons who feel that they have less wound edge control with skin tissue adhesives and prefer suture closures for this reason. There is a learning curve associated with the use of the skin tissue adhesives that may be a disadvantage in the user's early experience.

Use of skin tissue adhesives is contraindicated on mucosa or mucocutaneous junctions (lip), and in infected wounds or wounds in which a deep component or dead space cannot be adequately closed. Animal and human bites should not be closed with a skin adhesive as it has the potential to seal contaminants into the wound. Lacerations in hair-bearing areas such as the scalp or eyebrow should be closed with a suture. Wounds that have crushed or irregular edges should be debrided to a clean edge prior to closure. If this is not possible, then suture closure is recommended.

## Technique for Application of Tissue Adhesive

Application of the skin tissue adhesive should occur only after following proper wound care, hemostasis, and cleansing of the skin. Once the skin surface is clean and free of contaminants and can be easily approximated, the ampoule containing the adhesive is broken and the skin edges approximated. The adhesive is applied and held for 30 seconds to allow the adhesive to polymerize. Polymerization occurs when the monomer is exposed to moisture on the skin's surface. Once the initial application is complete and dry (after 30 seconds), a second application should be made. At least two layers should be applied to ensure adequate tensile strength to the closure and three to four layers are preferred. Once completed, the adhesive film should be undisturbed. It is particularly important to make sure that the patient does not scratch or pick at the film over the wound as this can cause premature sloughing of the adhesive. Showering or brief wetting of the film is permissible; however, soaking or swimming is not allowed. Ointments and medications should be avoided over the film as they may contribute to premature sloughing and provide no benefit as these agents are unable to reach the wound surface where they are intended. Sloughing of the film should occur spontaneously and without provocation and usually occurs in 5–10 days.

Studies comparing skin adhesive to both absorbable and nonabsorbable sutures have evaluated cosmetic outcomes in patients with lacerations over periods as long as a year and show no significant cosmetic differences when analyzed with a visual analog cosmesis scale.

## Long-Term Scar Care

There are a number of preparations available that are marketed to improve scar appearance and healing. In particular, Mederma, an onion extract, is marketed for this purpose and has been shown to be beneficial in improving scar appearance as compared to no treatment. However, when compared to plain petrolatum used in the same manner as Mederma, it offered no distinct advantage. Thus, one could infer that wound hydration that occurs with prolonged occlusive treatment as with either of these preparations is beneficial in enhancing scar appearance.

Silicone gel sheeting is beneficial in preventing the recurrence of these entities and should be strongly encouraged for at least 1 year or until thickening of the scar is no longer evident. Intralesional steroids also play a significant role in the routine postoperative management of hypertrophic scars and keloids. Not used routinely, but also beneficial, is postoperative radiation therapy in managing recurrent keloids, particularly those occurring on the earlobe that is amenable to radiation therapy without placing other structures at risk during radiation treatments.

## Scar Camouflage

Entire texts have been written on the subject of scar revision and camouflage techniques. However, there are a few simple nonsurgical measures that can be used to enhance scar appearance. One of the simplest is dermabrasion and can be employed as early as 6–8 weeks postoperatively. Surface irregularities associated with the initial wound healing can be addressed by removing the outer layers of the epidermis down to the level of the junction of the papillary and reticular dermis or just into the reticular dermis. Because dermabrasion is a cold technique, there is little risk of pigmentation problems, although they can occur and the patient should be warned about them. Most often they are mild in Fitzpatrick skin types 1–4 and can be easily treated. Laser treatments such as laser resurfacing are also helpful but run a greater risk of dyschromias post-treatment due to the concomitant thermal damage to the wound. Chemical peels can achieve a similar goal as laser resurfacing.

Depressed scars can be improved with nonablative laser treatments designed to stimulate collagen remodeling in the depth of the wound. This stimulates collagen synthesis and plumps up the depressed portion of the wound and results in a more even appearance to the wound and the surrounding skin. Several such lasers are available such as the Fraxel and the Affirm lasers, which use water as the target chromophore and operate at wavelengths of 1550 and 1440 nm, respectively.

Injectable filler materials are also useful in enhancing the appearance of depressed scars and there are a number of them on the market today. None of them offer a permanent correction of the problem and require retreatment on a periodic basis, the length of the interval depending on the nature of the filler material used. Autologous fat transfer and dermal fat grafts also represent an alternative method for augmenting depressed scars. In the experience of the author, reconstruction of defects with dermis fat grafts requires overcorrection as there is considerable resorption of the graft over time. Autologous fat is harvested and injected with approximately 50–60% of the graft persisting over time. The advantage of the autologous fat graft is that the material is readily available and can be repeated with ease. The obvious disadvantage is the necessity to repeat the procedure to achieve a 100% correction; however, this is no different than any other filler material, and it does offer the potential for a permanent correction with several procedures.

Flaps can develop trapdoor deformities that result from circumferential scar contraction around the perimeter of the flap. Other factors that contribute to the thickened appearance of the flap are chronic edema and having the apex of the flap in a dependent position. This can be treated with injection of the area by triamcinalone acetonide (Kenalog) 10mg/ml. If the flap is too bulky to be appropriately treated with Kenalog, it can be debulked with a minor procedure to undermine the flap and remove some of the subcutaneous fat. This should not be attempted until the flap has had an opportunity to establish an adequate blood supply from the recipient tissues. This is usually not an issue, however, as thickening does not usually develop until significant healing and contracture have occurred. Multiple small Z-plasties can be used to blend the flap edges with the native tissue as another alternative to break up the contracture.

## Scar Revision Techniques

There are a number of surgical scar revision techniques that can improve the appearance of a flap or incision. Underlying all of the possible techniques that can be used are the same principles that apply to the initial reconstruction, such as adherence to the esthetic units and relaxed skin tension lines.

The Z-plasty and the multiple Z-plasty are the most commonly used scar revision techniques when the scar needs to be lengthened or reoriented. The W-plasty will irregularize the scar but does not lengthen the scar. Perhaps the most commonly used technique is reexcision with meticulous closure of the incision. In most instances with proper execution of the initial reconstruction, surgical scar revision is not necessary. Most insurance companies do not reimburse for scar revision unless significant impairment of function can be established. Reimbursement is not usually approved for appearance-related scar revision surgery.

Essential to successful postoperative wound management is the understanding of wound-healing mechanisms (discussed in Chapters 2 and 3) and a motivated compliant patient. It is important to provide to the patient a written copy of the wound care instructions and to review them with the patient prior to discharge. It is also important to make sure that this is documented in the patient's chart. The patient and the surgeon must also understand that there are processes that occur during wound healing that can be influenced with our interventions and some that we have no control over. It is critical that the patient have confidence in the surgeon that he or she will do everything possible to achieve a positive outcome. Similarly, it is essential that the patient and physician feel comfortable discussing any issues that might arise during the course of treatment.

## References


1. Dunn DL, ed. *Wound Closure Manual*, Ethicon, Somerville, NJ, 2007.
2. Gabrielli F, Potenza C, Puddu P, et al. Suture materials and other factors associated with tissue reactivity, infection, and wound dehiscence among plastic surgery outpatients. *Plast Reconst Surg* 2001, 107(1), 38–45.
3. Holger JS, Wandersee SC, Hale DB. Cosmetic outcomes of facial lacerations repaired with tissue-adhesive, absorbable, and nonabsorbable sutures. *Am J Emerg Med* 2004, 22(4), 254–257.
4. Parell GJ, Becker GD. Comparison of absorbable with nonabsorbable sutures in closure of facial skin wounds. *Arch Facial Plast Surg* 2003, 5, 488–490.
5. Salthouse TN. Biologic response to sutures. *Otlaryngol Head Neck* 1980, 88, 658–664.
6. Quinn J, Wells G, Sutcliffe T, et al. A randomized trial comparing octycyanoacrylate tissue adhesive and sutures in the management of lacerations. *JAMA* 1997, 227(19), 1527–1560.
7. Bruns TB, Simon HK, McLario DJ, et al. Laceration repair using a tissue adhesive in a children's emergency department. *Pediatrics* 1996, 98, 673–675.
8. Singer AJ, Hollander JE, Valentine SM, et al. Prospective, randomized, controlled trial of tissue adhesive (2-octylcyanoacrylate) vs. standard wound closure techniques for laceration repair. *Acad Emerg Med* 1998, 5(2), 94–99.
9. Quinn J, Wells G, Sutcliffe T, et al. Tissue adhesive versus suture wound repair at 1 year: Randomized clinical trial correlating early, 3 month, and 1-year cosmetic outcome. *Ann Emerg Med* 1998, 32(6), 645–649.
10. Maas CS, ed. *Wound Management and Suturing Manual*, American Academy of Facial Plastic and Reconstructive Surgery, Alexandria, VA. 2001.

# 13

# Complications of Local Flaps: Prevention and Management

Michael J. Brenner, MD, FACS and Chad J. Sukut, MD

## Introduction

Complications associated with local flaps of the face are uncommon, but they are conspicuous when they occur. Although salvage or revision surgery is almost always an option, the emotional price for the patient—whether anxiety related to tissue loss, concern, and frustration with need for additional stages or fear regarding the eventual outcome—may be substantial. Many complications are preventable. A detailed knowledge of anatomy and a well-formulated plan for reconstruction are indispensable in facial reconstructive surgery. Surgeons familiar with potential complications are better able to steer clear of adverse outcomes and are also better equipped to take appropriate measures to manage complications when they occur.

Local flap complications are usually related to intrinsic patient factors, surgical technique, or suboptimal local flap design. Ensuring that there is no persisting cancer in the surgical field is a prerequisite for local flaps, as residual malignancy in a reconstructed bed is difficult to eradicate; steps required for managing residual carcinoma are likely to compromise aesthetics and function. The following discussion covers a range of complications and their management including ischemia, infection, hematoma, and disfigurement. Functional considerations discussed include strategies for avoiding nerve injury, nasal obstruction, and distortion to the lip, eyelid, and nose.

## Patient Factors

Relevant findings from the patient history and exam are easily overlooked, and failure to identify risk factors for flap complication may impose formidable obstacles to successful surgery. Patient-related risk factors may be broadly divided into modifiable and nonmodifiable risk factors for flap compromise. Among the modifiable risk factors are diabetes mellitus with poor glycemic control, hypothyroid state, malnutrition, and tobacco or alcohol usage. Tight glycemic control during the perioperative period decreases the risk for infection and wound-healing complications. Profound hypothyroidism also severely impedes wound healing, with 4–6 weeks required for normalization. Shorter periods of correction may still confer some benefit. Malnutrition, if related to chronic disease, may prove difficult to correct. Nonetheless, restoring nutritional reserves will help to ensure that the necessary building blocks are available to support wound healing and minimize risk of wound dehiscence and flap loss. Heavy alcohol use is associated with dilatation of blood vessels and alteration in platelet function, thereby increasing the risk for developing a hematoma.

Cigarette smoking is a major risk factor for flap complications and warrants special consideration. Patients should be counseled prior to surgery regarding the importance of minimizing tobacco consumption. Education is empowering for patients, and the time spent counseling patients on the profound effects of tobaccos products is effort well invested. It is preferable that smoking be discontinued 1–2 months prior to surgery, although shorter durations of cessation are beneficial as well. Cigarette smoking impairs flap viability through a variety of mechanisms. The vasoconstrictive effects of nicotine decrease flap perfusion. In addition, carbon monoxide, which has a high affinity for hemoglobin, displaces oxygen with carboxyhemoglobin. As a result, oxygen delivery is impaired. Additionally, toxic agents within tobacco smoke are hostile to the healing wound bed. The several-fold increase in flap necrosis in facelift patients who smoke cigarettes speaks to the potent effect of smoking on perfusion. Because facial reconstruction relies heavily on perfusion of transferred tissue with decreased blood flow, even small increases in perfusion related to smoking cessation are advantageous.

Another subset of patient-related factors is less modifiable and includes chronic impairment of the microcirculation of the head and neck, prior surgery that interferes with blood supply, and irreversible underlying disease. Among the factors that may impair the microcirculation of the head and neck are prior radiation therapy, a long history of poorly controlled diabetes, chronically elevated cholesterol levels, and long-standing tobacco consumption. Furthermore, individuals with very thin, frail skin lack a well-vascularized subcutaneous layer. Thin skin tolerates less ischemic stress. Prior surgery also influences reconstructive options, such as when a preferred donor site has been exhausted or when there has been transection of the axial pedicle supplying a desired flap. Chronic systemic illness, such as advanced cancer, also severely diminishes healing and should prompt a cautious approach. In patients with one or more of these factors, it is important to take a measured approach to reconstruction. It is advisable to counsel the patient regarding how underlying conditions may influence the selection of reconstructive approach and the prospects for successful repair.

## Surgical Technique

Many of the complications associated with local flaps are inherent to surgery. The nuances of perioperative technique, tissue handling, dissection, and hemostasis all influence reconstructive outcomes. In addition, avoidance of injury to adjacent structures assures satisfactory functional outcomes. These general principles can be applied to almost all reconstructive cases, and adherence to these principles is essential for ensuring the best possible result with surgery.

## Wound Infection

Although the rich blood supply of most facial tissues mitigates against infection, there are a number of risk factors for infection inherent to facial reconstructive surgery. Higher infection rates are observed with wounds closed in delayed fashion, as it is frequently necessary in Mohs reconstruction. Furthermore, the risk of infection dramatically increases in the setting of tissue ischemia, which is often present after flap transposition. Significant tissue manipulation and use of cautery may further increase risk of infection. Therefore, focal decreased blood supply is common. Maintaining tissue perfusion and oxygenation is extremely important in resisting bacterial colonization. Infections not only add to the overall morbidity of surgery, but they also impair wound healing potential and have detrimental effects on cosmetic outcomes.

A cascade of biochemical events occurs when the tissues involved in a facial reconstruction become infected. Free radicals and cytotoxic mediators are released in association with inflammatory edema. These events predispose to premature degradation of sutures, impaired collagen production, and increased risk of wound dehiscence. Infection may also cause thrombosis of the microvasculature, which in turn leads to increased tissue ischemia and necrosis. Subsequent healing by contraction is likely to leave widened, depressed scars with irregular texture. In rare cases, the infectious process may dissect aggressively through tissue planes and cause fasciitis, particularly when large cervical facial flaps are infected with aggressive bacteria.

Several factors can decrease the risk of infection, and early diagnosis and management is paramount. Standard skin preparation, scrubbing and draping, and prophylactic antibiotics are recommended. It is also helpful to minimize tissue trauma or charring intraoperatively. Appropriate wound care after surgery includes debridement of crusts, expressing any accumulated blood from the tissue bed, and timely removal of any drains. The presence of excessive pain, erythema, or drainage at the wound site may herald the presence of infection. These signs usually appears 3 days to 1 week after surgery. In some cases, it may be difficult to differentiate a topical reaction from true infection. Although the most severe infections tend to be those associated with *Staphylococcus aureus*, infections may also arise from streptococci, Gram-negative, and anaerobic organisms. In addition, viral and fungal infections occur occasionally. Patients undergoing dermabrasion or laser therapy should receive antiviral agents prophylactically to minimize the risk of infection, until the skin surface is reepithelialized.

## Dissection Plane and Tissue Handling

During dissection, preservation of subcutaneous perforators is vital to flap perfusion. One must remember that all blood supply to the skin arises from deeper vessels. Survival of any flap is a function of blood supply, either from the base of a flap, or directly from the undersurface of the flap. The commonly cited 3:1 length-to-width ratio is not a reliable parameter. Greater width of a pedicle does not necessarily translate into higher perfusion pressure. Perforating vessels along the flap's undersurface may be more important to the viability of the flap than blood traveling from the flap base. This is particularly true of the melolabial tissues, which are supplied by the angular vessels off the facial arteries. This principle is broadly applicable. For example, it is preservation of perforating vessels that allows pectoralis major flaps and free flaps to provide blood supply to skin paddles. A flap that is fully undermined is dependent upon the subdermal or subcutaneous plexus and vulnerable to ischemia. In contrast, a flap that also derives its blood supply from musculocutaneous or fasciocutaneous perforating vessels is more robust.

Atraumatic tissue handling minimizes ischemic stress and decreases tissue injury. Sharp dissection with a blade is generally preferable to blunt dissection, except when working near vascular pedicles that must be preserved. By avoiding crush injury, one ensures less damage to fragile capillaries and soft tissue. Use of skin hooks is, for the same reason, preferable to forceps. The tines of skin hooks are less prone to crush tissue or cause deepithelization. The plane of dissection is also important. A plane of dissection that is deep, and preserves the subdermal and subcutaneous plexus, affords greater blood flow than a shallow plane of dissection. Undermining should be sufficient to decrease tension, but care must be taken to avoid sacrifice of the blood supply arising from deep perforating vessels. Last, when possible, it is preferable to "push" tissue forward rather than "pull" on an already ischemic distal tip.

Meticulous tissue inset also improves flap viability. Often, surgeons will remove standing cutaneous cones at the conclusion of a procedure to achieve a smooth contour. However, redistribution of tension to inconspicuous sites is sometimes a better alternative, as it maximizes the base of the flap and decreases the risk of venous or arterial insufficiency. Also, it may be helpful to have tissues near the base of the flap assume much of the closure tension to minimize the risk of dehiscence. For example, preferential advancement of surrounding tissue relative to a flap beginning at the flap base minimizes tension at a relatively ischemic distal tip. Last, although it is tempting to close all defects, excessive wound tension is a common cause of tissue loss. In such cases, using a skin graft for a portion of the defect may minimize the risk of ischemia.

## Hemostasis

Bleeding is one of the most common complications of local flaps. The pooling of blood within a surgical bed is associated with more scarring, a greater risk for infection, and more deformity, due to poor obliteration of dead spaces. Common causes of bleeding are inadequate hemostasis at time of surgery, drug associated coagulopathy, and patient-related factors, such as hemophilia. Many drugs can contribute to bleeding risk, including nonsteroidal antiinflammatory medicines, aspirin containing products, vitamin E, and many herbal medicines. Clopidogrel and warfarin have a particularly potent inhibitory effect on coagulation, but the decision to hold these latter agents prior to surgery must be made discretely. There is a relatively high prevalence of coronary artery disease and coronary artery stents in patients requiring local flap reconstruction.

Several basic principles may decrease the likelihood of bleeding-related complications including using suture ligatures for larger vessels, and reserving bipolar electrocautery for small vessels. Monopolar cautery may result in a less precise hemostasis. Irrigating the wound with warm water allows for demonstration of vessels prone to bleeding, whereas cooler irrigation tends to cause vessel spasm and is less effective for showing sites of bleeding. The patient may be placed in a Trendelenburg position or have a Valsalva maneuver performed to stimulate potential sources of bleeding. For larger flaps, drains are helpful in obliterating "dead space" that cannot be readily addressed with compressive dressings. The patients are also counseled to keep their head elevated during the first 24–48 hours after surgery to minimize blood accumulation.

When hematomas do occur, they impair healing through a variety of mechanisms. One important factor is a decrease in local flap perfusion, related to stretching of the subdermal or subcutaneous plexus vessels. Hematomas also induce vasospasm, and elevation of the skin flap from the underlying tissue base decreases the opportunity for the flap to seat down and derive blood from deeper tissues. Hematoma strongly predisposes to infection, related to stasis of blood within the wound site; this infection may secondarily impair flap perfusion due to inflammatory edema and thrombosis. Last, the iron porphyrin element present in blood may contribute to free radical production, thereby further deteriorating flap viability and predisposing to necrosis.

Prompt treatment is critical to a satisfactory outcome once a hematoma is diagnosed. Classic findings include a tight, tense flap, often with ecchymosis of the surrounding tissues. Oozing may be present at suture lines, and the overlying tissue often assumes a pale bluish color. Small accumulations of blood may be aspirated with a large-bore needle, followed by placement of a compressive dressing for 48 hours. For larger collections of blood, evacuation in the operating room is necessary. If the blood is evacuated within hours, the likelihood of maintaining flap viability and avoiding skin slough is far more favorable. In contrast, beyond 48 hours, blood tends to clot or gel, subsequently undergoing fibrosis and scar formation. After fibrinolysis occurs, portions of the hematoma may liquefy, allowing repeat aspiration at 1-2 weeks.

## Avoidance of Nerve Injury

Motor nerve injury is among the most serious complications of facial reconstruction. The facial nerve is at risk during elevation of cutaneous flaps due to its relatively superficial course over the face and arborizing branches. Injury usually involves distal branches of the nerve, although extensive dissection in the preauricular region may also put the main trunk of the facial nerve at risk. Marginal mandibular, frontal, and buccal branches are all susceptible to injury. In the case of the marginal branch, injury is most common as the nerve descends just below the inferior rim of the mandible. Maintaining a plane of dissection superficial to the platysma, when possible, will minimize the risk of such injury. The buccal branch is susceptible to injury due to its relatively superficial course, and maintaining a plane of dissection superficial to the parotidomasseteric fascia will minimize risk of injury, as well as avoiding sialoceles. The frontal branch of the facial nerve is particularly susceptible to injury as it ascends over the zygomatic arch, where it is in the plane of the temporoparietal fascia just superficial to the periosteum of the zygoma. Last, great care must also be taken in dissecting over the posterior triangle where the spinal accessory nerve exits from behind the sternocleidomastoid muscle. Dissection in this area may be necessary when elevating large cervicofacial advancement flaps.

Sensory nerves are also susceptible to injury when dissecting the soft tissue planes of the face. The most common nerves at risk for injury are the great auricular nerve and the supraorbital and supratrochlear nerves. The great auricular nerve is prone to injury during subcutaneous dissection in the infraauricular area. Identification of this nerve as it crosses the superior aspect of the sternocleidomastoid muscle decreases the risk of injury. The supratrochlear and supraorbital nerves are at risk with dissection along the medial aspect of the superior orbital rim. The exit of these nerves in this region makes them prone to both traction as well as transection injuries during flap elevation. Injuries to these nerves can result in numbness, dysesthesias, and pain or itching. The supraorbital branch travels within the galea aponeurotica and may be traumatized with undermining in the subgaleal plane when attempting closure of a forehead donor site.

## Respect for Structural elements and Selection of Reconstruction

The osseocartilaginous framework of the nose is prone to buckling and susceptible to injury during nasal reconstruction. Care must be taken to avoid inducing nasal valve compromise or loss of support that will impede nasal airflow. Inadvertent injury to the cartilaginous lower two thirds of the nose structures can result in a variety of undesirable complications, including alar retraction, saddle nose deformity, tip asymmetries, and collapse of the internal or external nasal valve. Furthermore, failure to adequately reconstruct cartilage that was resected during tumor removal can result in any of these complications.

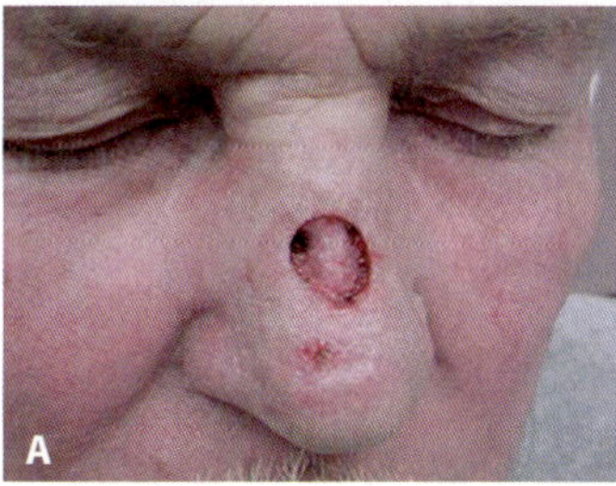

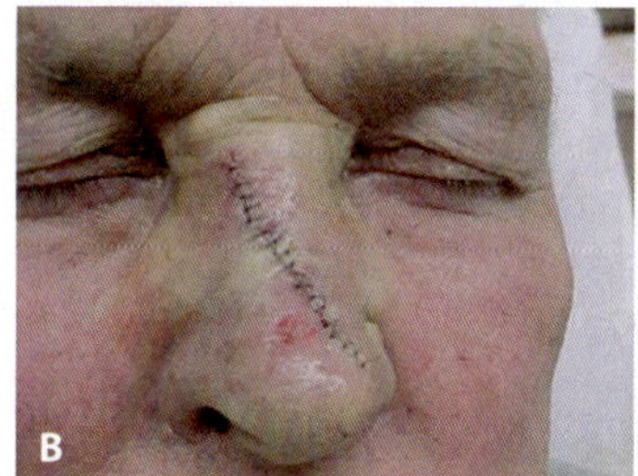

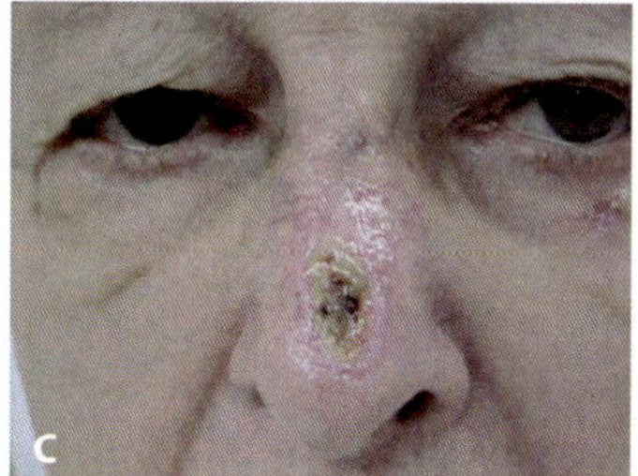


**Figure 13-1.** Ischemia with primary closure. (A) Initial defect. (B) Immediate appearance after primary closure under tension. (C) Dehiscence with tissue necrosis.

## Flap Design

Mastering the nuances of flap design allows one to dramatically decrease the incidence of complications. Whereas smoking cessation or use of sterile technique can be broadly applied, flap planning requires specific attention to the defect, surrounding structures, and available donor sites. This section outlines complications related to suboptimal flap design. For a large subset of facial defects, local flaps are the reconstructive option of choice due to favorable tissue color and texture. In addition, local flaps may decrease the tension across a closure, thereby decreasing risk of ischemia seen with primary closure (**Figure 13-1**). Skin grafts are effective for many shallow defects, but skin grafting deeper areas may result in less than ideal cosmesis (**Figures 13-2 and 13-3**).

### Ensuring Clear Margins

Before commencing reconstruction, one must establish that resection margins are clear of tumors. In cases where tumor margins are unclear—particularly in the case of melanoma or tumors with ill-defined borders—staging surgery and waiting for confirmation on final pathology should be considered. High-risk cases include large, recurrent,

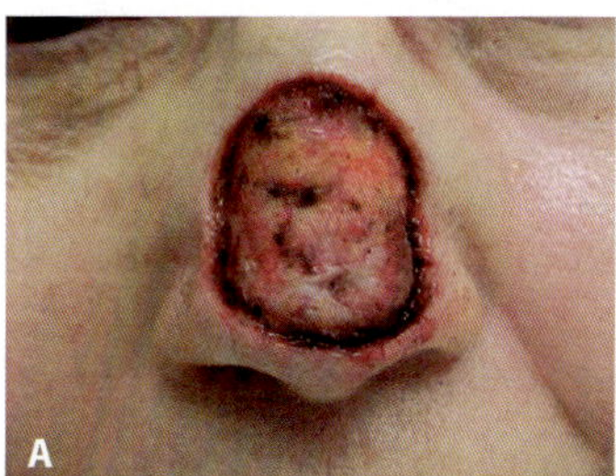

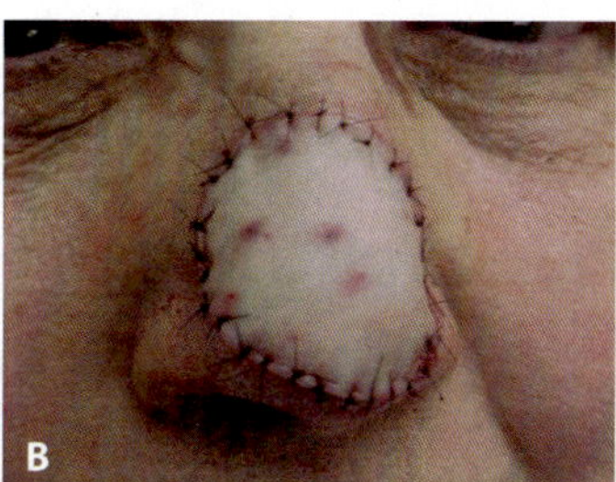

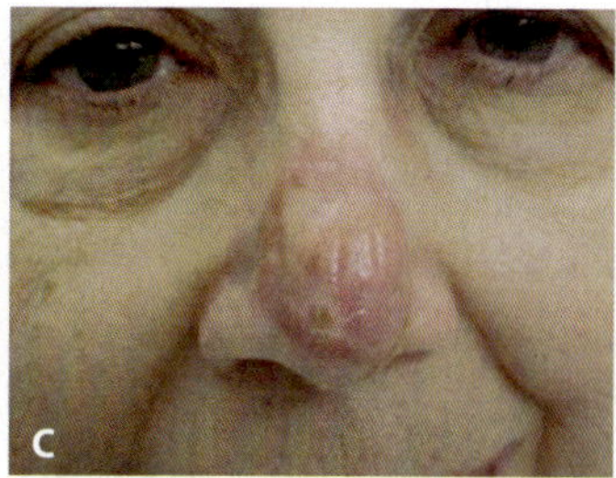


**Figure 13-2.** Unfavorable aesthetic outcome after skin graft to nasal tip. (A) Initial defect. (B) Immediate postoperative appearance. (C) Result after healing showing a patchlike appearance.

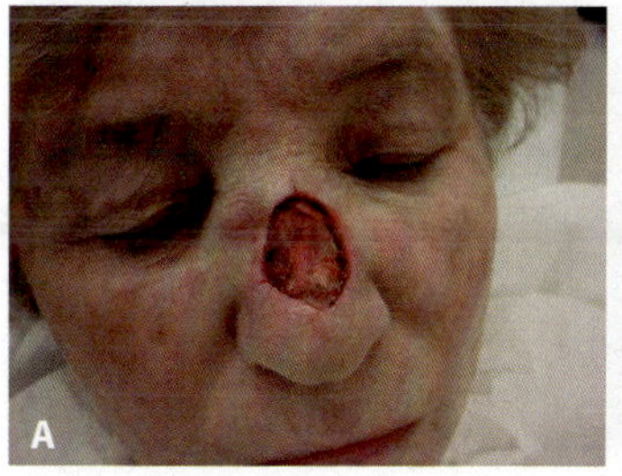

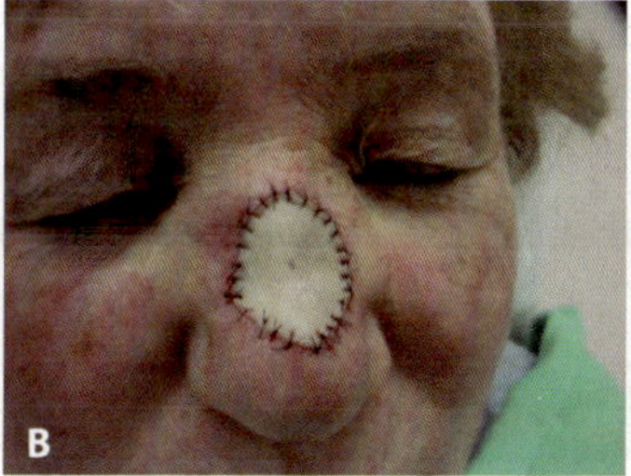

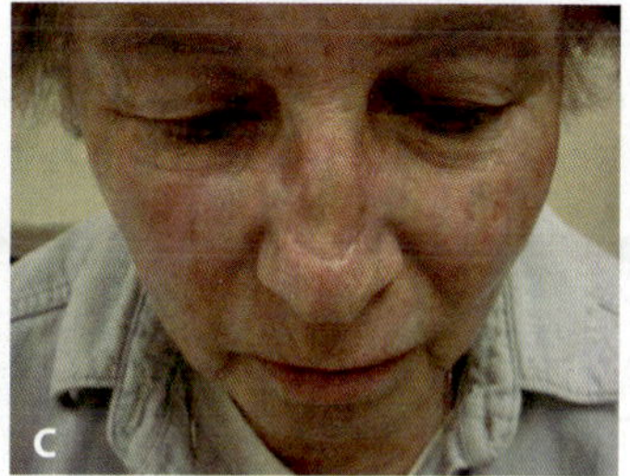


**Figure 13-3.** Outcome after skin graft to deep dorsal defect. (A) Initial defect. (B) Immediate postoperative appearance. (C) Result after healing showing contour deformity and mismatch.

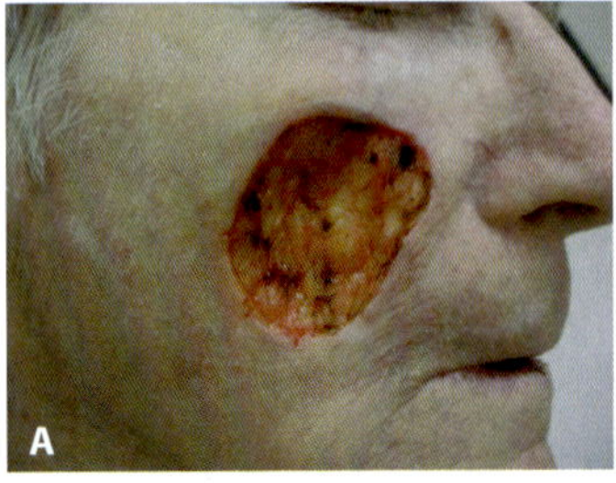
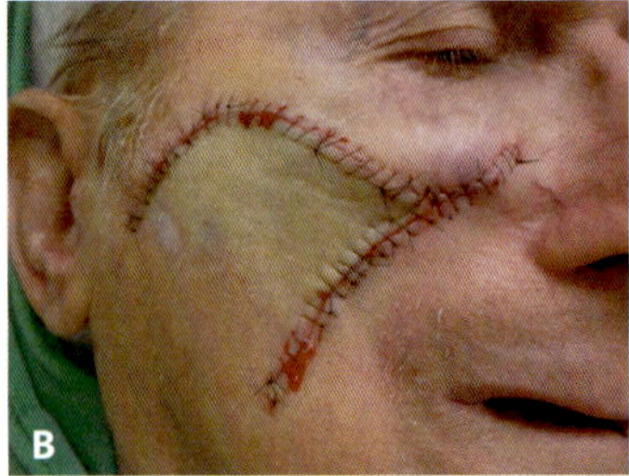
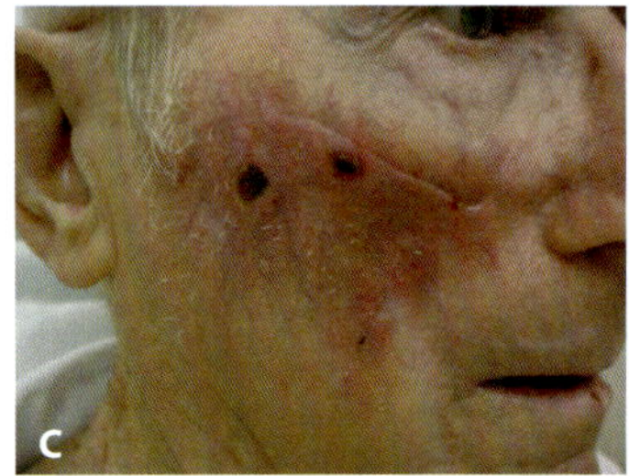

**Figure 13-4.** Ischemic cheek flap. (A) Initial defect. (B) Immediate postoperative appearance showing early signs of ischemia. (C) Postoperative result with scattered tissue loss.

infiltrative, or morpheaform tumors. Associated parasethesias or neural symptoms should raise suspicion for perineural invasion. Whereas standard hospital frozen sections are often unreliable, Mohs micrographic excision minimizes tissue loss and maximizes the prospects for successful tumor clearance. If flap reconstruction is undertaken and a positive margin later identified, reresection may prove difficult. Furthermore, subsequent reconstructive options are limited due to the prior procedure.

## Ischemia and Flap Loss

Flap ischemia refers to impaired delivery of blood, oxygen, and nutrients to tissues. Most tissues can survive with only a fraction of the usual blood flow, provided that neovascularization occurs to reduce dependency on the pedicle blood supply. However, sustained ischemia leads to tissue necrosis (**Figures 13-4–13-6**). Several factors conspire to increase the risk of ischemia in the local flaps—transection of small feeding vessels, torsion of vessels along the pedicle of the flap, and tension across suture lines. Transection of small sympathetic nerve branches induces release of catecholamines with resulting vasoconstriction. Thromboxane A is also released from small-platelet thrombi. The collective effect of these vasoactive substances is to decrease perfusion and increase the risk of flap loss. Overzealous flap

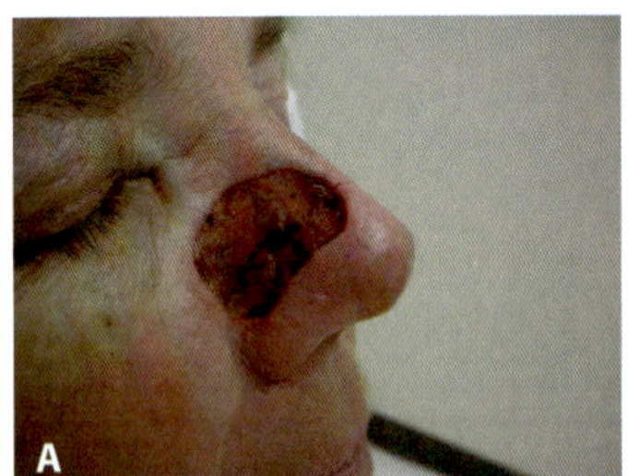
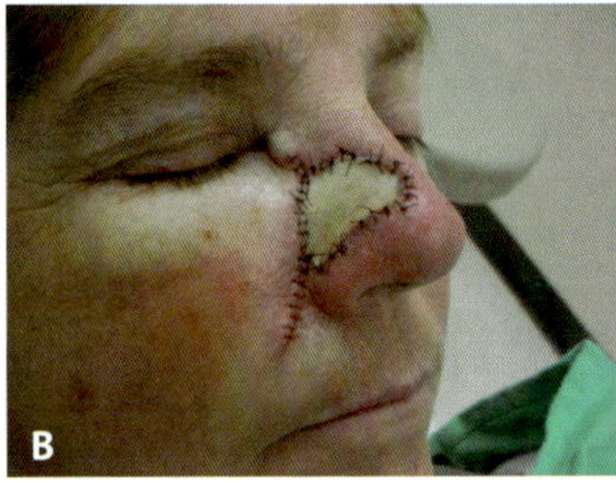
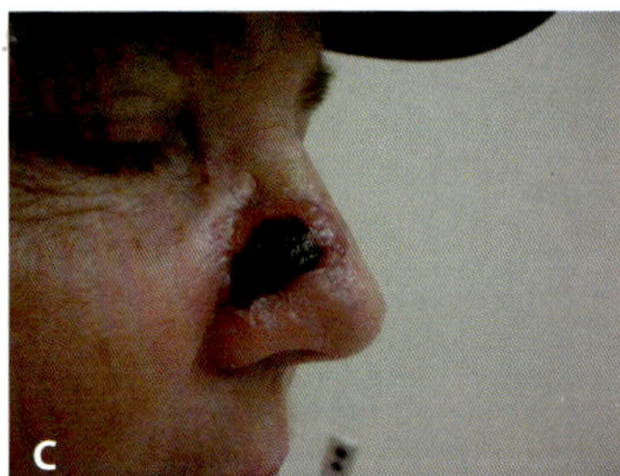

**Figure 13-5.** Ischemic nasal sidewall reconstruction with V-to-Y advancement. (A) Initial defect. (B) Immediate postoperative appearance showing ischemia. (C) Postoperative result with flap necrosis.

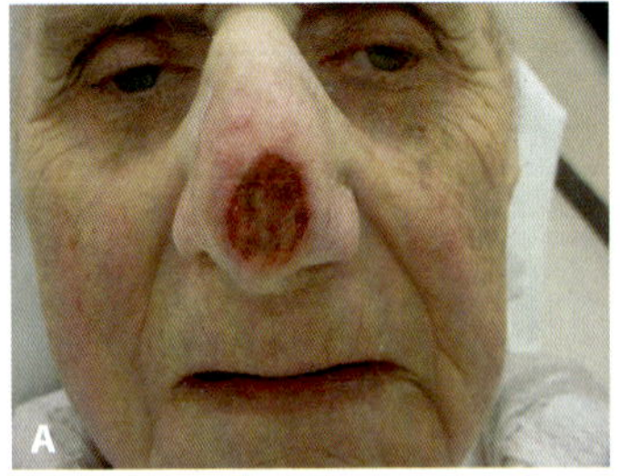
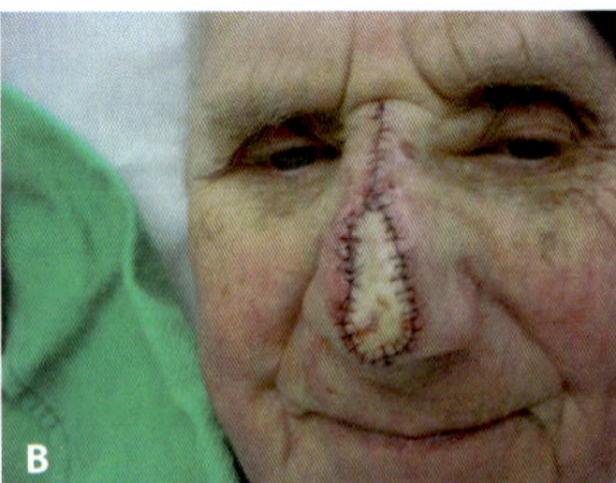
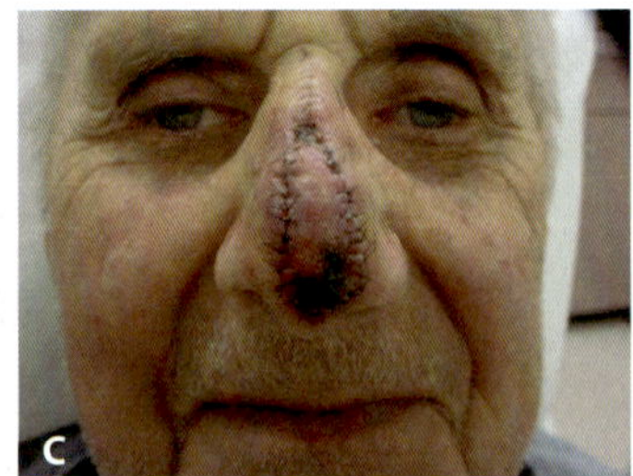

**Figure 13-6.** Ischemic nasal tip reconstruction based on nasalis. (A) Initial defect. (B) Immediate postoperative appearance with ischemia. (C) Partial local flap loss.

thinning, charring of tissues, and excessive tension across the wound closure all impair wound healing potential. Minimizing the impact of these factors during flap design and dissection will markedly diminish ischemic stress.

The signs of ischemia are easily recognizable. Reduced flap temperature, coupled with slow or absent bleeding on pinprick, is indicative of arterial insufficiency. Purple discoloration and bloated appearance to the flap with immediate bleeding on pinprick indicates venous congestion. Venous congestion is tolerated more poorly than arterial insufficiency, although either may cause flap demise. For arterial insufficiency, release of overly tight sutures may allow for salvage of the flap. Arterial insufficiency due to kinking of the flap pedicle or tight dressing is reversible, provided the diagnosis is made early. A flap showing arterial insufficiency may be returned to the donor bed for delay before performing the repair at a future time. This allows for enhanced blood supply to the flap, so that it may be more resistant to ischemia when reelevated. For venous insufficiency, suture release or medicinal leeching may allow for salvage. Antibiotic coverage with fluoroquinolones (ciprofloxacin) is recommended as a prophylaxis against *Aeromonas* infection if leeches are used. The same features of a hostile bed that predispose to local flap loss may also be associated with poor take of skin or composite grafts **(Figure 13-7)**.

Whenever possible, it is preferable to salvage as much of a threatened flap as possible. Once the extent of ischemia has demarcated, debridement should be performed. Removal of nonvital tissue decreases the risk of infection and allows for granulation. Devitalized tissue is removed with sharp dissection until bleeding tissue is encountered. Tissue that has good adherence to the underlying surgical bed is usually viable. If there is only partial-thickness loss, a debrided surgical bed can be left to granulate in preparation for secondary skin grafting. Inset of a new flap is likely to be necessary, however. Meticulous wound care, including use of moistening ointments, and either wet-to-dry dressings or peroxide promotes favorable healing.

## Unsightly and Malpositioned Scars

Full-thickness incisions invariably result in visible scars, but skillful placement of incisions and meticulous surgical technique minimize the incidence of unacceptable scars. Hypertrophic or keloid scars often benefit from steroid injection. In other cases, an abnormal appearance results from poor placement of incisions. Failure to respect facial aesthetic units invariably results in more conspicuous scars and abnormal appearance. One common example is blunting the crease of the alar sulcus, which forms a boundary between the nose, cheek, and upper lip. The use of interpolated cheek flaps for this area is preferred to advancement or transposition flaps, which tend to efface this aesthetic border **(Figure 13-8)**. It may be preferable to use separate flaps or a combination of a flap and skin graft to preserve normal boundaries and optimize cosmesis. For example, defects extending from the nose to the adjacent cheek are often best repaired with separate flaps. This approach allows for camouflage of the scar within a shadowed area while also preserving the normal concavity of the sulcus between the nose and cheek.

Patient-related factors also influence flap selection. Incisions that are made in thick, sebaceous skin are more likely to widen or leave depressed scars. Broader flaps, rather than intricate flap designs, minimize risk of unfavorable scars in such patients. Young patients heal differently than older patients. Although the risk of wound dehiscence is lower in young patients, younger patients have less tissue laxity and also often develop exaggerated erythema and hypertrophy. Applying sunscreen over a newly

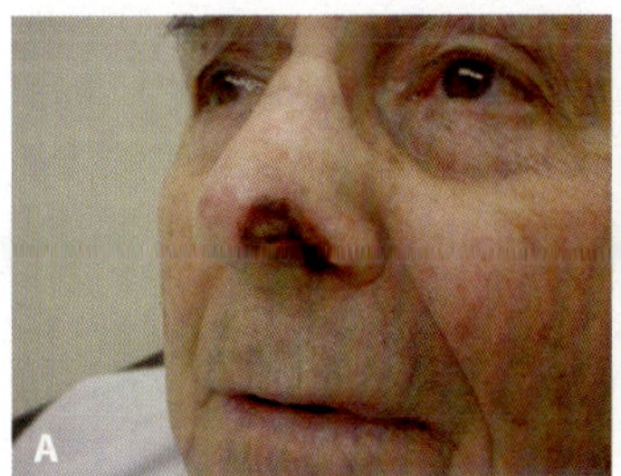

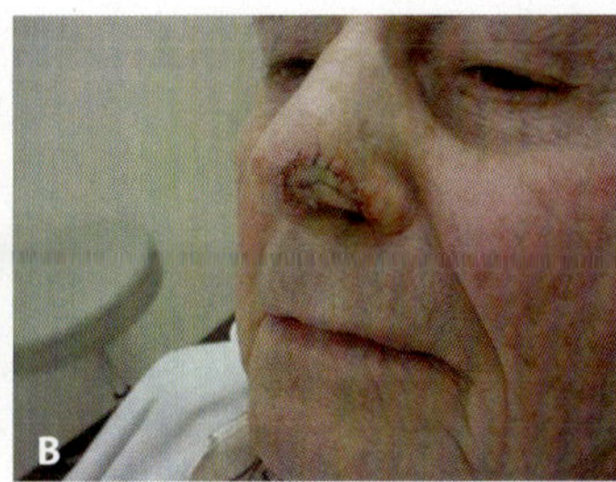

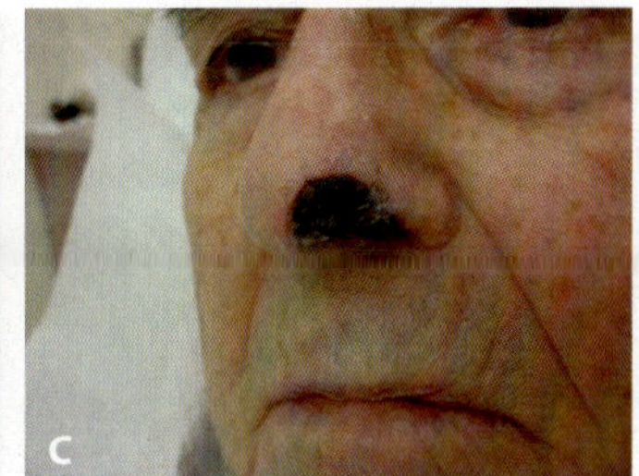


**Figure 13-7.** Necrosis of composite graft. (A) Initial defect. (B) Immediate postoperative result. (C) Necrotic graft at follow-up.

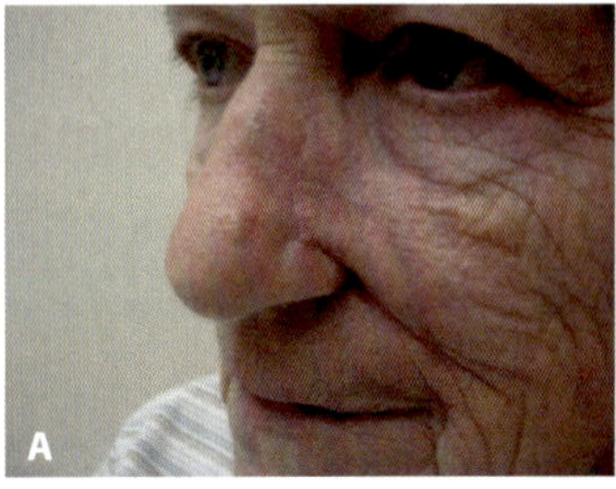
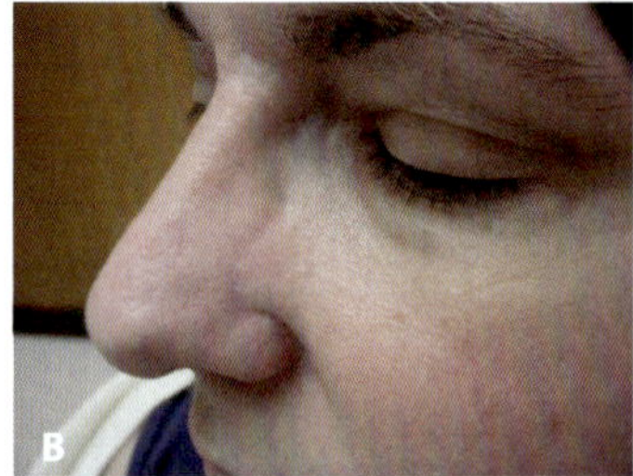
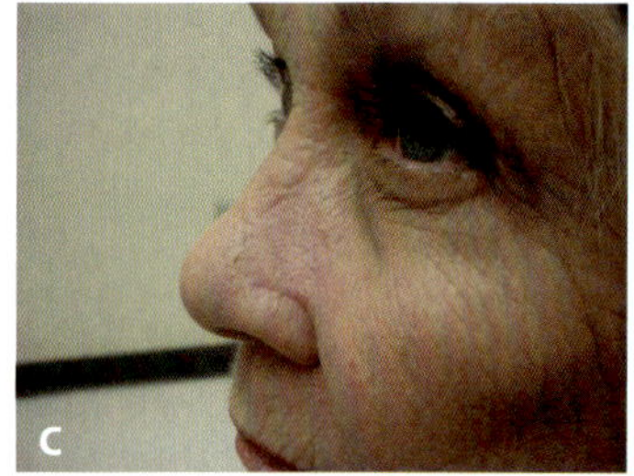

**Figure 13-8.** Blunting of melolabial sulcus with flap reconstruction. (A) Melolabial flap. (B) Cheek flap. (C) Cheek flap.

epithelialized surface minimizes postinflammatory hyperpigmentation. Due to the significant remodeling of scars in younger patients, it is preferable to delay revision in children for a year to allow time for spontaneous improvement. Patients with hyperflexibility possess more elastin and are therefore more likely to have widened scars. Gorlin's sign refers to the ability to touch the tongue to the nasal tip, and Beighton's sign refers to the capability to bend the thumb back to the flexor aspect of the forearm; both are signs of excessive or abnormal flexibility. These individuals are more prone to suboptimal scarring.

## Trap Door Deformity

Trap door deformity refers to the tendency of a flap to mushroom up or pincushion in its center, leaving a depressed scar around its periphery **(Figure 13-9)**. It results from persistent edema, poor lymphatic drainage, and accumulation of serum and hematoma deep to the flap. Flaps that have curved borders are particularly susceptible to this deformity. The cicatricial contraction of the edges of the flap results in central bulging. The scar sheet beneath the flap is thought to contribute to this deformity. Some degree of trap door is inevitable with most bilobed flaps due to the combination of dependent edema coupled with the curved shape of these flaps, especially when performed in patients with very sebaceous and thick skin. Generous undermining of the skin and soft tissues can reduce the tendency toward scar contracture. Superiorly based flaps are more prone to this problem due to venous congestion and disrupted lymphatic channels.

Although trap door deformity does tend to improve with the passage of time, a number of interventions may be helpful. Dermabrasion is useful for smoothing irregularities in nasal bilobe flaps and improves the blending of skin texture and contour. For more prominent trap door deformities, asteroid injection to the subcutaneous tissue may be performed initially. Usually low concentration triamcinolone acetonide (10 mg/mL) is preferred to minimize the risk of tissue atrophy. Not uncommonly, surgical revision proves necessary. In this case, correction involves incising the borders of the flap, removing subcutaneous fat and scar, and generous undermining followed by redraping with placement of Z-plasties, to minimize the risk of recurrence.

## Distortion of Mobile Structures

Distortion of mobile structures is another important consideration in a local flap reconstruction.

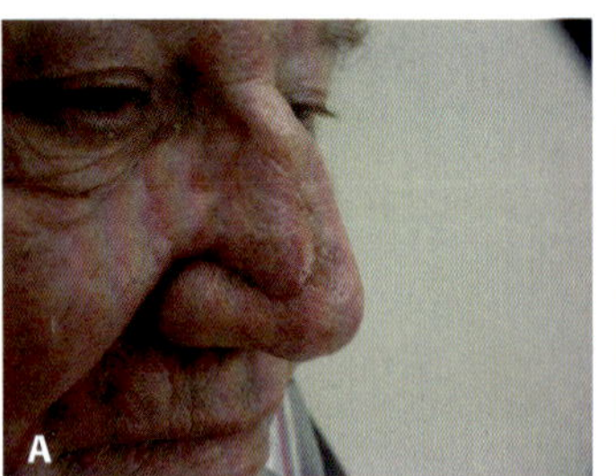
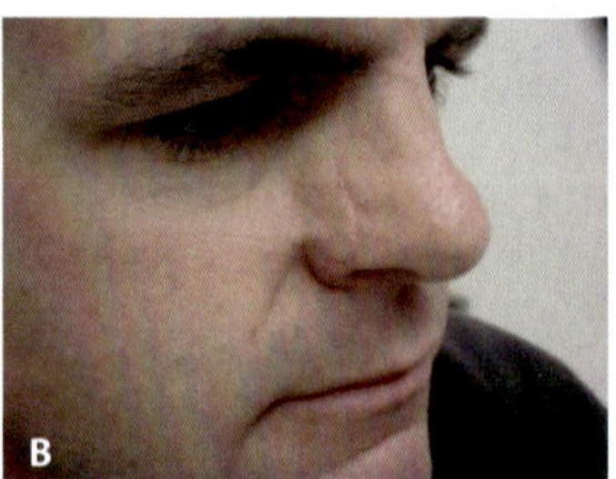
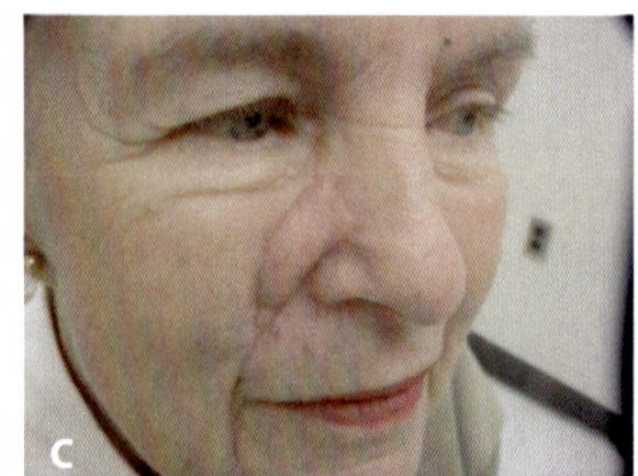

**Figure 13-9.** Trap door deformities, demonstrating pincushioning and dependent-flap lymphedema with venous stasis. (A) Cheek transposition flap. (B) Note flap (modified rhomboid flap). (C) Island melolabial flap.

Mobile structures include the eyelids, lips, earlobes, and nasal alar rim. Although such distortion may occur at time of initial reconstruction, it is more commonly observed as a late effect of healing. Because tissues heal by scar contraction, it is not uncommon for contractural forces to exert themselves on structures that are not rigidly anchored. Therefore, the potential for future tissue distortion is best identified at the time of initial surgery.

Eyelid malposition is a common—but generally preventable—problem after local flaps in the periorbital region. Distortion of the lower eyelid is more frequent than the upper eyelid due to the effect of gravity and senile laxity of the lower lid. Among the more common eyelid complications associated with local flaps are symptomatic dry eyes, lagophthalmos, lacrimal duct obstruction or avulsion, impairment of visual fields, or visual loss. Excessive tension on closure in the vertical dimension will predispose to eyelid retraction, with secondary effects on hydration of the cornea and risk for exposure keratitis. The ability of the eye to adequately generate a tear film is impaired with malposition of the puncta as well. Direct injury to the lid may also occur with surgery; therefore, it is important to be familiar with the cross-sectional anatomy of the upper and lower eyelids.

The lip, earlobes, and nose are also prone to distortion that creates a variety of functional and cosmetic difficulties. Distortion of the lip may include blunting of the lateral commissure, lip ectropion, or lip entropion. Distortion of the lips can result in cosmetic deformity, with an unacceptable appearance; but it may also have functional consequences. Abnormal distortion of the lip may interfere with speech, facial expression, and control of salivation. Excessive desiccation and aberrant salivation can also predispose to dental caries. Alar retraction is a significant risk when repairing nasal defects within a few millimeters of the alar rim with a local flap. Use of structural grafting and careful flap selection can avoid a vector of tension that is directed superiorly. Excessive tension on the earlobe may result in "pixie ear" where the earlobe is abnormally elongated.

## Nasal Lining Defects and Smoldering Infections

One of the more common oversights in nasal reconstruction is failure to adequately restore nasal lining. Because the nasal lining is difficult to visualize, inadequate reconstruction of this layer might seem to be a minor transgression. However, failure to resurface the nasal interior will doom an otherwise well-conceived nasal reconstruction due to late effects of scar contracture. The initial result of such a repair may be quite satisfactory, but the repair does not withstand the test of time. The undersurface of covering flaps contract as raw tissue surfaces heal secondarily, distorting the external shape of the nose and narrowing the nasal airway. Nasal lining flaps that are too thick, insufficiently pliable, or poorly vascularized yield poor results. Use of thin, vascularized flaps, usually vestibular skin or mucoperichondrium, avoids such distortion.

Nasal lining defects are also predisposed to chronic infection. Infections related to a hole in the nasal lining often present weeks after the original reconstruction and are usually heralded by drainage with erythema, edema, and warmth. With lining flaps that are torn or not fully viable, blood supply to the overlying cartilage may be tenuous. Fulminant infections may cause extensive lining necrosis with cartilage exposure and loss, but chronic smoldering infections are more common and tend to be more localized. Empiric antibiotics and a culture and sensitivity are helpful in decreasing the risk of loss of free grafts, but resurfacing of exposed tissue may be needed. If the response to antibiotics is not brisk, the wound should be explored and debrided as necessary. A few months thereafter, subsequent graft placement may be considered.

## Conclusion

The preponderance of complications in local flaps can be mitigated or prevented with careful planning and meticulous technique. If the surgeon ensures that blood is delivered to the tissues, the tissues will live and the risk of infection and unfavorable healing are dramatically reduced. Detailed knowledge of the relevant anatomy minimizes the risk of injury to adjacent structures and of distortion of mobile landmarks. Additional consideration of the nuances of aesthetic units and anticipation of late effects in wound healing helps ensure favorable healing.

## References

1. Angel MF, Ramasastry SS, Swartz WM, et al. The critical relationship between free radicals and degrees of ischemia: Evidence for tissue intolerance of marginal perfusion. *Plast Reconstr Surg* Feb 1988;81(2), 233–239.
2. Cutting C. Critical closing and perfusion pressures in flap survival. *Ann Plast Surg* Dec 1982;9(6), 524.

3. Diaz DD, Freeman SB, Wilson JF, Parker GS. Hematoma-induced flap necrosis and free radical scavengers. *Arch Otolaryngol Head Neck Surg* May 1992;118(5), 516–518.
4. Forrest CR, Pang CY, Lindsay WK. Dose and time effects of nicotine treatment on the capillary blood flow and viability of random pattern skin flaps in the rat. *Br J Plast Surg* May 1987;40(3), 295–299.
5. Gideroglu K, Yildirim S, Akan M, Akoz T. Immediate use of medicinal leeches to salvage venous congested reverse pedicled neurocutaneous flaps. *Scand J Plast Reconstr Surg Hand Surg* 2003;37(5), 277–282.
6. Jewett BS. Complications of local flaps. In: Baker SR, ed. *Local Flaps in Facial Reconstruction.* 2nd ed. New York: Mosby; 2007, 691–722.
7. Kaufman AJ, Kiene KL, Moy RL. Role of tissue undermining in the trapdoor effect of transposition flaps. *J Dermatol Surg Oncol* Feb 1993;19(2), 128–132.
8. Kinsella JB, Rassekh CH, Wassmuth ZD, Hokanson JA, Calhoun KH. Smoking increases facial skin flap complications. *Ann Otol Rhinol Laryngol* Feb 1999;108(2), 139–142.
9. Polk HC, Jr., Miles AA. Enhancement of bacterial infection by ferric iron: kinetics, mechanisms, and surgical significance. *Surgery* Jul 1971;70(1), 71–77.
10. Salasche SJ. Acute surgical complications: cause, prevention, and treatment. *J Am Acad Dermatol.* Dec
11. Salasche SJ, Grabski WJ. Complications of flaps. *J Dermatol Surg Oncol* Feb 1991;17(2), 132–140.
12. Sebben JE. Sterile technique and the prevention of wound infection in office surgery—Part I. *J Dermatol Surg Oncol* Dec 1988;14(12), 1364–1371.
13. Sebben JE. Sterile technique and the prevention of wound infection in office surgery—Part II. *J Dermatol Surg Oncol* Jan 1989;15(1), 38–48.
14. Utley DS, Koch RJ, Goode RL. The failing flap in facial plastic and reconstructive surgery: Role of the medicinal leech. *Laryngoscope* Aug 1998;108(8 Pt 1), 1129–1135.
15. Vural E, Key JM. Complications, salvage, and enhancement of local flaps in facial reconstruction. *Otolaryngol Clin North Am* Aug 2001;34(4), 739–751.

# Index

Information in figures and tables is indicated by *f* and *t*.

**G**



**H**

## S



## T